SECOND EDITION

Comprehensive Lactation Consultant Exam Review

Linda J. Smith, BSE, FACCE, IBCLC

Bright Future Lactation Resource Centre Ltd.
Dayton, Ohio

JONES AND BARTLETT PUBLISHERS

Sudbury, Massachusetts

BOSTON   TORONTO   LONDON   SINGAPORE

World Headquarters
Jones and Bartlett Publishers
40 Tall Pine Drive
Sudbury, MA 01776
978-443-5000
info@jbpub.com
www.jbpub.com

Jones and Bartlett Publishers Canada
6339 Ormindale Way
Mississauga, Ontario L5V 1J2
CANADA

Jones and Bartlett Publishers International
Barb House, Barb Mews
London W6 7PA
UK

Jones and Bartlett's books and products are available through most bookstores and online booksellers. To contact Jones and Bartlett Publishers directly, call 800-832-0034, fax 978-443-8000, or visit our website www.jbpub.com.

Substantial discounts on bulk quantities of Jones and Bartlett's publications are available to corporations, professional associations, and other qualified organizations. For details and specific discount information, contact the special sales department at Jones and Bartlett via the above contact information or send an email to specialsales@jbpub.com.

Image on CD-ROM for exam question A-134: Graph used with permission of Taylor & Francis AS

Library of Congress Cataloging-in-Publication Data
Smith, Linda J., 1946-
  Comprehensive lactation consultant exam review / Linda J. Smith. — 2nd ed.
    p. ; cm.
  Includes bibliographical references.
  ISBN-13: 978-0-7637-4029-0
  ISBN-10: 0-7637-4029-2
  1. Breastfeeding—Examinations, questions, etc. 2. Lactation—Examinations, questions, etc. I. Title.
  [DNLM: 1. Breast Feeding—Examination Questions. 2. Lactation—Examination Questions. 3. Lactation Disorders—Examination Questions. WS 18.2 S654c 2007]
  RJ216.S56 2007
  613.269'076—dc22

                          2006028730
6048

Production Credits
Executive Editor: Kevin Sullivan
Acquisitions Editor: Emily Ekle
Production Director: Amy Rose
Associate Editor: Amy Sibley
Editorial Assistant: Patricia Donnelly
Reprints Coordinator/Production Assistant: Amy Browning
Senior Marketing Manager: Katrina Gosek
Manufacturing and Inventory Coordinator: Amy Bacus
Interactive Technology Manager: Dawn Mahon Priest
Associate Marketing Manager: Rebecca Wasley
Composition: Northeast Compositors, Inc.
Cover Design: Kristin E. Ohlin
Cover Image: Anatomy of the Lactating Breast. © Medela AG, Switzerland, 2006.
Printing and Binding: Courier Stoughton
Cover Printing: Courier Stoughton
CD Duplication: Cycle Software

Printed in the United States of America
11 10 09 08 07   10 9 8 7 6 5 4 3 2

Dedication

This second edition is dedicated to the skilled and talented women and men who have knitted together a global network of support for breastfeeding and human lactation, studied this unique body of knowledge from many scientific perspectives, and advocated for mothers in diverse cultures and situations. Thank you all for your persistence, wisdom, and energy in promoting, protecting, and supporting breastfeeding.

I also dedicate this text to my children Edwin Smith and his wife Teri DeMarco, Hannah Smith Boswell and her husband Kim Boswell, and Carl Smith; my grandchildren Carrie Boswell, Wyatt Andrew Smith, and Cole Frederick Smith; and families everywhere who will benefit from the support created by lactation professionals worldwide.

ABOUT THE AUTHOR

Linda J. Smith, BSE, FACCE, IBCLC, is a lactation consultant, childbirth educator, author, and internationally known consultant on breastfeeding and birthing issues. A former La Leche League leader and Lamaze-certified childbirth educator, she has provided education and support to diverse families over three decades in nine cities in the United States and Canada. Linda has worked in a 3-hospital system in Texas, a public health agency in Virginia, and has served as breastfeeding coordinator for the Ohio Department of Health. Linda is one of the founders of the International Board of Lactation Consultant Examiners (IBLCE), a founder and past board member of the International Lactation Consultant Association (ILCA); she serves on the United States Breastfeeding Committee (USBC), and is ILCA's Liason to the Coalition for Improving Maternity Services (CIMS). She owns the Bright Future Lactation Resource Centre (BFLRC), whose mission is "Supporting the People who Support Breastfeeding" with lactation education programs, consulting services, and educational resources. BFLRC is on the Internet at www.BFLRC.com.

Linda's lactation management/exam preparation course is the longest-running course of its kind and the first to be based on the IBLCE exam blueprint. To date, more than 1500 students have taken the course.

ACKNOWLEDGMENTS

Thank you to the thousands of willing individuals who have participated in my lactation management and exam preparation courses over the past 14 years. You've taught me how to convey basic principles, new research, and fundamental attitudes in effective ways. Your input has helped me focus on topics and concepts that are central to understanding the breastfeeding mother–baby dyad.

Special thanks to Kevin Sullivan, Amy Sibley, Amy Browning, Amy Rose, and Patricia Donnelley at Jones and Bartlett, whose patience and prodding triggered this revision. Revising a book is far harder than writing it in the first place!

I greatly appreciate the collegial and professional friendship and support of Lois Arnold, Karin Cadwell, Carol Chamblin, Carol Dobrich, Madonna Fasimpaur, Hilary Flower, Catherine Watson Genna, Martha Grodrian, Lenore Goldfarb, Karen Kerkhoff Gromada, Cathy Holland, Kay Hoover, Greg Notestine, Cindy Turner-Maffei, Annie VerSteeg, Diane Wiessinger, and Barbara Wilson-Clay, who contributed advice, guidance, ideas, pictures, and/or test questions.

I am enormously grateful to the mothers and babies whose stories and photos bring life and realism to this book. I hope I've conveyed your collective persistence, courage, and strength.

I am grateful to my husband, Denny, and my now-adult children, Edwin, Hannah, and Carl, for teaching and supporting me as I experienced breastfeeding and mothering when breastfeeding was a minority activity in the United States. I hope this book helps you and your own children reap the fruits of skilled professional breastfeeding help.

Lastly, thanks especially to the dedicated and creative people who served on the boards of directors of ILCA and IBLCE. You have helped shape and guide this profession to where it is today: a network of nearly 20,000 professionals in 65 countries speaking 13 languages in support of breastfeeding mother–baby dyads worldwide.

INTRODUCTION TO THE SECOND EDITION

The second edition of *Comprehensive Lactation Consultant Exam Review* expands on the concept introduced in the first edition by providing a wealth of practice tests and practice questions in a well-referenced book and CD-ROM learning package that will help you review material that is tested on the international lactation consultant certification examination administered by the International Board of Lactation Consultant Examiners (IBLCE).

This edition contains one 200-question practice exam with unique questions that do not appear elsewhere in the book, a second 200-question practice exam compiled from questions included elsewhere in the book, and hundreds of practice questions grouped by discipline. This format allows the student to study each discipline separately and practice taking two complete exams. Clinical exercises for each discipline are included to help the student prepare in more depth for lactation consultant practice. The appendices contain information from IBLCE on test design and scoring, and from IBLCE and ILCA on professional practice responsibilities. The CD-ROM contains the full-color pictures needed to answer the questions in the clinical section of the practice tests. The images depict situations commonly encountered in lactation consultant practice and are used to test the candidate's clinical judgment.

The second edition is based on the IBLCE exam blueprint for the year 2000 and beyond. At this writing, a new task analysis is being conducted and a new blueprint will be published soon. Historically, there has been enough flexibility in the range of questions included on any year's exam to cover both the 2000 and future blueprint ranges of questions. This edition's grouping of the practice questions by discipline gives the student flexibility in studying and preparing. There is inevitable overlap in some of the disciplines, and some clinical situations could fall into more than one discipline. In this book, each question used will be assigned to only one discipline and one chronological period, which are identified in the answer sections.

Although an extensive body of research was used in preparing the practice questions, the references may not cover every possible concept that could appear on the IBLCE exam. When studying, use the most current editions of widely available texts and research articles published in relevant professional journals. If one reference contradicts another, look carefully for the common ground, or examine the cited primary research on the topic. The exam will test universal principles, not esoteric trivia. Many research articles can be downloaded in their entirety from the online version of the journals for free or for a small fee. In other cases, the abstract is available for free online. Most medical libraries provide public access to a wide selection of the journals cited.

- Knowledge areas are easily found in the recommended readings and bibliographies.
- Skills are learned through experience, preferably supervised, and are indirectly tested by the sample questions, especially the questions with accompanying photographs. The clinical exercises will help develop skills and deepen your understanding of each discipline.
- Attitudes are difficult to test with a paper-and-pencil examination, yet they are central to effective breast-feeding care. Listening to mothers' concerns and experiences is vital to understanding the supportive attitudes that emerge in the sample questions. Again, the clinical exercises should broaden your understanding in this area.

The sample questions may include signs and symptoms of various diseases, therapeutic treatments including antibiotics and other prescription medications, and other information related to the overall health or medical condition of the lactating mother or breastfed child. Inclusion of this information does not imply that the lactation consultant, on the basis of IBLCE certification alone, is qualified or legally allowed to diagnose medical conditions or recommend, prescribe, or determine medical treatments of the mother or child.

Although this book is intended to help you prepare for the IBLCE exam, no guarantees of passing the IBLCE exam are expressed or implied. This book is intended to augment lactation management or exam preparation courses, not replace them. Students in lactation management courses often find that coursework focuses their study, validates existing knowledge, and identifies weak areas. The book can also be used as a guide for self-study, formation of study groups, or to supplement academic courses.

Finally, every attempt was made to include sufficient questions similar in format to the IBLCE exam and that cover the depth and breadth of topics that might be tested on the IBLCE exam. The author has not had access to the actual exam questions except when she recertifies by examination, and she rigorously upholds the IBLCE policy on confidentiality. None of the questions in this book have been submitted to IBLCE for possible use. Some topics tested may be over- or underrepresented in this book. New research that expands, deepens, or even replaces earlier understandings will inevitably be published after this book is released. Therefore, this book's questions, references, and exercises should be considered a guide and starting point for study, not the final word on any topic or concept.

For more information and updates regarding IBLCE certification, contact the International Board of Lactation Consultant Examiners at 7245 Arlington Blvd., Suite 200, Falls Church VA 22042-3217, by phone at (703) 560-7330; by fax at (703) 560-7332; by e-mail at iblce@iblce.org; or on the Internet at www.IBLCE.org. IBLCE maintains regional offices in Australia and Europe.

PREPARING FOR THE PRACTICE EXAMS

EXAM STRUCTURE

- Each item (test question) has an introductory sentence or paragraph (stem). All the information necessary to answer the question is given in the stem and/or the response choices. Assume there are no additional complicating circumstances. Do not read more into the question than is provided, and don't waste time considering "what if." Each question is testing only one concept.
- Items 126 through 200 require viewing a picture or diagram in order to answer the question. Look for the obvious—what you need to see will be clearly visible, even if there are extraneous features in the picture.
- Some items refer to situations involving a mother and/or baby and ask what "you" should do. The "you" refers to your role as a lactation consultant. If you have another professional role that authorizes you to perform additional functions (such as medical diagnosis or prescribing medications), do not include these functions in the role of the lactation consultant for the purposes of this exam.
- Each item ends with a specific question, which should be read carefully to know what is being asked. A key word may be emphasized, such as "the most appropriate action" or "your first response." These represent the types of decisions that frequently occur in lactation consultant practice. For example, the lactation consultant may need to know which intervention is the most likely or least likely to be helpful or effective.
- Some questions will ask for the most (or least) likely cause or explanation for a situation. These test knowledge of the general principles of clinical practice. Still others will present several interventions, asking which should be suggested first. These are designed to test the lactation consultant's attitudes and skill.
- There is one correct answer for each question. Common misconceptions and outdated ideas are often used as incorrect responses.
- The questions in Exam A do not appear elsewhere in the book. Questions in Exam B are included in the practice questions grouped by discipline.
- The mother, obviously, is always referred to with female pronouns. Where a sample question refers to a specific baby, such as in a photograph, the matching gender pronouns are used. For questions simply referring to "a baby," male and female pronouns are used rather randomly, and any overemphasis on one gender is accidental.
- There is no penalty for guessing. If you can eliminate 1 or 2 choices as clearly wrong, but can't decide between the remaining choices, take a guess—you have a 50% chance of being right.

TAKING THE PRACTICE EXAMS

There are two complete and unique exams, each with unique questions. Answer all the questions. Each question has one and only one correct answer. No partial credit is given. There is no penalty for guessing. Use the answer sheets provided. Be sure to darken (fill in) the appropriate circle for each item on the answer sheets.

Allow yourself up to three hours for each 100 questions, then take a break of 30 minutes or more. The clinical photographs are on the enclosed CD-ROM. Look at the corresponding picture for *each* question to answer these test items. Everything you need to see to answer the question is clearly visible.

The answers for each exam follow each exam's questions. The answer section includes the correct answer, an explanation or rationale, the discipline and period, whether the question pertains to knowledge or application, and the degree of difficulty. Degree of difficulty is calculated by how closely the wrong answers approximate the correct answer. The easiest questions are rated 2; the most difficult are rated 5.

SCORING THE PRACTICE EXAMS

The passing grade for the practice exams is 65%, or 130 correct answers out of 200 questions. This score is approximately the average passing grade for IBLCE exams. All 200 questions are scored as one complete exam. To analyze your individual areas of strength and weakness, examine the disciplines and periods for each question to identify patterns.

If you disagree with an answer, read more about that topic in several of the resources, talk with experienced lactation consultants, and carefully examine the incorrect answers. On the actual IBLCE examinations each year, all questions are analyzed statistically after the test is administered. Questions that are ambiguous, mis-coded, or have other errors are identified by the psychometrician and discussed by the exam committee, and some are discarded before the final scoring. There is no mechanism for following this practice with this book.

CONSIDER USING THESE PROVEN SUCCESSFUL STRATEGIES

- Review your knowledge and skills about two to three days before the exam. Then put away all books and references until after the exam. Do not cram. Cramming does not help and increases anxiety.
- Do something relaxing and enjoyable on the two days prior to the test. Get some fresh air and a change of pace on the day before the test.
- Allow sufficient travel time to avoid feeling rushed. Get a good night's sleep and follow your normal routine as closely as possible. Wear comfortable clothes in layers.
- Eat normally and emphasize protein-rich foods that will help you stay alert and focused. Drink water, which facilitates brain and nerve function.
- Trust yourself. Give yourself positive affirmations and trust your knowledge of mothers and babies; for example, "I know how to help breastfeeding mothers and babies." "I am a good test taker."
- Use calming/centering techniques that have served you well in the past, such as taking a deep breath, closing your eyes, meditating, or focusing on your breathing. Visualize recalling all the wealth of your knowledge, passing the exam, and receiving your excellent score report.
- Anxiety isn't always a bad thing. Allow yourself to feel any anxiety that arises—it will pass, just as a labor contraction does, and you will feel normal afterward. A slight rise in adrenal hormones may sharpen your focus and concentration, even as the same hormones have the unpleasant side effect of making you feel testy.

- Carefully examine each question before answering. Read each question, especially the stem, very carefully before you answer.
- Never change an answer unless you are absolutely, positively sure the first answer was clearly wrong. If you are unsure, rely on your best guess and first hunch.
- Allow yourself to miss a few questions. Nobody has yet achieved a score of 100%.
- Review the *Candidate's Guide* one more time, paying attention to the structure and format of test items.

BE PATIENT AND CALM WHILE YOU WAIT FOR THE EXAM RESULTS

At lunch and after the exam, resist the temptation to discuss your answers with other candidates. This is a sure recipe for self-doubt and increased anxiety! All candidates are required to maintain the confidentiality of the exam by refraining from discussing specific questions, answers, or pictures. Remember that you only have to *pass.* Nobody has ever scored 100% in the entire history of the exam. If the worst happens and you don't get a passing grade, you can take the exam again in subsequent years. Use your score report to focus on areas of weakness. If necessary, take additional formal and informal educational courses, arrange mentoring experiences, and use the time to reflect on long-term goals and aspirations.

Keep reading to stay up to date, whether or not you pass the exam. New information that will either confirm or change existing practices is constantly appearing. Avail yourself of as many resources as possible, especially texts and reference books.

Plan your budget to purchase several new books and attend at least one major breastfeeding conference each year. Attend continuing educational programs in breastfeeding and related fields. Read the *Journal of Human Lactation* and other peer-reviewed journals. Search the Internet frequently for pertinent information.

Use your new credential proudly! Join ILCA and local coalitions or affiliate groups and participate as time allows. Continue building a support network for yourself as a lactation consultant. Just like the mothers you work with, lactation consultants need a support system, too!

Contents

PART 3. Additional Resources

PART 1 Practice Questions by Discipline

A. MATERNAL AND INFANT ANATOMY

In the 2000 exam blueprint, 19 to 33 questions are dedicated to maternal and infant anatomy.

SUBTOPICS INCLUDED IN THIS CATEGORY

1. Breast and nipple structure and development; blood, lymph, innervation, mammary tissue

   a. General development
   b. Changes during pregnancy
   c. Nipple variations
   d. Breast size variations
   e. Vascular, lymph, and nervous systems

2. Infant oral anatomy and reflexes; assessment; anatomical variations

   a. General, including embryology and fetal anatomy
   b. Gastrointestinal tract
   c. Head, neck, and oral anatomy
   d. Structures involved in suck-swallow-breathe

CORE READING

Textbooks

Auerbach K, Riordan J. *Clinical Lactation: A Visual Guide*. Sudbury, MA: Jones & Bartlett Publishers; 2000.

Clinical Protocol # 11: Neonatal Anklyoglossia. New Rochelle, NY: Academy of Breastfeeding Medicine; 2004.

Lawrence RA, Lawrence RM. *Breastfeeding: A Guide for the Medical Profession*. 6th ed. St. Louis: Elsevier Mosby; 2005.

Morbacher N, Stock J. *The Breastfeeding Answer Book*. 3rd ed. Schaumburg, IL: La Leche League International; 2003.

Morris SE, Klein MD. *Pre-Feeding Skills—A Comprehensive Resource for Mealtime Development*. 2nd ed. San Antonio: Therapy Skill Builders; 2000.

Netter FH. *Atlas of Human Anatomy*. Summit, NJ: CIBA-Geigy Corporation; 1989.

Riordan J. *Breastfeeding and Human Lactation*. Sudbury, MA: Jones & Bartlett Publishers; 2004.

Wilson-Clay B, Hoover K. *The Breastfeeding Atlas*. 3rd ed. Manchaca, TX: Lactnews Press; 2005.

Wolf LS, Glass RP. *Feeding and Swallowing Disorders in Infancy*. San Antonio: Therapy Skill Builders; 1992.

Key Research Articles

Nickell WB, Skelton J. Breast fat and fallacies: More than 100 years of anatomical fantasy. *J Hum Lact.* 2005;21(2):126–130.

Ramsay DT, Kent JC, Hartmann RA, Hartmann PE. Anatomy of the lactating human breast redefined with ultrasound imaging. *J Anat.* 2005;206(6):525–534.

Ramsay DT, Kent JC, Owens RA, Hartmann PE. Ultrasound imaging of milk ejection in the breast of lactating women. *Pediatrics.* 2004;113(2):361–367.

Ramsay DT, Mitoulas LR, Kent JC, Larsson M, Hartmann PE. The use of ultrasound to characterize milk ejection in women using an electric breast pump. *J Hum Lact.* 2005;21(4):421–428.

MATERNAL AND INFANT ANATOMY QUESTIONS

Notice on question numbering: A-000 means a basic question, with one correct answer and three wrong answers. AP-000, along with the camera icon, means there is a picture that needs to be viewed to answer the question. The pictures are located on the CD-ROM included with this book and are numbered to correspond with the questions. AN-000, along with the frowning face icon, means the question has a **NEGATIVE** stem, therefore read the entire question very carefully to find the one **WRONG** answer among the choices. APN-000, with both icons in the margin, means there is a picture associated with the question AND the question has a negative stem. See Appendix A for a fuller explanation of negative stem questions.

A-001. What is the average normal heart rate of a full-term infant?

a. 80–100 beats per minute
b. 100–120 beats per minute
c. 120–160 beats per minute
d. 160–200 beats per minute

A-002. A 4-year-old girl was hurt in an auto accident, and as part of her treatment, a chest tube was placed between her ribs below and distal to her right nipple. What is the most significant effect that this surgery might have on her ability to breastfeed?

a. damage to the ductal structure
b. damage to the blood vessels supplying the breast
c. severed nerve pathways to the nipple
d. cut blood vessels to the breast

A-003. You are asked to evaluate a baby's ability to breastfeed before discharge following an uncomplicated hospital birth 12 hours ago. The baby weighs 2700 grams, or 6 pounds. Which of the following characteristics of her sucking would lead you to suspect that this child was born slightly preterm (or near term)? The baby:

a. moves smoothly from rooting behavior to latch-on.
b. sucks, swallows, and breathes in a coordinated rhythm.
c. sucks in short bursts with pauses.
d. begins by sucking rapidly, then slows to a steady rhythm.

A-004.   For optimal breastfeeding, which best describes effective positioning at breast?

a.   The nipple is inside the baby's mouth.
b.   No areola is visible outside the perimeter of the baby's mouth.
c.   The baby's nose lightly touches the mother's breast.
d.   The baby's mouth is open to a wide (>120-degree) angle.

A-005.   A baby's tongue is pressing a mother's nipple against the baby's hard palate. Which cranial nerve was most responsible for this tongue movement?

a.   spinal accessory
b.   vagus
c.   hypoglossal
d.   trigeminal

A-006.   During breastfeeding, where is the infant's tongue usually placed?

a.   resting behind the alveolar ridge
b.   covering the alveolar ridge
c.   spread flat across the floor of the mouth
d.   extended past the lower lip

A-007.   At what point during gestation does the mammary ridge form?

a.   4–5 weeks
b.   14–15 weeks
c.   24–25 weeks
d.   34–25 weeks

A-008.   Which breast structure contains muscle fibers?

a.   lactiferous sinuses
b.   nipple-areola complex
c.   Montgomery's tubercles
d.   lobules

A-009.   A mother is uncertain about providing her own milk for her preterm baby and has been told that her milk helps nerve development. Which sensory system is most compromised by the absence of human milk?

a.   olfactory
b.   auditory
c.   taste
d.   visual

A-010. Which description best describes the configuration of milk ducts in the lactating breast?

a. deep in the breast, like the core of an apple
b. branching beginning posterior to the areolar margin
c. bulbous pea-shaped swellings near the areolar margin
d. superficial and easy to compress

A-011. What is thought to be the primary function of the Montgomery glands?

a. pigmented marker for visual targeting
b. lubricates the skin of the areola
c. secretes antibiotic substances
d. changes elasticity of areola skin

A-012. Which nodes collect most of the lymph drainage from the lactating breast?

a. axillary nodes
b. intermammary nodes
c. subclavicular nodes
d. mesenteric nodes

A-013. Which breast structure contains the cells that secrete milk?

a. lactiferous ducts
b. lobules
c. alveoli
d. nipple

AN-014. Which fetal presenting position is the **LEAST LIKELY** to affect the baby's ability to breastfeed?

a. left occiput anterior (LOA)
b. right occiput posterior (ROP)
c. left mentum anterior (LMA)
d. right sacrum posterior (RSP)

AP-015. This mother has a 2-week-old baby who has difficulty attaching to her smaller breast, has been fussy after feeds, and has not regained birth weight. She claims that she does not have enough milk. The most likely cause of this situation is:

a. the mother is not feeding her baby frequently enough.
b. the smaller breast has insufficient glandular tissue.
c. the baby is attached incorrectly to the breast.
d. the baby is sensitive to an allergen in his mother's milk.

AP-016.   What is the most likely reason this baby cannot make a good seal on the mother's breast?

a.   The tongue is trough-shaped.
b.   The tongue is too thick.
c.   The baby has a small mouth opening.
d.   The lingual frenulum is short and tight.

AP-017.   What is the most likely condition pictured?

a.   candida infection at the base of the nipple
b.   large, fibrous nipple
c.   nipple edema from excessive pumping
d.   scars from breast reduction surgery

AP-018.   What is the name of the stringlike structure under this baby's tongue?

a.   labial frenulum
b.   incisive papilla
c.   lingual frenulum
d.   mucous membrane

AP-019.   This baby is 1 day old. In this picture, what are the white structures in his mouth?

a.   Epstein's pearls
b.   natal teeth
c.   incisive papilla
d.   sucking blisters

AP-020.   This child's mother tried unsuccessfully to breastfeed, and her child now has difficulty eating. The most likely reason is that this child has:

a.   anklyoglossia.
b.   macroglossia.
c.   microglossia.
d.   micrognathia.

AP-021.   This baby's mother complains of clicking and smacking during breastfeeds. The most likely explanation is:

a.   the high domed palate prevents deep latch.
b.   tongue-tie prevents deep attachment.
c.   tongue shape causes intermittent loss of seal.
d.   buccal fat pads are interfering with tongue movement.

APN-022. The condition pictured appeared on day 4 postpartum. The mother might be experiencing a similar phenomenon in any of the following locations **EXCEPT**:

a. near the umbilicus.
b. upper, inner arm.
c. groin.
d. outer thigh.

A-023. When a baby is properly latched on, where is the tip of the mother's nipple located in the baby's mouth?

a. immediately behind the upper gum ridge
b. at the center of the hard palate
c. at the juncture of the hard and soft palates
d. at the center of the soft palate

A-024. In a lactating woman, the milk ducts act as:

a. secretory glands producing cleansing agents for the areola.
b. a visual signal for the baby to latch on.
c. channels for the milk to flow to the nipple.
d. milk-secreting glands.

A-025. What is the function of the infant's epiglottis during swallowing?

a. It prevents milk from entering the trachea.
b. It prevents air from entering the esophagus.
c. It propels the bolus of milk to the back of the mouth.
d. It traps the bolus of milk, triggering a swallow.

A-026. Which is the most common site of placental implantation in the uterus, which could affect the baby's intra-uterine position and labor complications?

a. anterior side, cervical region
b. anterior side, fundal region
c. posterior side, cervical region
d. posterior side, fundal region

A-027. What process is primarily responsible for the increase in breast size (volume) during pregnancy?

a. increase in fatty stores in the breast
b. development of the duct system
c. growth of secretory epithelial cells
d. growing uterus triggers rib cage expansion

A-028.   During breastfeeding, how long does the nipple extend beyond its resting length?

a.   one quarter resting length (25%)
b.   half again (50%)
c.   twice its length (100%)
d.   it does not extend at all (0%)

A-029.   Which position for laboring women is most likely to reduce blood flow to the uterus and affect the baby's well-being?

a.   sitting
b.   lying on the left side
c.   lying supine
d.   lying on the right side

A-030.   Which structure supports the breast on the chest wall?

a.   Bandl's fibers
b.   Cooper's ligaments
c.   mammary ligaments
d.   myoepithelial tissue

A-031.   Pooling or collection of fluid between the skin and cranial bones of the infant's head is called:

a.   caput succedaneum.
b.   cephalhematoma.
c.   periosteal swelling.
d.   hydrocephalus.

A-032.   During a difficult birth, a baby suffered damage to the hypoglossal nerve. What is the most likely effect on breastfeeding? The baby would be:

a.   unable to maintain latch at breast.
b.   unable to move tongue to collect milk.
c.   unable to swallow.
d.   unable to grasp breast with mouth/lips.

A-033.   How many stages are described in Tanner's phases of breast development?

a.   3
b.   4
c.   5
d.   6

AP-034.   This baby is having difficulty latching on and breastfeeding. The most likely reason is:

    a. the baby is crying too hard to latch well
    b. the lingual frenulum is restricting tongue movement
    c. the lips are too tense
    d. the baby's mouth is not open wide enough

AP-035.   Which structure in this baby's mouth is most likely to cause a breastfeeding problem?

    a. alveolar gum ridge
    b. philtrim
    c. lingual frenulum
    d. short tongue

AP-036.   Which statement most accurately describes this baby's oral anatomy?

    a. The fat pads are too small.
    b. The philtrim is too broad.
    c. The lips are too thin and tensed.
    d. All visible structures are normal.

AP-037.   What is the most accurate description of this nipple shape?

    a. normal
    b. flat
    c. conical
    d. inverted

AP-038.   This mother's baby was having trouble latching on and breastfeeding. The most likely maternal reason for the baby's difficulty is:

    a. her nipple is somewhat short and flat.
    b. her breast is engorged, preventing deep latch.
    c. her nipple is very small, and the baby couldn't feel it.
    d. her nipple is very large, and the baby was choking on it.

AP-039.   The pale-colored lumps on this mother's breast are most likely:

    a. lipomas.
    b. plugged pores.
    c. Montgomery's tubercles.
    d. warts.

AP-040. The most likely cause of this nipple wound is:

a. the baby was nursing on the nipple tip.
b. the baby is tongue-tied.
c. there was no nipple preparation during pregnancy.
d. the use of a pacifier between feeds.

AP-041. What is the most likely cause of the lumps on this woman's areola?

a. irritation from wet bra pads
b. infected Montgomery glands
c. poison ivy
d. normal anatomy

AN-042. Which of the following is **NOT** an important function of the nipple-areolar complex in breastfeeding?

a. visual cue for the baby to latch on
b. production of lubricants by sebaceous glands
c. delivery of milk through nipple lumen
d. nervous system stimulation of the milk-ejection reflex

AN-043. Which structure is **NOT** part of the fetal circulatory system?

a. ductus venosus
b. foramen ovale
c. ductus arteriosus
d. foramen magnum

AP-044. This mother is currently breastfeeding a 2-year-old. The condition pictured on her areola is most likely:

a. a herpes (viral) infection.
b. wounds from the child biting.
c. normal Montgomery glands.
d. urticaria (hives).

AP-045. This mother is only able to express a few drops of milk, and her mother is telling her to supplement her 8-day-old baby. Your first action would be to:

a. help her position her baby deeply onto her breast.
b. instruct her in use of a tube-feeding device to be used during feeds.
c. contact her physician for a prescription for a galactagogue.
d. explore her options for supplementing her baby.

AP-046. This mother is concerned about the condition shown in this picture. Which of the following is the most appropriate response?

a. You may have Reynaud's syndrome. Keep the room warm when you breastfeed.
b. The lumps are Montgomery glands, which help lubricate the skin. They're normal.
c. This appears to be an allergic reaction. Did you recently start wearing a new bra?
d. May I check your baby's mouth to see if he has a thrush infection?

AP-047. This mother is concerned about the appearance of her nipples. Your best response is:

a. you probably have a thrush infection.
b. a bacterial infection is a possibility.
c. don't breastfeed until the herpes lesion heals.
d. your breast appears normal.

AP-048. The nipple shown in this picture is:

a. inverted.
b. retracted.
c. folded.
d. flat.

APN-049. All of the following will improve this mother's breastfeeding success **EXCEPT**:

a. wearing breast shells several hours a day for a few weeks during her pregnancy.
b. learning non-pharmaceutical methods of pain relief for labor.
c. vigorously pulling and stretching her nipples several times a day.
d. arranging for 24-hour rooming-in starting at birth.

APN-050. During breastfeeding, this baby's mother has noticed loud clicking and smacking. The **LEAST LIKELY** reason for the clicking is:

a. prominent buccal fat pads compromising tongue motion.
b. oddly shaped tongue tip, causing loss of seal during sucking.
c. short, tight labial frenulum, preventing deep attachment at breast.
d. tight muscles around the mouth, causing overuse of lips to create a seal.

MATERNAL AND INFANT ANATOMY ANSWERS

The parenthetical material at the end of each answer includes the discipline and time period, indicates whether the question pertains to knowledge or application, and specifies the degree of difficulty.

A-001. The answer is C. Normal newborn heart rate is 120–160 beats per minute. Tachycardia (fast heart rate) or bradycardia (slow heart rate) can interfere with the baby's ability to breastfeed. (Anatomy; 1–2 days; Knowledge; Difficulty: 5)

A-002. The answer is C. Severing nerve pathways would be the worst consequence to lactation. (Anatomy; Prenatal; Application; Difficulty: 5)

A-003. The answer is C. Short sucking bursts with pauses is an indicator of immaturity. The other patterns are indicators of a mature infant. (Anatomy; 1–2 days; Application; Difficulty: 2)

A-004. The answer is D. A wide gape is the most important visible feature of effective positioning and latch. All of the nipple and a portion of the areola should be inside the infant's mouth, but not necessarily all of it, depending on the areola diameter. The nose may lightly touch the breast, or be close to it, not buried in the breast. (Anatomy; 1–2 days; Application; Difficulty: 2)

A-005. The answer is C. The hypoglossal is the primary motor nerve of the tongue. The other nerves listed are involved in suck-swallow-breathe but play a lesser role in tongue movement. (Anatomy; General Principles; Application; Difficulty: 5)

A-006. The answer is B. The tongue usually extends past the lower gum ridge (alveolar ridge) and is cupped around the breast. Occasionally, it will extend past the lower lip. (Anatomy; General Principles; Application; Difficulty: 4)

A-007. The answer is A. The mammary ridge forms at 4–5 weeks' gestation. (Anatomy; Preconception; Knowledge; Difficulty: 3)

A-008. The answer is B. Smooth muscle fibers are found in the nipple-areola complex. (Anatomy; General Principles; Knowledge; Difficulty: 3)

A-009. The answer is D. The visual system is the last sensory system to develop during gestation and is therefore the most affected by preterm nutrition. Human milk makes a significant difference in visual development of the preterm infant, partly because of fatty acid profiles. (Anatomy; Prematurity; Knowledge; Difficulty: 2)

A-010. The answer is D. Ultrasound research confirms that milk ducts are easily compressed, do not display typical sinuses, and are superficial to the breast surface. (Anatomy; General Principles; Knowledge; Difficulty: 4)

A-011. The answer is B. The Montgomery glands are sebaceous glands that produce oil to lubricate the nipple and areolar skin, and they may have other functions. (Anatomy; General Principles; Application; Difficulty: 4)

A-012. The answer is A. The axillary nodes collect most of the lymph fluid; the intermammary and subclavicular nodes collect some lymph from the breast. The mesenteric nodes are in the abdomen. (Anatomy; General Principles; Knowledge; Difficulty: 4)

A-013. The answer is C. The alveoli contain secretory cells that produce milk. (Anatomy; General Principles; Knowledge; Difficulty: 3)

AN-014. The answer is A. Left occiput anterior (LOA) is the most common fetal presentation and least likely to cause birth trauma that could affect the baby's ability to breastfeed. Posterior presentations are less common; mentum and sacrum presentations are rare. (Anatomy; Prenatal; Application; Difficulty: 2)

AP-015. The answer is B. The smaller breast has characteristics of insufficient glandular tissue. (Anatomy; 15–28 days; Application; Difficulty: 4)

AP-016. The answer is D. The baby's lingual frenulum is short and tight, attached at the tongue tip, and on the bottom (alveolar) gum ridge. This prevents the tongue from creating a good seal at the breast. (Anatomy; 3–14 days; Application; Difficulty: 4)

AP-017. The answer is B. This is a large, fibrous nipple with no abnormal conditions. (Anatomy; 3–14 days; Knowledge; Difficulty: 4)

AP-018.   The answer is C. The stringlike structure connecting the tongue to the floor of the mouth is the lingual frenulum (or frenum). The labial frenulum is on the upper (maxillary) gum ridge. The incisive papilla are behind the upper gum ridge, and mucus membrane covers most of the inside of the baby's mouth. (Anatomy; General Principles; Knowledge; Difficulty: 4)

AP-019.   The answer is B. The white structures in this newborn's mouth are natal teeth. (Anatomy; 1–2 days; Knowledge; Difficulty: 3)

AP-020.   The answer is A. This child is tongue-tied, a condition often referred to as ankyloglossia. The lingual frenulum is short and/or tight. Without full normal tongue mobility, breastfeeding and eating (and other activities involving movement of the tongue) are compromised. (Anatomy; > 12 months; Knowledge; Difficulty: 3)

AP-021.   The answer is C. This baby's tongue shape is unusual. This baby's other oral anatomic structures are normal. (Anatomy; 1–3 months; Application; Difficulty: 3)

APN-022.   The answer is D. Accessory mammary tissue may be found along the "milk lines" that run from the upper, inner arm to the inguinal region. Accessory mammary tissue develops during fetal development. (Anatomy; 3–14 days; Application; Difficulty: 4)

A-023.   The answer is C. The nipple tip extends to or close to the juncture of the hard and soft palates during normal latch and positioning. (Anatomy; 1–2 days; Application; Difficulty: 4)

A-024.   The answer is C. The milk ducts are channels that collect milk and direct it to the nipple. The ducts dilate during the milk-ejection reflex. Milk-secreting cells are in the alveolus; the areola is possibly a landmark for the baby; and the Montgomery glands (tubercles) secrete a substance that cleanses the areola. (Anatomy; General Principles; Knowledge; Difficulty: 3)

A-025.   The answer is A. The infant's epiglottis covers the trachea during swallowing, preventing milk from entering the airway. Between swallows, it prevents air from entering the esophagus. (Anatomy; General Principles; Knowledge; Difficulty: 4)

A-026.   The answer is D. The most common implantation site is the posterior side of the fundus. This is relevant to breastfeeding because placental implantation affects fetal maturity, position for delivery, and complications during labor including possible cesarean surgery, all of which affect the mother and the baby's ability to breastfeed. (Anatomy; Prenatal; Knowledge; Difficulty: 3)

A-027. The answer is C. Growth of the secretory epithelial cells (lactocytes) is the primary factor causing breast growth during pregnancy. (Anatomy; Prenatal; Application; Difficulty: 5)

A-028. The answer is C. The nipple stretches to twice its resting length (100%) during normal breastfeeding. (Anatomy; General Principles; Knowledge; Difficulty: 3)

A-029. The answer is C. In the supine position, the uterus can compress the inferior vena cava, causing maternal hypotension and reduced blood flow to the uterus. This is relevant to breastfeeding because a long, difficult labor can delay the onset of copious milk production. (Anatomy; Labor/Birth; Application; Difficulty: 3)

A-030. The answer is B. Cooper's ligaments support the breasts. Softening or stretching of these ligaments during pregnancy may contribute to sagging. (Anatomy; Prenatal; Knowledge; Difficulty: 3)

A-031. The answer is A. Caput succedaneum is the collection of fluid between the skin and cranial bone of the newborn, often associated with the use of vacuum extraction devices. Any head injury or insult may affect the infant's ability to breastfeed. (Anatomy; Labor/Birth; Knowledge; Difficulty: 3)

A-032. The answer is B. The hypoglossal nerve is the primary motor nerve of the tongue; therefore, an inability to move the tongue to gather or collect milk is the most likely result of damage to this nerve. (Anatomy; Labor/Birth; Application; Difficulty: 5)

A-033. The answer is C. Tanner described 5 phases in breast development from puberty until age 15–17 years. (Anatomy; Preconception; Knowledge; Difficulty: 4)

AP-034. The answer is B. The baby's short, tight frenulum is restricting proper tongue movement needed for latch and feeding. (Anatomy; 3–14 days; Application; Difficulty: 4)

AP-035. The answer is C. This baby's lingual frenulum, the stringlike tissue between the tongue and the floor of the mouth, is short and tight and likely to restrict tongue motion needed for effective feeding. (Anatomy; 1–2 days; Application; Difficulty: 3)

AP-036. The answer is D. This baby's oral anatomy is normal. (Anatomy; 3–14 days; Knowledge; Difficulty: 3)

AP-037. The answer is B. This nipple is flat. There is no distinct shank between the areola and nipple bud or tip. (Anatomy; 15–28 days; Knowledge; Difficulty: 4)

AP-038. The answer is A. This nipple is somewhat short and flat. Most babies would have no problem with this nipple. The breast is not engorged, and the nipple is in the normal range of sizes. (Anatomy; 3–14 days; Application; Difficulty: 3)

AP-039. The answer is C. The lumps are Montgomery's tubercles (Montgomery glands) and are entirely normal. (Anatomy; 7–12 months; Knowledge; Difficulty: 3)

AP-040. The answer is B. This wound was caused by a baby whose lingual frenulum was short and tight (tongue-tied). (Anatomy; 3–14 days; Application; Difficulty: 4)

AP-041. The answer is D. This is a normal breast. The slight pink color of the nipple and areola is normal for this woman. (Anatomy; 3–14 days; Application; Difficulty: 5)

AN-042. The answer is B. The nipple's sebaceous glands play a very minor, if any, role in lubrication. The nipple is a passageway for milk, is probably a visual cue for the baby, and contains many nerve endings involved in the milk-ejection reflex. (Anatomy; 1–2 days; Application; Difficulty: 2)

AN-043. The answer is D. The foramen magnum is the large opening in the cranium (skull) through which the spinal cord passes. The cranial nerves are involved in infant sucking. (Anatomy; Prenatal; Knowledge; Difficulty: 2)

AP-044. The answer is C. The raised areas on her areola are normal Montgomery glands. This is a normal breast. (Anatomy; 15–28 days; Application; Difficulty: 2)

AP-045. The answer is D. This mother's breasts are severely underdeveloped (hypoplastic) with very little visible glandular tissue and veining. At 8 days, she should be producing substantial quantities of milk. The first action is to assure the infant's nutrition while you and she explore other strategies for supporting her lactation. The metal disk is a U.S. 25-cent coin for size comparison. (Anatomy; 3–14 days; Application; Difficulty: 5)

AP-046. The answer is B. The pale-colored lumps on the areola are Montgomery's tubercles (Montgomery's glands) and are completely normal. (Anatomy; >12 months; Application; Difficulty: 2)

AP-047. The answer is D. This is a normal breast. (Anatomy; Prenatal; Application; Difficulty: 4)

AP-048. The answer is B. This nipple retracts upon compression at the areola. (Anatomy; Prenatal; Knowledge; Difficulty: 5)

APN-049. The answer is C. Vigorous pulling and stretching have not been shown to improve breastfeeding success for mothers with flat nipples and can actually damage tissue. The other actions will support her breastfeeding. (Anatomy; Prenatal; Application; Difficulty: 2)

APN-050. The answer is C. This baby's labial (upper) frenulum is normal. However, the other three choices are possible factors in the baby's clicking and smacking during breastfeeding. The buccal pads are exceptionally prominent. (Anatomy; 1–3 months; Application; Difficulty: 5)

Scoring:

Total number of questions in this section _____

Number of questions answered correctly _____

Percent correct (divide number correct by total number) _____

B. MATERNAL AND INFANT NORMAL PHYSIOLOGY AND ENDOCRINOLOGY

In the 2000 exam blueprint, 19 to 33 questions are dedicated to maternal and infant normal physiology and endocrinology.

SUBTOPICS INCLUDED IN THIS CATEGORY

1. Maternal/female hormones—general

   a. Milk production (milk synthesis—process)
     i. Lactogenesis
     ii. Endocrine/autocrine control of milk supply
     iii. Induced lactation and relactation
   b. Fertility
     i. Family planning, including Lactational Amenorrhea Method (LAM)
     ii. Sexuality
     iii. Breastfeeding during pregnancy; tandem nursing

2. Infant bodily functions

   a. Digestion, GI tract, and metabolism
   b. Hepatic, pancreatic, and renal function
   c. Placental nutrition to breastfeeding—evolution of infant nutrition
   d. Effect of complementary feeds
   e. Voiding and stool patterns; gut closure, gut micro⁻ora
   f. Process of suck-swallow-breathe

CORE READING

Textbooks

Clinical Protocol # 1: Hypoglycemia. New Rochelle, NY: Academy of Breastfeeding Medicine; 2006.

Clinical Protocol # 13: Contraception. New Rochelle, NY: Academy of Breastfeeding Medicine; 2005.

Clinical Protocol # 9: Use of galactogogues in initiating or augmenting maternal milk supply. New Rochelle, NY: Academy of Breastfeeding Medicine; 2004.

Guiding Principles for Complementary Feeding of the Breastfed Child. Washington, DC: Pan American Health Organization & World Health Organization; 2001.

Hypoglycaemia of the Newborn: Review of the Literature. Geneva, Switzerland: World Health Organization; 1998.

Lauwers J, Swisher A. *Counseling the Nursing Mother.* 4th ed. Sudbury, MA: Jones & Bartlett Publishers; 2003.

Lawrence RA, Lawrence RM. *Breastfeeding: A Guide for the Medical Profession*. 6th ed. St. Louis: Elsevier Mosby; 2005.

Morbacher N, Stock J. *The Breastfeeding Answer Book*. 3rd ed. Schaumburg, IL: La Leche League International; 2003.

Morris SE, Klein MD. *Pre-Feeding Skills—A Comprehensive Resource for Mealtime Development*. 2nd ed. San Antonio: Therapy Skill Builders; 2000.

Relactation: Review of Experience and Recommendations for Practice. Geneva, Switzerland: World Health Organization; 1998.

Riordan J. *Breastfeeding and Human Lactation*. Sudbury, MA: Jones & Bartlett Publishers; 2004.

Wilson-Clay B, Hoover K. *The Breastfeeding Atlas*. 3rd ed. Manchaca, TX: Lactnews Press; 2005.

Wolf LS, Glass RP. *Feeding and Swallowing Disorders in Infancy*. San Antonio: Therapy Skill Builders; 1992.

Key Research Articles

Caglar MK, Ozer I, Altugan FS. Risk factors for excess weight loss and hypernatremia in exclusively breast-fed infants. *Braz J Med Biol Res.* 2006;39(4):539–544.

Cregan MD, de Mello TR, Hartmann PE. Pre-term delivery and breast expression: Consequences for initiating lactation. *Adv Exp Med Biol.* 2000;478:427–428.

Cregan MD, de Mello TR, Kershaw D, McDougall K, Hartmann PE. Initiation of lactation in women after preterm delivery. *Acta Obstet Gynecol Scand.* 2002;81(9):870–877.

Cregan MD, Hartmann PE. Computerized breast measurement from conception to weaning: Clinical implications. *J Hum Lact.* 1999;15(2):89–96.

Cregan MD, Mitoulas LR, Hartmann PE. Milk prolactin, feed volume and duration between feeds in women breastfeeding their full-term infants over a 24 h period. *Exp Physiol.* 2002;87(2):207–214.

Cregan MD, Mitoulas LR, Hartmann PE. Variation in prolactin consumption by fully breastfed infants. *Adv Exp Med Biol.* 2004;554:431–433.

Daly SE, Kent JC, Owens RA, Hartmann PE. Frequency and degree of milk removal and the short-term control of human milk synthesis. *Exp Physiol.* 1996;81(5):861–875.

Daly SEJ, Hartmann PE. Infant demand and milk supply. Part 1: Infant demand and milk supply in lactating women. *J Hum Lact.* 1995;11:21–26.

Daly SEJ, Hartmann PE. Infant demand and milk supply. Part 2: The short-term control of milk synthesis in lactating women. *J Hum Lact.* 1995;11:27–31.

Daly SEJ, Kent JC, Huynh DQ, et al. The determination of short-term volume changes and the rate of synthesis of human milk using computerized breast measurement. *Exp Physiol.* 1996;77:79–87.

Hartmann P, Cregan M. Lactogenesis and the effects of insulin-dependent diabetes mellitus and prematurity. *J Nutr.* 2001;131(11):3016S–3020S.

Hartmann PE, Cregan MD, Ramsay DT, Simmer K, Kent JC. Physiology of lactation in preterm mothers: Initiation and maintenance. *Pediatr Ann.* 2003;32(5):351–355.

Kennedy KI, Visness CM. Contraceptive efficacy of lactational amenorrhoea. *Lancet.* 1992;339(8787):227–230.

Kent JC, Mitoulas L, Cox DB, Owens RA, Hartmann PE. Breast volume and milk production during extended lactation in women. *Exp Physiol.* 1999;84(2):435–447.

Kent JC, Mitoulas LR, Cregan MD, Ramsay DT, Doherty DA, Hartmann PE. Volume and frequency of breast-feedings and fat content of breast milk throughout the day. *Pediatrics.* 2006;117(3):e387–e395.

Kent JC, Ramsay DT, Doherty D, Larsson M, Hartmann PE. Response of breasts to different stimulation patterns of an electric breast pump. *J Hum Lact.* 2003;19(2):179–186; quiz 87–88, 218.

Labbok MH. Effects of breastfeeding on the mother. *Pediatr Clin North America.* 2001;48:143–158.

Metaj M, Laroia N, Lawrence RA, Ryan RM. Comparison of breast- and formula-fed normal newborns in time to first stool and urine. *J Perinatol.* 2003;23(8):624–628.

Mitoulas LR, Kent JC, Cox DB, Owens RA, Sherriff JL, Hartmann PE. Variation in fat, lactose and protein in human milk over 24 h and throughout the first year of lactation. *Br J Nutr.* 2002;88(1):29–37.

Ramsay DT, Mitoulas LR, Kent JC, et al. Milk flow rates can be used to identify and investigate milk ejection in women expressing breast milk using an electric breast pump. *Breastfeeding Med.* 2006;1(1):14–23.

Rogers IS. Relactation. *Early Hum Dev* 1997;49 Suppl:S75–81.

Viggiano D, Fasano D, Monaco G, Strohmenger L. Breast feeding, bottle feeding, and non-nutritive sucking; effects on occlusion in deciduous dentition. *Arch Dis Child.* 2004;89(12):1121–1123.

MATERNAL AND INFANT NORMAL PHYSIOLOGY AND ENDOCRINOLOGY QUESTIONS

Notice on question numbering: B-000 means a basic question, with one correct answer and three wrong answers. BP-000, along with the camera icon, means there is a picture that needs to be viewed to answer the question. The pictures are located on the CD-ROM included with this book and are numbered to correspond with the questions. BN-000, along with the frowning face icon, means the question has a NEGATIVE stem; therefore, read the entire question very carefully to find the one WRONG answer among the choices. BPN-000, with both icons in the margin, means there is a picture associated with the question AND the question has a negative stem. See Appendix A for a fuller explanation of negative stem questions.

B-001. The grandmother of a 4-week-old exclusively breastfed baby who has 5–6 profuse, yellow, loose stools every day is worried, and asks for an explanation. The most likely cause for stools of this kind is:

a. diarrhea.
b. infection with an intestinal parasite.
c. the mother recently ate bright yellow squash.
d. normal stools.

B-002. A healthy, full-term newborn is found to have a total bilirubin level of 14.2 mg/dL (245 μmol/L) on the fourth day of life. The BEST recommendation is:

a. breastfeed the baby at least 10 times a day.
b. feed artificial baby milk after breastfeedings.
c. feed artificial baby milk for 24 hours; maintain supply through pumping.
d. this level of bilirubin is rarely a problem.

B-003. A 27-year-old woman will give birth to her first baby in about 3 weeks. She asks her healthcare provider if she will be able to breastfeed after having a breast reduction with her nipple autotransplanted at the age of 19. The best response is:

a. there will be no problem breastfeeding.
b. it may be possible for the first 3 months.
c. you may not be able to breastfeed.
d. you should try and see what happens.

B-004. A mother calls about her 5-month-old infant, worried that she is losing her milk because her breasts are soft and her infant no longer seems content for 2 hours after feedings. He cries frequently and puts his fists to his mouth 45 minutes after feeding. The most likely cause for the situation she describes is:

a. her infant is experiencing a normal growth and behavior pattern.
b. offering bottles is interfering with breast milk production.
c. the development of colic in her infant.
d. her body is adapting well to her baby's demand for milk.

B-005. At 14-days postbirth, a mother tells you that she has bright red vaginal bleeding and that her baby (birth weight 9 lbs, 2 oz) seems constantly hungry. The most likely explanation for this is:

a. large-for-gestational age baby.
b. early return of menses.
c. uterine infection.
d. retained placenta.

B-006. After an unmedicated labor and birth, how soon is a baby most likely to be able and ready to breastfeed?

a. within the first 5 minutes
b. within the first hour
c. at approximately 6 hours
d. by 12 hours

B-007. A mother complains that her baby cries constantly. She has been feeding her baby on a strict schedule found in a popular parenting book. Your best response to her is:

a. it is acceptable to limit your baby's feeds to 10 minutes per breast.
b. you can give a pacifier to help your baby extend the time between feeds.
c. babies do best when there are no restrictions on length or frequency of breastfeeds.
d. giving water between feeds will get your baby onto a more regular feeding schedule.

B-008.   A mother calls on day 12 to obtain a breast pump to increase her milk supply. She had an emergency cesarean birth, did not breastfeed or pump for the first 3 days, and has been pumping 3–4 times a day since then. She has not been able to get the baby to latch and feed effectively. Which of the following is most likely to increase the rate of milk synthesis?

a.   Begin drinking 1/4 cup of fenugreek tea 3 times a day.
b.   Thoroughly drain the breasts every 2–3 hours by nursing, pumping, and/or expressing.
c.   Put the baby to breast every 2–3 hours to stimulate the breasts even if the baby does not feed well.
d.   Ask her physician to prescribe metaclopromide to increase prolactin.

B-009.   Cholecystokinin, which is released by sucking, has which of the following effects?

a.   arousal
b.   satiety
c.   agitation
d.   depression

B-010.   A mother asks why she can express an ounce of milk even after her baby finishes feeding. The most likely explanation for this is:

a.   the baby is not feeding effectively.
b.   babies normally do not take all of the milk available at a given feeding.
c.   she has an oversupply of milk.
d.   her baby does not like the taste of her milk.

B-011.   A 4-month-old, exclusively breastfed baby feeds about 8–10 times per day with 1–2 feeds at night. His mother is concerned that she cannot make enough milk because her neighbor had to increase the amount of formula for her baby at 4 months. Your best response to her is:

a.   your baby's feeding pattern indicates that he is ready for solids.
b.   your baby's milk needs are stable for at least another 2 months.
c.   your baby is clustering much of his milk intake at night, which is normal.
d.   your baby will take more milk from your breasts if he needs more.

B-012.   A laboring woman has received several bags of intravenous fluids during her labor. Her baby is now several hours old and is having trouble latching on to her. The most likely explanation for this is:

a.   her breasts are edematous from the IV fluids.
b.   the labor affected the baby's ability to suck.
c.   her milk tastes unpleasant because of the fluids given.
d.   the drug reduced the colostrum available, and the baby is frustrated.

B-013. The mother of a premature baby needs to express milk for her baby. She has relatively small breasts. Which expressing pattern is most likely to result in abundant supply?

a. 6 times a day for 30 minutes per breast
b. every 3–4 hours for 10 minutes per breast
c. every 2–3 hours until the milk flow ceases
d. every 1–2 hours during the day and once at night

B-014. A 2-day-old baby feeds from one breast for about 25 minutes, then falls asleep and releases the breast. A few minutes later, he wakes and feeds on the second breast for about 10 minutes, then falls asleep and releases the breast. The most likely explanation for this behavior is:

a. the mother does not yet have enough milk to satisfy the baby.
b. the baby is not latched deeply onto the breast.
c. the baby is sleepy and poorly coordinated as a result of labor medications.
d. this is a normal pattern for this age baby.

BN-015. A woman had an emergency hysterectomy at 37 weeks' gestation. Which of the following statements is **LEAST** relevant to her ability to breastfeed?

a. The mother may have difficulty establishing a full milk supply if she experienced excessive blood loss.
b. The mother will be unable to produce milk if her ovaries were removed along with her uterus.
c. The baby may nurse poorly due to the effects of the mother's anesthetics.
d. The baby's first nursing may be delayed for several hours.

BN-016. Which of the following statements about the effect of human milk on the child's immune system is **FALSE**?

a. Human milk stimulates baby to begin making his own SigA and other antibodies.
b. Exclusively breastfed babies have better response to immunizations.
c. Mother's own milk provides passive immunity between placentally acquired immunity and autonomous immune protection.
d. The breastfed baby has a higher risk of infection because he relies on mother's immune protection during breastfeeding.

BN-017. When a baby cannot breastfeed, advantages of using a small cup or spoon include all of the following **EXCEPT**:

a. inexpensive; readily available.
b. suck response may diminish.
c. avoids bottle/teat use.
d. easy to clean.

BN-018. A 34-week-old, premature infant is being discharged to his parents' care. Breastfeeding discharge teaching should include all of the following **EXCEPT**:

a. he should be fed in a position that supports his head, neck, and shoulders.
b. his sucking bursts should be regular and rhythmic.
c. any supplements to direct breastfeeding should be mother's own expressed milk.
d. he needs to be fed at least every 2–3 hours around the clock.

BN-019. All of the following developmental processes are interrupted by premature birth **EXCEPT**:

a. bone mineralization.
b. gut maturation.
c. deposition of fat.
d. hearing and taste.

BP-020. This baby feeds for 30–45 minutes at each breast, each feeding, in the exact position shown in this picture. The most likely cause of this behavior is:

a. normal behavior.
b. disorganized sucking.
c. mother has low milk supply.
d. delayed clearing of labor drugs.

BP-021. Which of these practices most supports the baby's ability to crawl to the breast immediately after birth?

a. Avoiding washing off the amniotic fluid from baby's hands.
b. Bathing the mother immediately so her perspiration does not offend the baby.
c. Giving narcotics epidurally during the labor so the mother is pain-free at this stage.
d. Suctioning the baby to clear his airway of mucus.

BP-022. Which hormone is especially high in this mother–baby dyad immediately postbirth?

a. adrenaline
b. oxytocin
c. estrogen
d. prolactin

BP-023. To minimize physiologic stress to the infant from this procedure, the best strategy would be:

a. warm the room to prevent the infant from becoming chilled.
b. clamp the cord while the baby is resting skin-to-skin on mother's body.
c. have the mother's partner or helper hold the baby while the cord is clamped.
d. ask the mother to breastfeed the baby while the cord is being clamped.

 BP-024. At this postdelivery stage, which statement is most accurate?

a. Too many visitors can interfere with feeding.
b. The mother is getting ready to go back to work.
c. The baby can't consume all the milk that the mother is making.
d. The baby is sleeping 6–8 hours at night.

B-025. Which method of family planning would most interfere with breastfeeding?

a. tubal ligation
b. progestin-only oral contraceptives
c. intrauterine devices
d. natural family planning (periodic abstinence)

B-026. A mother wants to continue breastfeeding her 18-month-old child during a subsequent pregnancy. A neighbor told her to wean so that the toddler's breastfeeding does not trigger premature labor. Your best response is:

a. suggest she immediately wean the older baby.
b. tell her breastfeeding during a normal pregnancy is not harmful to either child.
c. suggest she use lanolin during the pregnancy to prevent nipple pain.
d. recommend that she discontinue sexual relations so that uterine contractions do not jeopardize the pregnancy.

B-027. A mother is concerned about her baby's feeding pattern. The baby nurses 10–30 minutes on one breast and then self-detaches. Your best response to her is:

a. this is a normal, common pattern.
b. babies get all they need in the first 10 minutes.
c. your baby has a sucking problem.
d. your let-down reflex is too slow.

B-028. How much milk does a newborn obtain at the breast each day during the first week if breastfeeding is on cue (unrestricted)?

a. 3–4 oz (90–120 ml) per day of colostrum
b. increasing amounts each day as milk volume increases
c. less than needed for adequate hydration until day 5
d. 25 ounces (750 ml) per day from day 2 onward

B-029. The husband of a breastfeeding woman is eager for his wife to be as amorous as she was before his son was born 3 months ago. He asks you for some suggestions that will help her feel more eager for his lovemaking. Your best response is:

a. you'll just have to learn to live with it. When the baby weans, your relationship will get better.
b. try helping her with the baby, housework, and cooking. She would probably consider that as great foreplay.
c. it would be more appropriate for me to talk directly with your wife about this subject.
d. you may want to use some lubricant, time your lovemaking around the baby's sleep and nursing pattern, and take your time to help her get into the mood.

B-030. A 5-month-old exclusively breastfed baby is recovering from hernia surgery. Which is the most likely breastfeeding pattern for this child?

a. the same as before the hospitalization
b. more frequent nursing sessions to quench thirst
c. longer nursing sessions for the comforting of slow milk flow
d. less frequent sessions because milk supply has decreased

B-031. Which of the following complementary family planning methods is most effective and compatible with breastfeeding?

a. condoms
b. implanted progestin
c. combined oral contraceptives
d. Lactational Amenorrhea Method

BN-032. A cesarean birth is likely to affect breastfeeding in all of the following ways **EXCEPT**:

a. increased maternal pain.
b. need for maternal medications.
c. delayed lactogenesis II.
d. more separation of mother and infant.

BN-033. Which statement regarding the timing of Lactogenesis II is **FALSE**?

a. It begins 30–40 hours after delivery of the placenta.
b. It may initially go unnoticed by the mother.
c. It may be delayed 10–20 hours if the mother has diabetes.
d. The timing is dependent on breast stimulation by the baby.

BP-034. This mother–infant dyad needs to be carefully assessed for:

a. duration of feeds.
b. thrush.
c. nipple shield use.
d. latch-on technique.

BP-035. This picture was taken 3 hours after the baby fed on this breast. The condition pictured is most likely:

a. infectious mastitis in the upper, outer quadrant.
b. galactocele on the lateral side (toward the mother's arm).
c. moderate postfeed breast fullness.
d. edema caused by milk stasis.

BP-036. The behavior exhibited by this baby often occurs about 2 hours after the last breastfeed. What is your best recommendation to the mother?

a. Offer the baby a pacifier to satisfy her need to suck.
b. Breastfeed her again, now.
c. Let her cry a bit so her feedings get spaced out.
d. Give her some water to tide her over until the next feed.

BP-037. What is the most likely conclusion you could draw from the appearance of this lactating woman's breasts?

a. The smaller breast has insufficient glandular tissue.
b. The larger breast is making much more milk than the smaller.
c. The baby most recently nursed on the smaller breast.
d. Lactation and breastfeeding are proceeding smoothly for her and her baby.

BP-038.   What is the first suggestion you would give this mother?

a.   Use a nipple shield during feeds.
b.   Have your baby's suck evaluated immediately.
c.   Keep up the good work—everything looks great.
d.   Bring your baby deeper onto your breast.

BP-039.   What neurodevelopmental state is this baby in?

a.   drowsy
b.   quiet alert
c.   active alert
d.   REM sleep

BP-040.   This baby's mother complains about clicking and smacking during breastfeeds, which have continued since the baby was a newborn. She has just begun taking solid food. The first action you would do is:

a.   check for a cleft of the soft palate.
b.   observe a full breastfeeding session.
c.   have the baby's doctor diagnose or rule out thrush infection.
d.   ask the mother to record what foods the baby has taken in the past 24 hours.

BP-041.   Upon seeing this 14-day-old infant, the first question you would ask the mother about her own health status is:

a.   are you getting enough rest?
b.   are you eating a well-balanced diet?
c.   do you have a fever?
d.   what color and quantity is your vaginal discharge?

BP-042.   The condition pictured appeared suddenly 3 days postbirth. The first suggestion you would give to this mother is:

a.   try massaging the plug of milk toward your nipple.
b.   see whether the lump changes size after you nurse your baby.
c.   put hot compresses on the swollen area.
d.   make an appointment with a breast surgeon for a biopsy.

BP-043. This mother is 4 days postbirth. What is the most likely cause of the condition pictured?

a. plugged milk duct
b. infected sweat gland in axilla
c. mastitis in the tail of Spence
d. milk stasis in accessory breast tissue

 BP-044. This mother is worried that her left breast is larger than her right. Your first response should be:

a. the left breast appears to have mastitis.
b. different breast sizes are very common.
c. what size were your breasts before pregnancy?
d. the left will clearly make more milk than the right.

 BP-045. This mother calls you to find a solution for sudden and persistent sore nipples that have not responded to standard remedies. She had a menstrual period 10 weeks ago but has not had once since. Your first comment/question should be:

a. you'll need to wean your toddler because continued breastfeeding might cause a miscarriage.
b. the tenderness is likely because of pregnancy hormones. How much of a problem is this for you?
c. is your toddler teething? His saliva may be irritating to your nipples now.
d. have you or he recently taken an antibiotic?

 BN-046. A mother delivered a preterm baby at 28 weeks' gestation. All of the following will be helpful to establish and maintain an adequate milk supply **EXCEPT**:

a. beginning to express or pump within the first 12 hours following birth.
b. expressing the breasts fully for 2 minutes after the flow of drops ceases.
c. expressing or pumping every 2–4 hours around the clock.
d. pumping every 2 hours during the day and getting a good night's sleep at night.

MATERNAL AND INFANT NORMAL PHYSIOLOGY AND ENDOCRINOLOGY ANSWERS

The parenthetical material at the end of each answer includes the discipline and time period, indicates whether the question pertains to knowledge or application, and specifies the degree of difficulty.

B-001. The answer is D. Stools of exclusively breastfed babies in the first month are exactly as described. (Physiology; 15–28 days; Application; Difficulty: 3)

B-002. The answer is A. It is always appropriate to make sure the baby is feeding well as the first strategy. While that level of bilirubin is rarely a problem for a healthy, full-term newborn, the lactation consultant should always make sure the baby is effectively feeding as a top priority. (Physiology; 3–14 days; Application; Difficulty: 3)

B-003. The answer is D. No assumptions can be made about her ability to breastfeed after breast surgery, although she should be followed closely in the first week postbirth because surgery can disrupt ducts and nerve pathways needed for adequate milk synthesis. (A. Anatomy; Prenatal; Application; Difficulty: 3)

B-004. The answer is A. Her infant is experiencing a normal growth and behavior pattern, possibly a sudden increase in appetite. Initial breast edema is resolved, and the breasts are becoming calibrated to produce enough milk for her baby without feeding him until he is overfull. The behavior she describes is a normal pattern for breastfed babies. (Physiology; 1–3 months; Application; Difficulty: 4)

B-005. The answer is D. Bright red lochia at 14 days with signs of low milk supply suggest that retained placental fragments are suppressing the onset of Lactogenesis II. (Physiology; 3–14 days; Application; Difficulty: 3)

B-006. The answer is B. The Baby-Friendly Hospital Initiative Step 4 states, "Place babies in skin-to-skin contact with their mothers immediately following birth for at least an hour and encourage mothers to recognize when their babies are ready to breastfeed, offering help if needed." Some babies get to the breast and are nursing well in the first 5–10 minutes. Many unmedicated babies are nursing well by 30 minutes, while some babies take an hour or longer to accomplish their first feed. (Physiology; 1–2 days; Application; Difficulty: 4)

B-007. The answer is C. Babies feed for varying lengths and at varying intervals according to their hunger, emotional needs, growth and developmental stages, and other physiological factors. Placing restrictions on length or frequency, or offering substitutes, disrupts the breastfeeding relationship and interferes with fulfillment of infant needs. (Physiology; 15–28 days; Application; Difficulty: 2)

B-008. The answer is B. Thorough removal of milk will increase the *rate* of milk synthesis. Stimulation without removal is not effective because milk stasis slows the rate of milk synthesis. Galactagogues are not well researched. Metaclopromide™ will increase prolactin, but needs to be combined with adequate milk removal. (Physiology; 3–14 days; Application; Difficulty: 5)

B-009. The answer is B. The release of cholecystokinin causes satiety and relaxation. (Physiology; General Principles; Knowledge; Difficulty: 2)

B-010. The answer is B. Babies consume about 2/3 of the available milk in a breast during any given feeding. (Physiology; 15–28 days; Application; Difficulty: 3)

B-011. The answer is D. Babies deliberately leave some milk in the breasts, consuming about 2/3 of the available milk volume at a given feed. Milk volumes consumed are relatively stable from the first week or so until at least 6 months. The normal range varies widely. Artificially fed babies may need more milk as they get older because the nutrients are less available for growth. (Physiology; 4–6 months; Application; Difficulty: 4)

B-012. The answer is A. Overhydration during labor may cause breast, nipple, and areolar edema, making latch-on difficult for the baby. To date, little research has investigated this issue. (Physiology; Labor/Birth; Application; Difficulty: 5)

B-013. The answer is C. Small breasts usually have less storage capacity than larger breasts, so frequent expression triggers a high rate of milk synthesis. The rate of synthesis is highest when the breasts are emptiest, so expressing until the flow ceases will also maximize the rate of milk synthesis. (Physiology; Prematurity; Application; Difficulty: 4)

B-014. The answer is D. This is a normal pattern on day 2. The baby's appetite, interest, and ability to feed will determine whether one or both breasts are taken at a given feeding. This pattern would be described as a paired breastfeed. (Physiology; 1–2 days; Application; Difficulty: 5)

BN-015. The answer is B. Ovarian function postbirth is not related to lactation. The other statements are relevant. (Physiology; Prematurity; Application; Difficulty: 2)

BN-016. The answer is D. Breastfeeding triggers and enhances maturation of the baby's own immune system. (Physiology; General Principles; Application; Difficulty: 5)

BN-017. The answer is B. Some believe that cup-feeding for an extended time may reduce the baby's sucking urge. (Physiology; Prematurity; Application; Difficulty: 2)

BN-018. The answer is B. Premature babies often exhibit an irregular and arrhythmic sucking pattern, which improves as they mature. All the other statements are accurate and appropriate. (Physiology; Prematurity; Application; Difficulty: 2)

BN-019. The answer is D. Hearing and taste develop early in gestation. All the other processes are compromised by preterm birth. (Physiology; Prematurity; Knowledge; Difficulty: 2)

BP-020. The answer is B. A common sign of disorganized sucking is the baby feeds for extended periods with its eyes closed. Feeding for 30–45 minutes per breast is not normal behavior for this healthy 3-week-old. Mother's milk supply cannot be ascertained by infant feeding behavior, and the effect of most labor drugs would have diminished by this time. (Physiology; 15–28 days; Application; Difficulty: 5)

BP-021. The answer is A. The baby finds his way to the breast partly by smell. Placing the unwashed baby on the mother's unwashed body facilitates the baby's ability to self-attach to the breast. The other practices listed would interfere with this natural process. (Physiology; Labor/Birth; Knowledge; Difficulty: 3)

BP-022. The answer is B. Oxytocin is especially high in the immediate postbirth period, which helps mother and baby develop trust in one another. (Physiology; Labor/Birth; Knowledge; Difficulty: 4)

BP-023. The answer is B. Skin-to-skin contact is calming and soothing for the infant. Most procedures can be done while the baby is resting skin-to-skin on the mother's body. In theory, the mother might be breastfeeding during this procedure. However, holding the baby skin-to-skin would be more realistic and not depend on the infant's readiness to feed. (Physiology; Labor/Birth; Application; Difficulty: 5)

BP-024.   The answer is C. Many mothers have more milk than their baby needs in the first 2 weeks. Supply gradually adjusts to the baby's needs over the first 6 weeks or so. (Physiology; 3–14 days; Application; Difficulty: 4)

B-025.   The answer is B. Use of progestin-containing contraceptives can diminish milk supply if given prior to 8 weeks postbirth. (Physiology; 1–3 months; Knowledge; Difficulty: 4)

B-026.   The answer is B. There is no documented harm to either the fetus or older baby by continuing to breastfeed. Nipple pain during pregnancy is hormonally based and may be unavoidable. (Physiology; Prenatal; Application; Difficulty: 4)

B-027.   The answer is A. Research and experience show that a range of 7–30 minutes per breast is normal and common. About 30% of babies always feed from only one breast (always unpaired feeds). (Physiology; 15–28 days; Application; Difficulty: 3)

B-028.   The answer is B. On days 1–3, the baby gets about 30 ml/day of colostrum. As lactogenesis II occurs, the baby obtains more per day as milk volume rapidly rises to 600 ml/day or more by day 5. (Physiology; 1–2 days; Knowledge; Difficulty: 4)

B-029.   The answer is D. Libido varies widely among breastfeeding women. Men/fathers should be helped to find new ways to please the mother that are compatible to the biology and psychology of the breastfeeding period. (Physiology; 1–3 months; Application; Difficulty: 3)

B-030.   The answer is C. Longer nursing sessions are most likely, although a baby who was recently hospitalized may also nurse more frequently, but not necessarily to quench thirst. It is highly unlikely that a child would want the same or less frequent breastfeeding than prior to the hospitalization. (Physiology; 4–6 months; Application; Difficulty: 2)

B-031.   The answer is D. Lactational Amenorrhea Method is the most compatible with breastfeeding. Condoms are also a first choice but less reliable. Progestin-only methods are second choices, and methods containing estrogen are third choices. (Physiology; 4–6 months; Knowledge; Difficulty: 4)

BN-032. The answer is C. The timing of Lactogenesis II is not affected by the mode/route of delivery. (Physiology; Labor/Birth; Knowledge; Difficulty: 3)

BN-033. The answer is D. Lactogenesis II, or the onset of copious milk secretion, is not dependent on breast stimulation by the baby. All the other statements are true. (Physiology; Labor/Birth; Knowledge; Difficulty: 3)

BP-034. The answer is D. The location of the abrasions suggests that the baby is nursing on the nipple tips instead of taking a large, deep grasp of the nipple/areola complex. (Physiology; 15–28 days; Application; Difficulty: 5)

BP-035. The answer is C. This is an entirely normal breast with moderate fullness. There are no visual indications of mastitis, galactocele, or edema. (Physiology; 15–28 days; Knowledge; Difficulty: 5)

BP-036. The answer is B. Babies should be breastfed when they show signs of hunger. Crying, as shown in the picture, is a late hunger cue. The other options do not meet the baby's need for frequent feedings. (Physiology; 15–28 days; Application; Difficulty: 3)

BP-037. The answer is D. These lactating breasts are entirely normal. The mother's baby is 13 months old and thriving. A is false. B and C may be true but cannot be determined solely from breast appearance. (Physiology; > 12 months; Application; Difficulty: 4)

BP-038. The answer is D. The compression stripe from 1:00 to 7:00 indicates a shallow latch. The first intervention should be correcting the positioning and latch during feeds. (Physiology; 3–14 days; Application; Difficulty: 5)

BP-039. The answer is B. This baby is in the quiet alert state. (Physiology; 15–28 days; Knowledge; Difficulty: 4)

BP-040. The answer is B. Observing a full breastfeeding is always recommended and appropriate, especially before a more complicated assessment is done. (Physiology; 7–12 months; Application; Difficulty: 5)

BP-041. The answer is D. This mother still had bright red vaginal bleeding and a very low milk supply. This situation strongly suggests a retained placenta, which suppresses the onset of Lactogenesis II. (Physiology; 3–14 days; Application; Difficulty: 4)

BP-042. The answer is B. Feeding the baby and noticing any changes related to milk flow is the first action to take. If the swelling decreases after nursing, it is likely that the accessory breast tissue in the axilla has an outlet. (Physiology; 3–14 days; Application; Difficulty: 4)

BP-043. The answer is D. The swelling is accessory breast tissue that is producing milk in the immediate postbirth period. (Physiology; 3–14 days; Knowledge; Difficulty: 5)

BP-044. The answer is B. Uneven breast size is very common. Total milk production is not related to breast size. (Physiology; 3–14 days; Application; Difficulty: 4)

BP-045. The answer is B. Many mothers experience tender nipples if they become pregnant while breastfeeding. The tenderness is related to high levels of pregnancy hormones and does not respond to the usual remedies. (Physiology; Prenatal; Application; Difficulty: 3)

BN-046. The answer is D. Long periods without collecting milk may cause milk stasis, which will suppress Lactogenesis II. Frequent and thorough removal of milk is essential. (Physiology; Prematurity; Application; Difficulty: 5)

Scoring:

Total number of questions in this section   _____

Number of questions answered correctly   _____

Percent correct (divide number correct by total number)   _____

C. MATERNAL AND INFANT NORMAL NUTRITION AND BIOCHEMISTRY

In the 2000 exam blueprint, 10 to 16 questions are dedicated to maternal and infant normal nutrition and biochemistry.

SUBTOPICS INCLUDED IN THIS CATEGORY

1. Definitions of breastfeeding (exclusive—partial—token)

2. Milk synthesis and compositional changes

    a. Milk components
    b. Function and effect on baby
    c. Comparison with other products/milks
    d. Risks and hazards of other foods for infants
    e. Ritual and traditional foods

3. Introduction of foods other than human milk (the "what" of other foods)

    a. Family (solid) foods
    b. Feeding patterns and intake over time
    c. Cultural beliefs; inappropriate foods

4. Maternal diet and nutrition

    a. Normal weight gain and loss patterns
    b. Special diets; supplements
    c. Maternal ritual and traditional foods

CORE READING

Textbooks

Global Strategy for Infant and Young Child Feeding: A Joint WHO/UNICEF Statement. Geneva, Switzerland: World Health Organization; 2003.

Guidelines for Appropriate Complementary Feeding of Breastfed Children 6–24 Months of Age—Facts for Feeding. Washington, DC: Linkages Project/AED; 2004.

Guiding Principles for Complementary Feeding of the Breastfed Child. Washington, DC: Pan American Health Organization; 2003.

Hanson LA. *Immunobiology of Human Milk: How Breastfeeding Protects Babies.* Amarillo, TX: Pharmasoft (Hale) Publishing; 2004.

Jensen RG. *Handbook of Milk Composition.* San Diego: Academic Press; 1995.

Koletzko B, Michaelson KF, Hernell O. *Short and Long Term Effect of Breastfeeding on Child Health*. New York: Kluwer Academic/Plenum Publishers; 2000. *Advances in Experimental Medicine and Biology;* vol. 478.

Lauwers J, Swisher A. *Counseling the Nursing Mother*. 4th ed. Sudbury, MA: Jones & Bartlett Publishers; 2003.

Lawrence RA, Lawrence RM. *Breastfeeding: A Guide for the Medical Profession*. 6th ed. St. Louis: Elsevier Mosby; 2005.

Mohrbacher N, Stock J. *The Breastfeeding Answer Book*. Schaumburg, IL: La Leche League International; 2003.

Nutrient Adequacy of Exclusive Breastfeeding for the Term Infant During the First Six Months of Life. Geneva, Switzerland: World Health Organization; 2002.

Riordan J. *Breastfeeding and Human Lactation*. Sudbury, MA: Jones & Bartlett Publishers; 2004.

Roepke J. *Introduction of Complementary Foods for the Exclusively Breastfed Infant*. Schaumburg, IL: La Leche League International; 2005.

Anti-inflammatory characteristics of milk, http://www.pediatricresearch.org/talks/brmlkinf/.

Anti-microbial & other factors in human milk, http://www.latrobe.edu.au/www/microbio/milk.html.

Key Research Articles

Agostoni C, Marangoni F, Grandi F, et al. Earlier smoking habits are associated with higher serum lipids and lower milk fat and polyunsaturated fatty acid content in the first 6 months of lactation. *Eur J Clin Nutr*. 2003;57(11):1466–1472.

Goldman AS, Goldblum RM, Garza C. Immunologic components in human milk during the second year of lactation. *Acta Paediatr Scand*. 1983;72(3):461–462.

Hartmann PE, Cregan MD, Ramsay DT, Simmer K, Kent JC. Physiology of lactation in preterm mothers: Initiation and maintenance. *Pediatr Ann*. 2003;32(5):351–355.

Hartmann PE, Rattigan S, Saint L, Supriyana O. Variation in the yield and composition of human milk. *Oxf Rev Reprod Bio.l* 1985;7:118–167.

Horne RS, Parslow PM, Ferens D et al. Comparison of evoked arousability in breast and formula fed infants. *Arch Dis Child*. 2004;89(1):22–25.

ILCA. *Clinical Guidelines for the Establishment of Exclusive Breastfeeding*. Raleigh, NC: International Lactation Consultant Association; 2005.

Kent JC, Arthur PG, Retallack RW, Hartmann PE. Calcium, phosphate and citrate in human milk at initiation of lactation. *J Dairy Res*. 1992;59(2):161–167.

Kent JC, Mitoulas L, Cox DB, Owens RA, Hartmann PE. Breast volume and milk production during extended lactation in women. *Exp Physiol*. 1999;84(2):435–447.

Kent JC, Mitoulas LR, Cregan MD, Ramsay DT, Doherty DA, Hartmann PE. Volume and frequency of breastfeedings and fat content of breast milk throughout the day. *Pediatrics*. 2006;117(3):e387–e395.

Kramer MS, Kakuma R. Optimal duration of exclusive breastfeeding. *Cochrane Database Syst Rev*. 2002(1):CD003517.

Kunz C, Lonnerdal B. Re-evaluation of the whey protein/casein ratio of human milk. *Acta Paediatr.* 1992Feb; 81(2):107–112.

Labbok MH. Effects of breastfeeding on the mother. *Pediatr Clin North America.* 2001;48:143–158.

Labbok MH, Clark D, Goldman AS. Breastfeeding: Maintaining an irreplaceable immunological resource. *Nat Rev Immunol.* Jul2004;4(7):565–572.

Mandel D, Lubetzky R, Dollberg S, Barak S, Mimouni FB. Fat and energy contents of expressed human breast milk in prolonged lactation. *Pediatrics.* 2005;116(3):e432–e435.

Mitoulas LR, Kent JC, Cox DB, Owens RA, Sherriff JL, Hartmann PE. Variation in fat, lactose and protein in human milk over 24 h and throughout the first year of lactation. *Br J Nutr.* 2002;88(1):29–37.

Mizuno K, Ueda A. Antenatal olfactory learning influences infant feeding. *Early Hum Dev.* 2004;76 (2):83–90.

Neville MC, Allen JC, Archer PC, et al. Studies in human lactation: Milk volume and nutrient composition during weaning and lactogenesis. *Am J Clin Nutr.* 1991;54:81–92.

Onyango AW, Receveur O, Esrey SA. The contribution of breast milk to toddler diets in western Kenya. *Bull World Health Organ.* 2002;80(4):292–299.

Picciano MF. Nutrient composition of human milk. *Pediatr Clin North Am.* 2001;48:53–67.

Saint L, Smith M, Hartmann PE. The yield and nutrient content of colostrum and milk of women from giving birth to 1 month post-partum. *Br J Nutr.* 1984;52(1):87–95.

Scammon R, Doyle L. Observations on the capacity of the stomach in the first ten days of postnatal life. *American Journal of Diseases of Children.* 1920;20:516–38.

Zangen S, Di Lorenzo C, Zangen T et al. Rapid maturation of gastric relaxation in newborn infants. *Pediatr Res.* 2001;50(5):629–632.

Zeskind PS, Goff DM, Marshall TR. Rhythmic organization of neonatal heart rate and its relation to atypical fetal growth. *Dev Psychobiol.* 1991;24(6):413–429.

MATERNAL AND INFANT NORMAL NUTRITION AND BIOCHEMISTRY QUESTIONS

Notice on question numbering: C-000 means a basic question, with one correct answer and three wrong answers. CP-000, along with the camera icon, means there is a picture that needs to be viewed to answer the question. The pictures are located on the CD-ROM included with this book and are numbered to correspond with the questions. CN-000, along with the frowning face icon, means the question has a **NEGATIVE** stem; therefore, read the entire question very carefully to find the one **WRONG** answer among the choices. CPN-000, with both icons in the margin, means there is a picture associated with the question AND the question has a negative stem. See Appendix A for a fuller explanation of negative stem questions.

C-001. Which of the following protective components of milk is destroyed by freezing?

a. lysozyme
b. lymphocytes
c. secretory IgA
d. lactoferrin

C-002. Compared to term milk, preterm milk is higher in which component?

a. protein
b. lactose
c. phosphorus
d. iron

C-003. Fat levels in mother's milk are highest:

a. when the milk ejection reflex is strong.
b. during the night.
c. when the mother eats a high-fat diet.
d. when the breast is relatively empty.

C-004. Which of the following statements best describes fetal nutrition?

a. The umbilical cord delivers nutrients directly to the fetal gut.
b. The fetus swallows and digests amniotic fluid.
c. The fetus absorbs nutrients from the amniotic fluid through his skin.
d. The fetus has no digestive enzymes of his own until after 40 weeks.

C-005. Which nutrient is most difficult for premature babies to digest?

a. carbohydrate
b. protein
c. fats
d. minerals

C-006. Which component of human milk is most variable?

a. proteins
b. lipids
c. carbohydrates
d. minerals

C-007. Researchers have found that inguinal hernia and some other disorders of the urogenital tract are less common in breastfed babies. Which of the following components has the most significant role in tissue maturation of the infant?

a. epidermal growth factor
b. nerve growth factor
c. secretory IgA
d. lactoferrin

C-008. Which of the following components of mother's milk varies the most with the infant's feeding pattern?

a. proteins
b. minerals
c. fat-soluble vitamins
d. lactose

C-009. Which nutritional recommendation is most relevant to a breastfeeding mother?

a. Drink a large glass of water whenever you breastfeed.
b. Avoid spicy or gas-producing foods.
c. Increase your caloric intake to make enough milk.
d. Follow your usual dietary practices.

C-010. Which hormone in the milk is most responsible for anti-inflammation activity?

a. prolactin
b. prostaglandins
c. oxytocin
d. relaxin

CN-011. Lactoferrin in human milk has all of the following functions **EXCEPT**:

a. nutrition.
b. nerve myelinization.
c. iron transport.
d. anti-inflammatory agency.

CP-012. The most likely result of this mother's dietary practices would be:

a. her milk will contain more vitamin A.
b. her milk supply will increase.
c. the baby's breath may smell like cantaloupe.
d. the baby will reject the cantaloupe-flavored milk.

CP-013. At this stage of lactation, which of the following components of human milk is most increased over newborn-period levels?

a. lactoferrin
b. lactose
c. whey
d. casein

CPN-014. To help prevent rickets in this child, you would recommend all of the following **EXCEPT**:

a. expose the child's face to sunlight for 20 minutes every day.
b. the mother should take a vitamin D supplement.
c. the mother should expose her face and head to sunlight for 2 hours a week.
d. give the child a vitamin D supplement regardless of symptoms.

C-015. Which statement is most accurate about the variation in composition of human milk?

a. Fat levels vary within a feed.
b. Zinc levels increase over time.
c. Lactose levels are related to time of day.
d. Vitamin K is lowest in colostrum, then increases.

C-016. A breastfeeding mother who follows a strict vegetarian diet (no animal protein whatsoever) should take a supplement containing which of the following vitamins?

a. vitamin A
b. vitamin B$_{12}$
c. vitamin C
d. vitamin K

C-017. Which milk component causes the stools of exclusively breastfed babies to have a mild, yeast-like odor?

a. glycopeptides
b. *Candida albicans*
c. phospholipids
d. bifidus factor

C-018. A breastfeeding mother needs to be sure that her diet includes:

a. additional B vitamins.
b. plenty of liquids to assure sufficient milk volume.
c. an extra 1000 calories per day.
d. her normal intake of food and drink.

C-019. Manufacturers of artificial feeding products have attempted to increase the protective properties in their products by adding which of the following nonprotein nitrogen compounds found in human milk?

a. polyamines
b. nucleic acids
c. nucleotides
d. creatinine

C-020. Which of the following statements best describes the difference in fat content of colostrum vs. mature milk?

a. Colostrum has 4–5 g/100 ml, and mature milk has 2–3 g/100 ml of fat.
b. Colostrum has 2–3 g/100 ml, and mature milk has 4–5 g/100 ml of fat.
c. Colostrum has roughly 1/4 the fat content of mature milk.
d. Colostrum has 10 cc of fat, and mature milk has 20 cc of fat.

C-021. Pregnant vegan mothers would need to supplement their plant-foods-only diet by taking:

a. vitamin B_{12}.
b. calcium.
c. fat-soluble vitamins A, D, E, and K.
d. iron.

C-022. Research has shown that babies who received human milk have higher scores in cognitive development and vision. Which of the following milk components is most likely to explain this difference?

a. long-chain fatty acids
b. short-chain fatty acids
c. phospholipids
d. sterols

C-023. Anemia in the exclusively breastfed baby is rare because of the bioavailability of which trace element found in human milk?

a. manganese
b. fluoride
c. iodine
d. iron

C-024.   A mother wants to know how soon she will return to her prepregnancy weight after her baby is born. Which is the best of the following responses?

a.   Most breastfeeding mothers lose 2–3 lb (0.9–1.4 kg) per week.
b.   Making milk uses 1000 calories a day from your diet.
c.   Gradual weight loss preserves your health and energy.
d.   Restrict your food intake intake to 1500 calories a day.

C-025.   Compared to mature milk, colostrum is higher in:

a.   lactose.
b.   immunofactors.
c.   volume.
d.   hormones.

C-026.   A mother is hesitant to breastfeed because she has heard that she needs to eat a high-calorie, nutrient-rich diet during lactation. Your best response is:

a.   women living under a wide variety of circumstances are capable of fully nourishing their infants by breastfeeding.
b.   refer her to a supplemental food program to assure adequate nutrient intake.
c.   provide her with a multivitamin and mineral supplement.
d.   discourage her from breastfeeding, as her current circumstances make it doubtful that she is eating adequately.

C-027.   Which mineral is particularly difficult for the premature (preterm) infant to absorb?

a.   zinc
b.   iron
c.   sodium
d.   chromium

C-028.   Human milk is often a bluish-white color because:

a.   the whey:casein ratio of human milk is 80:20.
b.   the whey:casein ratio of human milk is 20:80.
c.   secretory IgA is a blue color.
d.   human casein does not bind calcium.

C-029. Compared to milk from mothers who deliver at term, milk from mothers who deliver preterm is:

a. higher in lactose, vitamins, and minerals.
b. higher in protein, sodium, and chloride.
c. lower in calcium, magnesium, and phosphorus.
d. equivalent in immunologic properties.

C-030. Which of the following components of human milk protects the baby by binding nutrients needed by pathogens in the baby's gut?

a. lactoferrin
b. lysozyme
c. mucins
d. oligosaccharides

C-031. Compared with milk from mothers who deliver at term, preterm milk is higher in:

a. macrophages.
b. milk volume.
c. zinc.
d. B vitamins.

 CP-032. Approximately how much milk does an average full-term baby receive in the first week postbirth?

a. The baby gets about 150 ml/day (5 oz/day) of colostrum.
b. The baby gets increasing amounts each day as milk volume increases.
c. The baby needs a supplement until day 5 when the mom's supply is sufficient.
d. The baby gets 750 ml/day (25 oz/day) from day 2 onward.

C-033. Which aspect of lipid composition varies most in human milk?

a. ratio of unsaturated to saturated fats
b. profile of fatty acids (chain length)
c. percent of fat in a given feed
d. ratio of triglycerides to cholesterol

CN-034. The ease with which human milk fat is digested by the infant is explained by all of the following **EXCEPT**:

a. unsaturated fats comprise 57% of total lipids.
b. lipases are present in the milk.
c. lipids are encased in membranes (globules).
d. cholesterol is the predominant lipid in human milk.

CN-035. Prelacteal ritual feeds of butter, herbs, etc. increase the risk of all of the following **EXCEPT**:

a. oversupply of milk
b. infection with pathogens
c. alteration of gut flora
d. reduced availability of colostrum

CN-036. Which attribute of anti-infectious properties in human milk is **NOT CORRECT**?

a. They decrease over the duration of lactation.
b. They remain stable over the duration of lactation.
c. They are stable to heating or freezing.
d. They interact in inhibiting or killing pathogens.

CN-037. Which carbohydrate is **NOT** found in human milk?

a. lactose
b. oligosaccharides
c. sucrose
d. gluconjugates

CN-038. The whey protein alpha-lactalbumin has all of the following properties **EXCEPT**:

a. it regulates milk synthesis.
b. mucins in this protein bind pathogens in vitro.
c. it is similar to the alpha-lactalbumin in cow's milk.
d. it promotes gastric emptying.

CN-039. All of the following components of human milk provide anti-inflammatory properties EXCEPT:

a. complement.
b. prostaglandins.
c. lactoferrin.
d. secretory IgA.

CN-040. Growth hormones and other factors in human milk support optimal growth and maturation in all of the following body systems **EXCEPT** the:

a. respiratory system.
b. urogenital system.
c. gastrointestinal system.
d. skeletal system.

CN-041. You are helping a woman who has a documented allergy to dairy products (cow's milk). Which of the following foods would **NOT** provide the nutrients contained in dairy products?

a. rice and potatoes
b. split peas and lentils
c. kale and cabbage
d. corn tortillas soaked in lime

CN-042. The benefits of human donor milk remain similar to those of real-time breastfeeding **EXCEPT**:

a. species specificity.
b. allergy prevention.
c. bioavailability.
d. HIV prevention.

CN-043. Lactose in human milk has all of the following properties **EXCEPT**:

a. it contains a supply of 40% of infants' energy needs.
b. it aids absorption of phosphorus and manganese.
c. it protects the gastrointestinal tract from pathogens.
d. it supports the central nervous system (CNS) and cognitive development.

CN-044. Fresh human milk can be instilled in the eye to treat infections. Components in milk that are beneficial for this use include all of the following **EXCEPT**:

a. lactose.
b. fatty acids.
c. lysozyme.
d. mucins.

CN-045. All of the following are properties of lysozyme **EXCEPT**:

a. it destroys *E. coli* and other bacteria.
b. it increases in milk after 6 months' lactation.
c. it is destroyed by pasteurization.
d. it is active against inflammation.

CN-046. All of the following components are missing in artificial feeding products **EXCEPT**:

a. calcium.
b. cholesterol.
c. alpha-lactalbumin.
d. leukocytes.

CN-047. A breastfeeding mother is also pregnant. She is worried about her bones being depleted of calcium due to the overlap. All of the following are appropriate responses by the lactation consultant **EXCEPT**:

a. the added burden of pregnancy overlapping with breastfeeding requires an extra 400 mg of calcium a day.
b. women ages 19–50 need the same amount of calcium regardless of whether they are breastfeeding or pregnant.
c. an overlap of breastfeeding and pregnancy actually triggers accretion of bone mineral.
d. if you are avoiding dairy, you will want to focus on bio-available calcium sources such as calcium-fortified water and orange juice.

CN-048. A breastfeeding mother is also pregnant. She asks what it takes to "eat for three" while she's pregnant. All of the following are appropriate responses by the lactation consultant **EXCEPT**:

a. you need to wean; breastfeeding while pregnant will rob the fetus of needed nutrients.
b. eat enough calories of a basic mixed diet.
c. make sure you are gaining weight within the same parameters as if you were pregnant and not breastfeeding.
d. do you ordinarily have special dietary needs (for example, do you avoid dairy, causing you to need alternative sources of calcium)?

CN-049. Soluble components of human milk that have immunologic significance include all of the following **EXCEPT**:

a. interferon.
b. fibronectin.
c. estrogen.
d. lactoferrin.

CN-050. A 7-month-old child is beginning to turn away when her mother tries to breastfeed while eating her own dinner. All of the following are possible explanations for this behavior, **EXCEPT**:

a. the child is ready to begin self-feeding family foods.
b. the mother's milk does not provide sufficient fat and calories.
c. the child's gut has matured to handle family foods.
d. the child is bored with breastfeeding and wants to play with the mother's food.

C-051. Lactoferrin in the mother's milk is beneficial to the baby because it:

a. binds iron needed by pathogens in the baby's gut.
b. attacks and kills pathogenic bacteria in the baby's gut.
c. promotes the absorption of lactose.
d. provides nutrients for *Lactobacillus bifidus* in the gut.

C-052. Bacterial counts in human milk, expressed 1 hour ago, are most likely to be:

a. lower, because the milk is being held at a lower temperature.
b. lower, because macrophages in the milk are actively phagocytic.
c. higher, because antibacterial properties of human milk work best at body temperature.
d. higher, because human milk is a rich medium for bacterial growth.

C-053. Why do the breastfed baby's stools become firmer over time, even before the addition of solid foods?

a. Casein increases in proportion to whey over time.
b. There is less liquid in proportion to minerals in the milk over time.
c. Breast milk supplies inadequate fluids over time, necessitating adding other drinks.
d. The baby perspires more, using more of the liquid in milk for metabolism.

C-054. A pregnant woman follows a vegan diet and intends to breastfeed. You should advise her that:

a. her milk supply may be compromised by her diet.
b. she should take a vitamin B_{12} supplement.
c. her baby will need a multivitamin supplement.
d. she will have to change her diet if she wants to breastfeed.

CN-055. The species specificity of human milk is characterized by all of the following **EXCEPT**:

a. milk components match 50% of the baby's genetic material.
b. milk is 75% bioavailable to the infant.
c. the 200+ identified components have nutritive and immune functions.
d. milk components meet all the physiological needs of the infant.

MATERNAL AND INFANT NORMAL NUTRITION AND BIOCHEMISTRY ANSWERS

The parenthetical material at the end of each answer includes the discipline and time period, indicates whether the question pertains to knowledge or application, and specifies the degree of difficulty.

C-001. The answer is B. Freezing destroys living white cells such as T- and B-lymphocytes. The other components are not significantly affected by freezing. (Biochemistry; General Principles; Knowledge; Difficulty: 5)

C-002. The answer is A. Preterm milk is higher in protein and similar to term milk in lactose, phosphorus, iron, and most other components. (Biochemistry; Prematurity; Knowledge; Difficulty: 2)

C-003. The answer is D. Research in Australia has found that the relative fullness of the breast accounts for about 70% of the fat variation in milk. (Biochemistry; General Principles; Knowledge; Difficulty: 4)

C-004. The answer is B. Amniotic fluid provides protein and other nutrients to the fetus in addition to nutrients present in the cord blood vessels. (Biochemistry; Prenatal; Knowledge; Difficulty: 3)

C-005. The answer is C. Fats are most difficult for preterm babies to digest. Human milk fat is released simultaneously with digestive enzymes, making it optimal for preterm babies. (Biochemistry; Prematurity; Knowledge; Difficulty: 4)

C-006. The answer is B. Lipids are the most variable of the components listed. The proportion of fat in milk increases as the breast empties, and there is a slight variation in fatty acid profiles with maternal diet. The others are very stable across women, over the course of a day, and over the duration of breastfeeding. (Biochemistry; General Principles; Knowledge; Difficulty: 3)

C-007. The answer is A. Epidermal growth factor plays a major role in gut maturation. Lactoferrin also promotes tissue maturation. (Biochemistry; General Principles; Knowledge; Difficulty: 5)

C-008. The answer is C. Fat-soluble vitamin intake is related to fat levels in milk, which vary with several factors. Protein, minerals, and lactose do not vary with infant feeding patterns. (Biochemistry; General Principles; Knowledge; Difficulty: 2)

C-009. The answer is D. Mothers' dietary practices have very little effect on lactation. Following good dietary practices is important for the breastfeeding mother's general health. (Biochemistry; General Principles; Application; Difficulty: 5)

C-010. The answer is B. Prostaglandins in the milk have anti-inflammatory properties that protect all tissues, especially the infant gut. (Biochemistry; General Principles; Knowledge; Difficulty: 4)

CN-011. The answer is B. Lactoferrin has no known function relative to nerve myelinization or growth. It is a major protein source, it is an iron transport agent, and it reduces/prevents inflammation. (Biochemistry; General Principles; Knowledge; Difficulty: 5)

CP-012. The answer is C. Mother's milk contains traces of flavors present in the mother's food choices, which helps the baby learn and enjoy family food preferences. Shortly after this picture was taken, the baby's breath smelled faintly of cantaloupe. (Biochemistry; 3–14 days; Application; Difficulty: 3)

CP-013. The answer is D. Casein in milk increases in proportion to whey over time. Lactose and lactoferrin increase slightly over time. (Biochemistry; 7–12 months; Knowledge; Difficulty: 4)

CPN-014. The answer is D. Routine supplementation of all breastfed babies is not justified by the prevailing research. Supplementation should be based on history and a case-by-case basis. (Biochemistry; 4–6 months; Application; Difficulty: 2)

C-015. The answer is A. Fat levels vary within a feed, between feeds, and in proportion to the relative fullness or emptiness of the breast. The other statements are false. Zinc levels decrease over time; lactose levels are unrelated to the time of day, and vitamin K is highest in colostrum. (Biochemistry; General Principles; Knowledge; Difficulty: 3)

C-016. The answer is B. Water-soluble vitamins such as B_6 and B_{12} in milk are strongly dependent on maternal dietary intake. These nutrients are essential to the baby. (Biochemistry; General Principles; Knowledge; Difficulty: 2)

C-017. The answer is D. Bifidus factor supports gut colonization with *Lactobacillus bifidus*, a friendly bacteria that protects the gut mucosa from pathogens. Bifidus factor is not found in the milk of other animals. (Biochemistry; 15–28 days; Knowledge; Difficulty: 3)

C-018.   The answer is D. Most breastfeeding mothers can follow the eating and fluid intake patterns of an average woman in a developed country. Fluid intake is unrelated to milk volume; excess calories are unnecessary, and B vitamins are found in many animal-based foods. (Biochemistry; General Principles; Knowledge; Difficulty: 4)

C-019.   The answer is C. Manufacturers are experimenting with the addition of nucleotides to increase the protective properties of their products. However, even with nucleotides added, the manufactured products fall far short of human milk's protective properties. (Biochemistry; General Principles; Knowledge; Difficulty: 2)

C-020.   The answer is B. Colostrum has 2–3 g/100 ml; mature milk has 4–5 g/100 ml of fat. (Biochemistry; 1–2 days; Knowledge; Difficulty: 3)

C-021.   The answer is A. Women who eat no animal products need a dietary source of vitamin B_{12}. The other nutrients listed can be obtained from plant foods. (Biochemistry; Prenatal; Application; Difficulty: 5)

C-022.   The answer is A. Omega-3 fatty acids DHA and AA are especially important in development of the central nervous system and are found in abundance in human milk. (Biochemistry; General Principles; Knowledge; Difficulty: 3)

C-023.   The answer is D. Iron in human milk is highly bioavailable. Exclusively breastfed babies are very unlikely to become anemic. (Biochemistry; General Principles; Knowledge; Difficulty: 2)

C-024.   The answer is C. Gradual weight loss preserves health and energy. About 500 calories are utilized in making milk per day. (Biochemistry; Prenatal; Knowledge; Difficulty: 4)

C-025.   The answer is B. The most important function of colostrum is to protect the baby from pathogens. Colostrum is especially high in secretory IgA and white cells. (Biochemistry; Labor/Birth; Knowledge; Difficulty: 3)

C-026.   The answer is A. A well-balanced diet with adequate calories is important for the mother's overall health. Most milk components are not substantially related to mother's dietary intake. (Biochemistry; Prenatal; Application; Difficulty: 4)

C-027. The answer is B. Preterm infants are often unable to absorb iron effectively. Iron in human milk is more easily absorbed than iron from other sources. (Biochemistry; Prematurity; Knowledge; Difficulty: 4)

C-028. The answer is A. Human milk whey-casein ratio is about 80:20 in the early weeks. The casein portion binds calcuim and scatters light, therefore appears white; the whey portion is slightly blue. Cow's milk has a whey-casein ratio of 20:80, which means the high portion of casein causes the white opaque color of cow's milk. (Biochemistry; General Principles; Knowledge; Difficulty: 2)

C-029. The answer is B. Preterm milk is higher in protein, sodium, and chloride than milk from mothers who deliver at term. (Biochemistry; Prematurity; Knowledge; Difficulty: 3)

C-030. The answer is A. Lactoferrin binds to iron, which starves pathogenic bacteria of the iron needed to proliferate. (Biochemistry; General Principles; Knowledge; Difficulty: 5)

C-031. The answer is A. Preterm milk is higher in white cells, especially macrophages, than term milk. Milk volume, zinc, and B-vitamin levels are similar. (Biochemistry; Prematurity; Knowledge; Difficulty: 4)

CP-032. The answer is B. On days 1–3, the baby gets about 30 ml/day (1 oz/day) of colostrum. As lactogenesis II progresses, the baby obtains more per day as milk volume rapidly rises to about 600 ml/day (20 oz/day) or more by day 5. (Biochemistry; 1–2 days; Knowledge; Difficulty: 5)

C-033. The answer is C. The major variation in fat content is related to the relative emptiness of the breast. The proportion of fat increases as the breast drains. Ratios of unsaturated to saturated fats and triglycerides to cholesterol are relatively stable. Fatty acid profiles change slightly with changes in maternal diet. (Biochemistry; General Principles; Knowledge; Difficulty: 4)

CN-034. The answer is D. Triglycerides are the predominant lipids in human milk. Human milk fat is far more easily digested, especially by premature babies, than any other source of lipids. (Biochemistry; General Principles; Knowledge; Difficulty: 5)

CN-035. The answer is A. Ritual feeds increase the risk of infections and illnesses and interfere with breastfeeding. (Biochemistry; 1–2 days; Knowledge; Difficulty: 5)

CN-036. The answer is A. Immune factors form a layer in milk that is the first to appear in the colostral phase and the last to disappear during weaning. Some factors even increase over time; some are stable to heating or freezing; and most interact to inhibit or kill pathogens. (Biochemistry; General Principles; Knowledge; Difficulty: 3)

CN-037. The answer is C. Sucrose is not found in human milk. The other carbohydrates play an important role in infant growth and immune function. (Biochemistry; General Principles; Knowledge; Difficulty: 3)

CN-038. The answer is C. Cow's (bovine's) milk does not contain alpha-lactalbumin. (Biochemistry; General Principles; Knowledge; Difficulty: 2)

CN-039. The answer is A. A complement is a biochemical pathway for inflammation and is poorly represented in human milk. (Biochemistry; General Principles; Knowledge; Difficulty: 5)

CN-040. The answer is D. As of this writing, research has not yet documented improved skeletal development in breastfed babies over those artificially fed. Some long-term skeletal advantages of breastfeeding are beginning to appear in the literature. (Biochemistry; General Principles; Knowledge; Difficulty: 5)

CN-041. The answer is A. She needs a dietary source of calcium, which is high in all of the choices except rice and potatoes. (Biochemistry; General Principles; Knowledge; Difficulty: 2)

CN-042. The answer is D. Pasteurized donor milk from screened donors does not transmit the HIV virus. Pasteurization kills the virus. (Biochemistry; General Principles; Knowledge; Difficulty: 2)

CN-043. The answer is B. Lactose aids absorption of calcium and iron. (Biochemistry; General Principles; Knowledge; Difficulty: 5)

CN-044. The answer is A. Lactose does not appear to be protective against inflammation or pathogens. Fatty acids disrupt cell membranes of some viruses. Lysozyme kills bacteria by disrupting cell walls. Mucins adhere to pathogens, preventing their attachment to mucous membranes. (Biochemistry; General Principles; Application; Difficulty: 5)

☹ **CN-045.** The answer is C. Lysozyme is stable at temperatures used for pasteurization. All of the other properties are true. Lysozyme is especially important for premature babies. (Biochemistry; Prematurity; Knowledge; Difficulty: 2)

☹ **CN-046.** The answer is A. Calcium is found in artificial feeding products. The other components listed are not found in manufactured foods for infants. (Biochemistry; General Principles; Knowledge; Difficulty: 2)

☹ **CN-047.** The answer is A. During pregnancy, even for malnourished mothers, extra calcium is excreted with the urine; instead the body acquires the needed calcium through intrinsic processes such as enhanced uptake. The other three responses are appropriate for helping her assess her needs. (Biochemistry; Prenatal; Application; Difficulty: 5)

☹ **CN-048.** The answer is A. If a mother is gaining weight within healthy parameters, there is no reason to think that breastfeeding is taking away from the fetus. The other three responses are appropriate for helping her assess her specific needs. (Biochemistry; Prenatal; Application; Difficulty: 5)

☹ **CN-049.** The answer is C. Estrogen in human milk does not appear to have an immunologic function. (Biochemistry; General Principles; Knowledge; Difficulty: 5)

☹ **CN-050.** The answer is B. Human milk contains sufficient and even increased fat and calories in the second 6 months of lactation. The other statements are true. (Biochemistry; 7–12 months; Application; Difficulty: 2)

C-051. The answer is A. Lactose promotes the absorption of iron. Lactoferrin indirectly helps establish intestinal flora by keeping the pathogenic population in check, but it does not directly promote the growth of beneficial bacteria in the gut. (Biochemistry; 3–14 days; Knowledge; Difficulty: 5)

C-052. The answer is B. Macrophages and possibly neutrophils and T-lymphocytes actively kill microbes by phagocytosis. (Biochemistry; 1–2 days; Knowledge; Difficulty: 4)

C-053. The answer is A. The whey-casein ratio changes from 90:10 in the newborn period to closer to 60:40 around 6 months. (Biochemistry; 1–3 months; Knowledge; Difficulty: 3)

C-054. The answer is B. A vegan diet includes no animal sources and is thus deficient in vitamin B_{12}. A supplement taken by the mother will provide adequate B_{12} to the baby through her milk. (Biochemistry; Prenatal; Application; Difficulty: 4)

CN-055. The answer is B. Human milk is 99% bioavailable to the infant, leaving very little residue in the gut. (Biochemistry; General Principles; Knowledge; Difficulty: 2)

Scoring:

Total number of questions in this section _____

Number of questions answered correctly _____

Percent correct (divide number correct by total number) _____

D. MATERNAL AND INFANT IMMUNOLOGY AND INFECTIOUS DISEASE

In the 2000 exam blueprint, 11 to 19 questions are dedicated to maternal and infant immunology and infectious disease.

SUBTOPICS INCLUDED IN THIS CATEGORY

1. Protection against infection

    a. Antibodies and immune factors in milk
    b. Immune systems
    c. Anti-inflammatory properties
    d. Long-term protective factors

2. Cross-infection

    a. Bacteria and viruses in milk
    b. Maternal infections
    c. HIV and AIDS issues

3. Allergies and food sensitivities

    a. Etiologies; triggers
    b. Manifestations
    c. Management

CORE READING

Textbooks

Hanson, L. *Immunobiology of Human Milk: How Breastfeeding Protects Infants.* Amarillo, TX: Hale Publishing (Pharmasoft Publishing); 2004.

HIV and Infant Feeding: A Guide for Health Care Managers and Supervisors and Guidelines for Decision Makers. Geneva, Switzerland: World Health Organization; 2002.

Koletzko B, Michaelson KF, Hernell O. *Short and Long Term Effect of Breastfeeding on Child Health.* New York: Kluwer Academic/Plenum Publishers; 2000. *Advances in Experimental Medicine and Biology*; vol. 478.

Lawrence RA, Lawrence RM. *Breastfeeding: A Guide for the Medical Profession.* 6th ed. St. Louis: Elsevier Mosby; 2005.

Riordan J. *Breastfeeding and Human Lactation.* Sudbury, MA: Jones & Bartlett Publishers; 2004.

Walker M. *Breastfeeding Management for the Clinician: Using the Evidence.* Sudbury, MA: Jones & Bartlett Publishers, 2006.

WHO/UNICEF. *Global Strategy for Infant and Young Child Feeding: A Joint WHO/UNICEF Statement.* Geneva, Switzerland: World Health Organization; 2003.

WHO Child Growth Standards. Geneva: World Health Organization, 2006. http://www.who.int/childgrowth/en

HIV and Infant Feeding: Infant Feeding Options and Guidelines for Decision-Makers. Geneva: World Health Organization; 1998.

Food Allergy and Anaphylaxis Network. http://www.foodallergy.org/

Australasian Society of Clinical Immunology and Allergy (ASCIA). http://www.allergy.org.au/

Key Research Articles

Ball TM, Wright AL. Health care costs of formula-feeding in the first year of life. *Pediatrics.* 1999;103(4):870–876.

Basile LA, Taylor SN, Wagner CL, Horst RL, Hollis BW. The effect of high-dose Vitamin D supplementation on serum Vitamin D levels and milk calcium concentration in lactating women and their infants. *Breastfeeding Medicine.* 2006;1(1):27–35.

Beaudry M, Dufour R, Marcoux S. Relation between infant feeding and infections during the first six months of life. *J Pediatr.* 1995;126–191–7.

Benn CS, Michaelsen KF. Does the effect of breast-feeding on atopic dermatitis depend on family history of allergy? *J Pediatr.* 2005;147(1):128–129; author reply 129.

Bottcher MF, Fredriksson J, Hellquist A, Jenmalm MC. Effects of breast milk from allergic and non-allergic mothers on mitogen- and allergen-induced cytokine production. *Pediatr Allergy Immunol.* 2003;14(1):27–34.

Buescher ES. Host defense mechanisms of human milk and their relations to enteric infections and necrotizing enterocolitis. *Clin Perinatol.* 1994–6; 21(2):247–262.

Burr ML, Limb ES, Maguire MJ, et al. Infant feeding, wheezing, and allergy: A prospective study. *Arch Dis Child.* 1993;68(6):724–728.

Businco L, Bruno G, Giampietro PG. Soy protein for the prevention and treatment of children with cow-milk allergy. *Am J Clin Nutr.* 1998;68(6 Suppl):1447S–52S.

Butte NF, Goldblum RM, Fehl LM, Loftin K, Smith EO, Garza C, et al. Daily ingestion of immunologic components in human milk during the first four months of life. *Acta Paediatr Scand.* 1984;73(3):296–301.

Cavataio F, Iacono G, Montalto G, et al. Clinical and pH-metric characteristics of gastro-oesophageal reflux secondary to cow's milk protein allergy. *Archives of Diseases of Childhood.* 1996;75:51–56.

Chantry CJ, Howard CR, Auinger P. Full breastfeeding duration and associated decrease in respiratory tract infection in US children. *Pediatrics.* 2006;117(2):425–432.

Chen A, Rogan WJ. Breastfeeding and the risk of postneonatal death in the United States. *Pediatrics.* 2004;113(5):e435–439.

Coutsoudis A, Pillay K, Huhn L, Spooner E, et al. Method of feeding and transmission of HIV-1 from mothers to children by 15 months of age: Prospective cohort study from Durban, South Africa. *AIDS.* 2001; 15:379–387.

Davis D, et al. Infant feeding practices and occlusal outcomes: A longitudinal study. *J Can Dent Assoc.* 1991; 57(7):593–594.

Dewey KG, Heinig J, Nommsen-Rivers L. Differences in morbidity between breastfed and formula-fed infants. *J Pediatr.* 1995;126:696–702.

Di Pietro J, et al. Behavioral and heart rate pattern differences between breastfed and bottle-fed neonates. *Develop Psych.* 1988;23(4):467–474.

Duncan B, Ey J, Holberg CJ, et al. Exclusive breast-feeding for at least 4 months protects against otitis media. *Pediatrics.* 1993;91:867–872.

Edmond KM, Zandoh C, Quigley MA, Amenga-Etego S, Owusu-Agyei S, Kirkwood BR. Delayed breastfeeding initiation increases risk of neonatal mortality. *Pediatrics.* 2006;117(3):e380–386.

Falth-Magnusson K. Breast milk antibodies to foods in relation to maternal diet, maternal atopy and the development of atopic disease in the baby. *Int Arch Allergy Appl Immunol.* 1989;90(3):297–300.

Friedman NJ, Zeiger RS. The role of breast-feeding in the development of allergies and asthma. *J Allergy Clin Immunol.* 2005;115(6):1238–1248.

Gerstein HC. Cow's milk exposure and type I diabetes mellitus: A critical overview of the clinical literature. *Diabetes Care.* 1994;17(1):13–18.

Goldman AS. The immunological system in human milk: The past—a pathway to the future. *Adv Nutr Res.* 2001;10:15–37.

Goldman AS, Goldblum RM, Garza C. Immunologic components in human milk during the second year of lactation. *Acta Paediatr Scand.* 1983;72(3):461–462.

Goldman AS, et al. Evolution of immunologic functions of the mammary gland and the postnatal development of immunity. *Pediatr Res.* 1998;Feb;43(2):155–162.

Goldman AS, et al. Transfer of maternal leukocytes to the infant by human milk. *Curr Top Microbiol Immunol.* 1997;222:205–213.

Goldman AS. Immunologic system in human milk. *J Pediatr Gastroenterol Nutr.* 1986 May–Jun;5(3):343–345.

Goldman AS. The immune system of human milk: Antimicrobial, antiinflammatory and immunomodulating properties. *Pediatr Infect Dis J.* 1993 Aug;12(8):664–671

Gray RH, Campbell OM, Apelo R, et al. Risk of ovulation during lactation. *Lancet.* 1990;335:25–29.

Groer M, Davis M, Steele K. Associations between human milk SIgA and maternal immune, infectious, endocrine, and stress variables. *J Hum Lact.* 2004;20(2):153–158; quiz 159–163.

Hahn-Zoric M, et al. Antibody responses to parenteral and oral vaccines are impaired by conventional and low protein formulas as compared to breastfeeding. *Acta Paediatr Scand.* 1990,79:1137–1142.

Hanson LA, Ceafalau L, Mattsby-Baltzer I, Lagerberg M, Hjalmarsson A, Ashraf R, et al. The mammary gland-infant intestine immunologic dyad. *Adv Exp Med Biol.* 2000;478:65–76.

Hanson LA, et al. Protective factors in milk and the development of the immune system. *Pediatrics.* 1985 Jan;75(1 Pt 2):172–176.

Hanson LA, et al. The immune response of the mammary gland and its significance for the neonate. *Ann Allergy.* 1984 Dec;53(6 Pt 2):576–582.

Hanson LA, Korotkova M, Haversen L, Mattsby-Baltzer I, Hahn-Zoric M, Silfverdal SA, et al. Breast-feeding, a complex support system for the offspring. *Pediatr Int.* 2002;44(4):347–352.

Hanson LA, Korotkova M, Lundin S, Haversen L, Silfverdal SA, Mattsby-Baltzer I, et al. The transfer of immunity from mother to child. *Ann N Y Acad Sci.* 2003;987:199–206.

Hanson LA, Korotkova M. The role of breastfeeding in prevention of neonatal infection. *Semin Neonatol.* 2002;7(4):275–81.

Hanson LA, Silfverdal SA, Korotkova M, Erling V, Strombeck L, Olcen P, et al. Immune system modulation by human milk. *Adv Exp Med Biol.* 2002;503:99–106.

Hanson LA. Protective effects of breastfeeding against urinary tract infection. *Acta Paediatr.* 2004;93(2):154–156.

Hanson LA. The mother-offspring dyad and the immune system. *Acta Paediatr.* 2000;89(3):252–258.

Hanson LA, Korotkova M, Telemo E. Breast-feeding, infant formulas, and the immune system. *Ann Allergy Asthma Immunol.* 2003;90(6 suppl 3):59–63.

Hartmann SU, Berlin CM, Howett MK. Alternative modified infant-feeding practices to prevent postnatal transmission of human immunodeficiency virus type 1 through breast milk: Past, present, and future. *J Hum Lact.* 2006;22(1):75–88; quiz 89–93.

Hartmann SU, Berlin CM, Howett MK. Response to heat treating breast milk as an infant feeding option. *J Hum Lact.* 2006;22(3):268.

Hasselbalch H, Jeppesen DL, Engelmann MDM, Michaelsen KF, Nielsen MB. Decreased thymus size in formula-fed infants compared with breastfed infants. *Acta Paediatrica.* 1996;85:1029–1032

Host A. Importance of the first meal on the development of cow's milk allergy and intolerance. *Allergy Proc.* 1991;10:227–232.

Host A, Halken S. Hypoallergenic formulas—when, to whom and how long: After more than 15 years we know the right indication! *Allergy.* 2004; 59 Suppl 78:45–52.

Howie PW, Forsyth JS, Ogston SA, Clark A, Florey C. Protective effect of breastfeeding against infection. *Br Med J.* 1990;300:11–16.

Iacono G, Carroccio A, Vatataio F, et al. Gastroesophageal reflux and cow's milk allergy in infants: A prospective study. *J Allergy Clinical Immunology.* 1996;97:822–827.

Iliff PJ, Piwoz EG, Tavengwa NV, et al. Early exclusive breastfeeding reduces the risk of postnatal HIV-1 transmission and increases HIV-free survival. *Aids.* 2005;19(7):699–708.

Inoue N, Sakashita R, Kamegai T. Reduction of masseter muscle activity in bottle-fed babies. *Early Human Development.* 1995;42:185–193.

Institute of Medicine (Subcommittee on Nutrition during Lactation, Food and Nutrition Board). *Nutrition during Lactation.* Washington DC: National Academy of Sciences; 1991.

Israel-Ballard K, Chantry C, Dewey K, Lonnerdal B, Sheppard H, Donovan R, et al. Viral, nutritional, and bacterial safety of flash-heated and pretoria-pasteurized breast milk to prevent mother-to-child transmission of HIV in resource-poor countries: A pilot study. *J Acquir Immune Defic Syndr.* 2005;40(2):175–181.

Jeffery BS, Mercer KG. Pretoria pasteurization: A potential method for the reduction of postnatal mother-to-child transmission of the human immunodeficiency virus. *J Trop Pediatr.* 2000;46:219–223.

Kostraba JH, Cruickshanks KJ, et al. Early exposure to cow's milk and solid foods in infancy, genetic predisposition, and risk of IDDM. *Diabetes.* 1993;42:288–295.

Kramer M, Chalmers B, Hodnett E, Sevkovskaya Z, Dzikovich I SS, Collet JP, Vanilovich I, Mezen I, Ducruet T, Shishko G, Zubovich V, Mknuik D, Gluchanina E, Dombrovskiy V, Ustinovitch A, Kot T, Bogdanovich N, Ovchinikova L, Helsing E, (Trial). PSGPoBI. Promotion of breastfeeding intervention trial (PROBIT): A randomized trial in the Republic of Belarus. *JAMA 2001.* 2001;285(4).

Kramer MS, Kakuma R. The optimal duration of exclusive breastfeeding: A systematic review. *Adv Exp Med Biol.* 2004;554:63–77.

Labbok MH, Clark D, Goldman AS. Breastfeeding: Maintaining an irreplaceable immunological resource. *Nat Rev Immunol.* 2004;4(7):565–572.

Labbok MH, Hendershot GE. Does breastfeeding protect against malocclusion? An analysis of the 1981 child health supplement to the National Health Interview Survey. *Am J Prev Med.* 1987;3(4):227–232.

Lanting CE, Fidler V, Huisman M, Touwan BD, Boersma ER. Neurological differences between 9-year-old children fed breastmilk or formula-milk as babies. *Lancet,* 1994;344(8933):1319–1322.

Lawrence R. *A Review of the Medical Benefits and Contraindications to Breastfeeding in the United States* (Maternal and Child Health Technical Information Bulletin). Arlington, VA: National Center for Education in Maternal and Child Health; October 1997.

Lawrence RA, Howard CR. Given the benefits of breastfeeding, are there any contraindications? *Clin Perinatol.* 1999;26(2):479–90,viii.

Liles C., Tompson M. Breastfeeding in the context of HIV/AIDS: Where is the evidence base supporting policy recommendations? Toronto, ON: *XVI Int'l AIDS Conference,* 2006 poster session.

Lucas A., Morley R, Cole TJ, Gore SM. A randomized multicentre study of human milk versus formula and later development in preterm infants. *Arch Dis Child.* 1994;70(2 Spec no);F141–46.

Machida HM, Catto Smith AG, Gall DG, Travenen C, Scott RB. Allergic colitis in infancy: Clinical and pathologic aspects. *J Pediatr Gastroenterol Nutr.* 1994;19:22–26.

Merrett TG, Burr ML, Butland BK, et al. Infant feeding and allergy: twelve-month prospective study of 500 babies in allergic families. *Ann Allergy.* 1988;61(6 pt 2):13–20.

Mestecky J, ed. *Immunology of Milk and the Neonate.* New York: Plenum Press; 1991.

Montgomery SM, Ehlin A, Sacker A. Breast feeding and resilience against psychosocial stress. *Arch Dis Child.* 2006.

Muraro A, Dreborg S, Halken S, et al. Dietary prevention of allergic diseases in infants and small children. Part III: Critical review of published peer-reviewed observational and interventional studies and final recommendations. *Pediatr Allergy Immunol.* 2004;15(4):291–307.

Newburg DS, Ruiz-Palacios GM, Morrow AL. Human milk glycans protect infants against enteric pathogens. *Annu Rev Nutr.* 2005;25:37–58.

Oddy WH, Li J, Landsborough L, Kendall GE, Henderson S, Downie J. The association of maternal overweight and obesity with breastfeeding duration. *J Pediatr.* 2006;149(2):185–191.

Oddy WH, Pal S, Kusel MM, Vine D, de Klerk NH, Hartmann P, et al. Atopy, eczema and breast milk fatty acids in a high-risk cohort of children followed from birth to 5 yr. *Pediatr Allergy Immunol.* 2006;17(1):4–10.

Oddy WH, Scott JA, Graham KI, Binns CW. Breastfeeding influences on growth and health at one year of age. *Breastfeed Rev.* 2006;14(1):15–23.

Oddy WH, Sherriff JL, de Klerk NH, Kendall GE, Sly PD, Beilin LJ, et al. The relation of breastfeeding and body mass index to asthma and atopy in children: A prospective cohort study to age 6 years. *Am J Public Health.* 2004;94(9):1531–1537.

Oddy WH. A review of the effects of breastfeeding on respiratory infections, atopy, and childhood asthma. *J Asthma.* 2004;41(6):605–621.

Paradise JL, Elster BA, Tan L. Evidence in infants with cleft palate that breast milk protects against otitis media. *Pediatrics.* 1994;94:853–860.

Prescott SL, Tang ML. The Australasian Society of Clinical Immunology and Allergy position statement: Summary of allergy prevention in children. *Med J Aust.* 2005;182(9):464–467.

Raisler J, Alexander C, O'Campo P. Breastfeeding and infant illness: A dose-response relationship? *Am J Pub Health.* 1999;89:25–30.

Rapp D. *Is This Your Child? Discovering and Treating Unrecognized Allergies in Children and Adults.* New York: Quill William Morrow; 1991.

Saarinen UM, Kajosaari M. Breastfeeding as prophylaxis against atopic disease: Prospective follow-up study until 17 years old. *Lancet.* 1995;346:1065–1069.

Scariati PD, Grummer-Strawn LM, Fein SB. A longitudinal analysis of infant morbidity and the extent of breastfeeding in the US. *Pediatrics.* 1997;99(6):e5.

Schwartz RH, Amonette MS. Cow milk protein hydrolysate infant formulas no always "hypoallergenic." *J Pediatr.* 1991; ltr118:839.

Setchell KDR, Zimmer-Nechemias L, Cai J, Heubi JE. Exposure of infants to phyto-oestrogens from soy-based infant formula. *Lancet.* 1997;350:23–27.

Stuebe AM, Rich-Edwards JW, Willett WC, Manson JE, Michels KB. Duration of lactation and incidence of Type 2 diabetes. *JAMA.* 2005;294(20):2601–2610.

Tanoue Y, Oda S. Weaning time of children with infantile autism. *Journal of Autism and Developmental Disorders.* 1989;19(3):425–434.

Thior I, Lockman S, Smeaton LM, et al. Breastfeeding plus infant zidovudine prophylaxis for 6 months vs formula feeding plus infant zidovudine for 1 month to reduce mother-to-child HIV transmission in Botswana: A randomized trial: The Mashi Study. *JAMA.* 2006;296(7):794–805.

Tompson M, Personal correspondence with Lawrence M. Gartner, MD, Professor Emeritus, University of Chicago, 5/18/00.

van Odijk J, Kull I, Borres MP, et al. Breastfeeding and allergic disease: A multidisciplinary review of the literature (1966–2001) on the mode of early feeding in infancy and its impact on later atopic manifestations. *Allergy.* 2003;58(9):833–843.

Walker M. *Selling Out Mothers and Babies: Marketing Breastmilk Substitutes in the USA.* Weston, MA: NABA REAL; 2001.

Wilson AC, Forsyth JS, Greene SA, et al. Relation of infant diet to childhood health: 7 year follow-up of cohort of children in Dundee infant feeding study. *Br Med J.* 1998;316:21–25.

Zeiger RS. Dietary aspects of food allergy prevention in infants and children. *J Pediatr Gastroenterol Nutr.* 2000;30:S77–S86.

Zoppi G, et al. Diet and antibody response to vaccinations in healthy infants. *Lancet.* 1983–7–2:11–14.

MATERNAL AND INFANT IMMUNOLOGY AND INFECTIOUS DISEASE QUESTIONS

Notice on question numbering: D-000 means a basic question, with one correct answer and three wrong answers. DP-000, along with the camera icon, means there is a picture that needs to be viewed to answer the question. The pictures are located on the CD-ROM included with the book and are numbered to correspond with the questions. DN-000, along with the frowning face icon, means the question has a NEGATIVE stem;

therefore, read the entire question very carefully to find the one WRONG answer among the choices. DPN-000, with both icons in the margin, means there is a picture associated with the question AND the question has a negative stem. See Appendix A for a fuller explanation of negative stem questions.

D-001. Bacterial counts 1 hour after expression are lower than immediately after collection. The most likely explanation for this is:

a. the cooler temperature in the container is unsuitable for growth of bacteria.
b. macrophages in milk are actively phagocytic.
c. gangliosides in milk disrupt the cell walls of bacteria.
d. bifidus factor starves the bacteria of nutrients.

D-002. A pregnant woman with many allergies asks about infant feeding. Your best response is:

a. a baby is never allergic to its mother's milk, but he may be sensitive to foods in the mother's diet.
b. since many allergic tendencies are inherited, there is nothing you can do to reduce your baby's chances of being allergic.
c. the hypoallergenic formulas will prevent any allergic reaction in your baby.
d. whether you breastfeed or not, you should delay solid foods until 6 months or later to help your baby avoid allergies.

D-003. Which of the infant's host defense systems are most effective at birth?

a. ability to cough
b. low pH of the stomach contents
c. innate defensins in the baby's skin and vernix
d. complement system and phagocytes

D-004. Which of these statements BEST describes the mucosal defense system?

a. A microbe is taken up by the mother's B cells and passed to M cells.
b. Helper T cells break down the pathogens.
c. The mother's secretory immune system provides targeted protection.
d. The infant's mucosal membranes provide passive immunity.

D-005. An exclusively breastfed baby's risk of food allergies is:

a. decreased, because few food allergens pass through the mother's milk.
b. decreased, because the mother's milk makes passage of allergenic proteins through the baby's gut less likely.
c. increased, because allergens pass readily through the mother's milk.
d. increased, because the mother's milk increases the permeability of the baby's gut.

DN-006. Medical uses for donor human milk include all of the following conditions **EXCEPT**:

a. postsurgical nutrition.
b. skin treatment of burns.
c. solid organ transplants.
d. allergies and feeding intolerance.

DN-007. A 3-week-old, exclusively breastfed baby with a strong family history of allergy has a severe reaction the first time he is fed with a cow's-milk-based formula. The **LEAST LIKELY** explanation for this is:

a. the baby was sensitized by intact cow's milk protein that passed into his mother's milk.
b. the baby was given a bottle of formula in the hospital nursery.
c. the mother consumed large amounts of dairy products during pregnancy.
d. the allergic reaction was more likely due to the latex in the bottle nipple than the cow's milk.

DN-008. Women who do not breastfeed their babies are at higher risk for all of the following conditions related to reproduction **EXCEPT**:

a. postpartum hemorrhage.
b. delayed return to prepregnancy weight.
c. menstrual irregularities and pain.
d. closely spaced pregnancies.

DP-009. Why would you want to discourage this practice in the first few hours postbirth?

a. The grandmother might drop the baby or fail to support its head sufficiently.
b. The clothing used to wrap the baby may be unclean or unsterile, risking an infection.
c. It's more important that the baby's father and grandfather be the first to hold the baby.
d. The grandmother's bacterial flora is foreign to the baby and prevents colonization with the mother's flora.

DP-010. Which of the following is most likely to be found in the mouth of this mother's baby?

a. dried milk on the tongue
b. normal tongue
c. oral thrush (*Candida*)
d. strep throat

DP-011. What is the most likely cause of the condition pictured?

a. acidic urine from human milk feedings
b. yeast infection (*Candida*)
c. allergic reaction to cow's-milk protein passing through the mother's milk
d. sensitivity to chemicals in disposable diapers

DP-012. Why is this position for birth beneficial for the newborn's health?

a. The grandmother can be the first to view the baby, thus enhancing bonding.
b. The attendant cannot pull on the newborn's head, thus avoiding head and neck trauma.
c. The mother can lift the baby out of her body herself, thus empowering her.
d. The baby is exposed to the mother's normal gut flora in her feces, thus colonizing with beneficial bacteria.

DP-013. The mother of this infant is most likely to complain of:

a. difficulty getting baby to latch on.
b. stinging, burning nipples.
c. vaginal discharge.
d. plugged ducts.

DP-014. Which of the following is the most likely cause of the condition pictured?

a. cold temperature in the room
b. supplements of cow's-milk-based formula
c. supplements of rice cereal
d. the baby's recent tetanus immunization

DP-015. Which immunofactor in human milk is at its highest level at this point in time?

a. SIgA
b. lactose
c. lysozyme
d. complement

DPN-016. When this condition is seen in a breastfeeding infant, all of the following recommendations are appropriate **EXCEPT**:

a. simultaneous treatment of the baby and the mother's breast should begin.
b. unless the mother has signs of infection, treat only the baby's mouth with an antifungal medication.
c. check the mother's nipples for signs or symptoms of infection.
d. assume that the mother's nipples, all infant sucking objects, and possibly other infant areas are infected until proven otherwise.

D-017. Which method of family planning is most likely to interfere with breastfeeding?

a. progestin-containing drugs
b. estrogen-containing drugs
c. cervical cap or diaphragm
d. natural family planning (periodic abstinence)

D-018. Which of the following descriptions of the protective aspects of breastfeeding is true?

a. effective as long as the baby is directly breastfeeding
b. the same whether the child is directly breastfed or given breast milk in a bottle
c. dose related for the baby, extending well past the time of direct breastfeeding
d. available only to the baby, not the mother

D-019. A mother contracts rubella while breastfeeding her 2-month-old baby. Which of the following actions is most appropriate?

a. The mother should continue breastfeeding.
b. The mother should immediately stop breastfeeding.
c. The baby should be isolated from the mother.
d. The mother and the baby should immediately receive the rubella vaccine.

D-020. Giving iron-rich foods to an infant under 6 months may increase infection because:

a. lactoferrin is bound in solution by added foods.
b. the foods may be contaminated with pathogens.
c. the iron-binding function of lactoferrin is overwhelmed.
d. iron makes the infant gut more permeable to pathogens.

D-021. When a breastfeeding mother becomes ill:

a. her milk supply often decreases.
b. she can transmit many diseases to her baby via her milk.
c. she can usually continue breastfeeding.
d. she is likely to be more sick than if she were not breastfeeding.

D-022. Which birth practice results in the most immune protection for the baby?

a. cesarean surgery under sterile conditions
b. lying down with a clean cloth or sheet under the mother's pelvic area
c. assisting the mother to birth in a supported squatting position
d. administering an enema to remove any feces from the lower bowel

D-023. Which type of bacteria is most dangerous for the newborn?

a. anaerobic bacteria in the gut
b. *Enterococcus* bacteria in the feces
c. *Staphylococcus epidermis* on the skin
d. aerobic bacteria on the mucous membranes

D-024. How long does it take for a baby's intestinal microflora to return to normal after being treated with an antibiotic?

a. Antibiotics have no effect on the infant's gut bacterial flora.
b. One day is sufficient for the breastfed baby to recover normal flora.
c. The microflora return to normal in 7–10 days for the breastfed child; 2–3 weeks for the formula-fed child.
d. Several weeks are necessary for the breastfed child's microflora to return to normal.

D-025. Which is the most prevalent antibody on mucosal membranes and in human milk?

a. IgA
b. IgE
c. IgG
d. IgM

D-026. What statement best describes the thymus gland's role in the infant's immune system?

a. A large thymus gland may be related to increased risk of SIDS.
b. Breastfed infants have smaller thymus glands than formula-fed children.
c. The larger the thymus gland, the lower the infant mortality rate.
d. A small thymus gland at birth is related to prematurity and prenatal nutrition.

D-027. Which type of cell in human milk gives rise to antibodies targeted against specific microbes?

a. neutrophils
b. B-lymphocytes
c. macrophages
d. granulocytes

DN-028. Artificially fed (formula-fed) children are at higher risk for all of the following gastrointestinal illnesses **EXCEPT**:

a. short-gut syndrome.
b. diarrhea.
c. necrotizing enterocolitis (NEC).
d. Crohn's disease.

DN-029. Which of the following respiratory conditions is **LEAST LIKELY** to be related to infant feeding?

a. otitis media (ear infections)
b. bronchitis and bronchiolitis
c. tuberculosis
d. wheezing/reactive airway disease

DN-030. All of the following conditions have been shown to be more common in people who were artificially fed as infants **EXCEPT**:

a. multiple sclerosis.
b. insulin-dependent diabetes mellitus.
c. coronary heart disease.
d. childhood cancers.

DN-031. Secretory IgA in mother's milk has all of the following functions **EXCEPT**:

a. binding of microbes in the baby's gut.
b. active destruction of bacteria.
c. anti-inflammatory action.
d. stimulating the infant's immune system.

DN-032.   Viral fragments that appear in mother's milk have all of the following features **EXCEPT**:

a.   they often cause infant illness.
b.   they act as a vaccination against disease.
c.   they are not whole-virus particles.
d.   they can be killed by heat treatments.

DN-033.   Research has identified artificial feeding as a risk factor in suboptimal neurological development, as manifested in all of the following **EXCEPT**:

a.   gross muscle coordination.
b.   cognitive development (IQ).
c.   visual acuity.
d.   reading and school performance.

DN-034.   Which of the following diseases is **LEAST LIKELY** to be related to artificial feeding?

a.   ulcerative colitis
b.   osteoarthritis
c.   eczema
d.   respiratory infections

DN-035.   A pregnant woman and her husband both have many allergies. She asks whether there is anything she can do to reduce her child's risks of allergic disease. Your responses should include all of the following **EXCEPT**:

a.   avoid common allergens such as cow's milk during your pregnancy.
b.   exclusively breastfeed for at least 6 months.
c.   continue breastfeeding to 24 months or longer if your child is willing.
d.   take steroid medications to strengthen your immune system.

DN-036.   A mother with influenza asks if she should continue breastfeeding her 5-month-old, exclusively breastfed child. Your responses would include all of the following **EXCEPT**:

a.   yes, because your milk will quickly obtain specific antibodies to lessen the chance that your child with get this infection.
b.   yes, because your milk contains white cells that will help your baby fight this infection, if he gets it at all.
c.   yes, because you will get well quicker if you don't have the additional burden of preparing artificial feeds.
d.   yes, because lactation speeds up your own production of antibodies so you won't get as sick.

DN-037. All of these statements accurately describe the protective role of breastfeeding **EXCEPT**:

a. the interaction of anti-inflammatory and anti-infective factors is more than the sum of its parts.
b. the unique components of milk protect the mammary gland and the recipient infant from many diseases.
c. once lactation and breastfeeding cease, the mother and infant are just as vulnerable to disease as anyone else.
d. protections associated with breastfeeding extend past the time of direct breastfeeding.

DN-038. Breastfeeding protects the infant from allergy by all of the following methods **EXCEPT**:

a. limiting the baby's exposure to nonhuman proteins.
b. slowing or preventing the absorption of allergens through the baby's gut.
c. protecting the baby's gut from inflammation, which weakens the mucosal barrier.
d. providing white cells in milk, which attack the allergens directly.

DN-039. The risk of which of the following maternal reproductive cancers is **NOT** reduced by breastfeeding?

a. cervical cancer
b. premenopausal breast cancer
c. ovarian cancer
d. endometrial cancer

DP-040. What is the most important reason to support a mother using this position to give birth?

a. Her feces will colonize her baby with normal beneficial bacterial flora.
b. Her milk will change from colostrum to mature milk sooner.
c. Her support person will be able to hold the baby immediately.
d. The baby will rotate to an easier position for birth.

DP-041. The rash on this baby's face appeared when he began receiving supplements of cow's-milk-based artificial baby milk. What is the most likely cause of the rash?

a. normal infant acne
b. reaction to nonhuman protein in the artificial baby milk
c. presence of bovine antigen in the mother's milk
d. allergic reaction to latex in the bottle teat

DP-042. This exclusively breastfed baby is gaining well and is otherwise healthy. For the condition pictured, your best recommendation to the mother is:

a. Try eliminating dairy products from your diet for a week to rule out an allergic response.
b. Give the baby water in between breastfeeds because her urine is too concentrated.
c. Start supplementing with soy formula because your milk supply is inadequate.
d. Ask the baby's pediatrician to prescribe an antifungal ointment for the baby's skin.

MATERNAL AND INFANT IMMUNOLOGY AND INFECTIOUS DISEASE ANSWERS

The parenthetical material at the end of each answer includes the discipline and time period, indicates whether the question pertains to knowledge or application, and specifies the degree of difficulty.

D-001. The answer is B. Macrophages and possibly neutrophils and T-lymphocytes actively kill microbes by phagocytosis. (Immunology; General Principles; Knowledge; Difficulty: 5)

D-002. The answer is A. Exclusive breastfeeding for about 6 months is the best strategy to reduce the baby's risk. The mother's avoidance of known allergens during pregnancy may also reduce the baby's risks of allergy. It is more important that the mother exclusively breastfeed for about 6 months than other actions she should be considering at this time. Delaying solid foods does not address the baby's more likely early exposure to cow's milk and soy proteins, which are very common allergens in humans. (Immunology; Prenatal; Knowledge; Difficulty: 3)

D-003. The answer is C. Innate defensins on the baby's skin and in the vernix provide a measure of protection to the newborn. The other systems are not fully mature at birth. Breast milk compensates for and enhances the development of other host defense systems. (Immunology; General Principles; Knowledge; Difficulty: 5)

D-004. The answer is C. The mother's secretory immune system provides targeted protection through the entero-mammary and broncho-mammary pathways. (Immunology; General Principles; Knowledge; Difficulty: 5)

D-005. The answer is B. Breast milk optimizes the environment in the baby's gut. Allergens may be present in breast milk and may create problems for a sensitive baby, but the risk of allergies is significantly reduced through breastfeeding. (Immunology; 4–6 months; Application; Difficulty: 4)

DN-006. The answer is B. As of this writing, donor milk has not been prescribed for skin treatment of burns. (Immunology; General Principles; Knowledge; Difficulty: 5)

DN-007. The answer is D. Although sudden, severe latex allergies are possible, the reaction is more likely to be caused by an ingested allergen, especially cow's-milk protein. All of the other choices are possible sources or routes of sensitization. (Immunology; 15–28 days; Application; Difficulty: 2)

DN-008. The answer is C. Menstrual irregularities and pain are not known to be related to whether the woman breastfed her children. (Immunology; Preconception; Knowledge; Difficulty: 2)

DP-009. The answer is D. Colonization with the mother's flora sets up the optimal microbial environment for the newborn. When anyone else holds the baby, there is a greater risk of colonization with less friendly organisms. (Immunology; Labor/Birth; Application; Difficulty: 3)

DP-010. The answer is C. The shiny, reddened color of this mother's nipple and areola is typical of thrush (*Candida*) infection. Her baby's mouth is likely to show white plaques that do not rub off and are typical of oral thrush/fungal (*Candida*) infections. (Immunology; 15–28 days; Application; Difficulty: 4)

DP-011. The answer is C. The reddened skin is only found on the genitalia and anal opening, suggesting an allergic response. Yeast infections are characterized by blisters or papules. Acidic urine does not result from human milk feedings, and chemical sensitivities would likely appear under the entire diaper area. This baby was in fact allergic to dairy products ingested by her mother. (Immunology; 15–28 days; Application; Difficulty: 3)

DP-012. The answer is D. The newborn is born sterile. Exposure to the mother's feces colonizes the infant with her beneficial gut bacteria, which helps avoid colonization with harmful pathogens from the environment. (Immunology; Labor/Birth; Knowledge; Difficulty: 5)

DP-013. The answer is B. This baby has oral thrush, which easily transfers to the mother's nipples. Although a mother may have a vaginal *Candida* infection, it is most likely that she will have symptoms of thrush on her nipples. (Immunology; 1–3 months; Application; Difficulty: 3)

DP-014. The answer is B. This was diagnosed as eczema, an allergic reaction that began soon after this baby was given supplements of cow's-milk-based formula. Rice cereal is a less common allergen. It is unlikely that cold temperature or a tetanus immunization triggered this response. (Immunology; 15–28 days; Application; Difficulty: 3)

DP-015. The answer is A. Secretory IgA in milk/colostrum is 10 times higher on the first postpartum day than at any other time during lactation. Lactose is low at this time because lactose is low in colostrum. (Immunology; Labor/Birth; Application; Difficulty: 4)

DPN-016. The answer is B. Mother–baby cross-infection is likely when the baby has an oral infection. Assume that the mother's nipples are also infected with the same organism, as well as other infant body parts and any/all sucking objects. (Immunology; 1–3 months; Application; Difficulty: 2)

D-017. The answer is B. Use of estrogen-containing contraceptives will nearly always diminish milk supply. Progestin-containing drugs may also lower milk supply in some women, especially if taken prior to 8 weeks postbirth. The other methods do not use hormones and are highly compatible with breastfeeding. (Immunology; 1–3 months; Knowledge; Difficulty: 3)

D-018. The answer is C. Protection against many short- and long-term diseases is well established, even though the specific mechanisms are still poorly understood as of this writing. (Immunology; >12 months; Knowledge; Difficulty: 3)

D-019. The answer is A. The mother's milk contains rubella-specific antibodies very quickly after maternal exposure. The baby has already been exposed; therefore, continued breastfeeding helps protect the baby. Maternal rubella infection is not a contraindication for breastfeeding. (Immunology; 1–3 months; Application; Difficulty: 3)

D-020. The answer is C. Lactoferrin binds iron in milk and makes it available to the infant. Adding additional sources of dietary iron overwhelms the lactoferrin, leaving the iron available to pathogenic bacteria for growth. (Immunology; 4–6 months; Knowledge; Difficulty: 4)

D-021. The answer is C. With very rare exceptions, breastfeeding should continue if the mother is ill at the time of birth or if she becomes ill during breastfeeding. (Immunology; General Principles; Application; Difficulty: 3)

D-022. The answer is C. According to Dr. Lars Hanson, "Human babies, like all mammals, are delivered next to their mother's anus. This insures exposure to the mother's normal and beneficial intestinal bacteria." All the other procedures listed actually reduce the baby's immune protection because the infant is exposed to other bacteria in the environment, instead of the mother's beneficial gut bacteria. (Immunology; Labor/Birth; Application; Difficulty: 5)

D-023. The answer is D. Aerobic bacteria require oxygen and are potentially more harmful than anaerobic bacteria, which do not require oxygen. The mucous membranes are the most common route for infections of the newborn. (Immunology; General Principles; Knowledge; Difficulty: 4)

D-024. The answer is D. Antibiotic treatments severely reduce the number of anaerobic bacteria, allowing the growth of pathogenic aerobic strains including *Klebsiella* and *Enterobacter*. It takes several weeks for the breastfed child's gut to recover, and much longer for the child who is deprived of human milk. (Immunology; General Principles; Knowledge; Difficulty: 4)

D-025. The answer is A. Secretory IgA is the main antibody appearing on mucous membranes and in the GI tract. SIgA binds microbes and blocks them from entering tissues; thereby the immune system in tissues is not triggered. IgM and IgG neutralize toxins, but they trigger an inflammatory reaction. IgE is elevated during allergic reactions. (Immunology; General Principles; Knowledge; Difficulty: 4)

D-026. The answer is C. A fully breastfed baby's thymus gland is twice the size of that of a formula-fed baby. A small thymus at birth is related to low birth weight, malnutrition, and higher infant mortality. An old and false myth alleged that SIDS was due to a large thymus. Prenatal infections are a common cause of fetal death and are associated with smaller thymus glands. (Immunology; General Principles; Knowledge; Difficulty: 4)

D-027. The answer is B. B-lymphocytes produce targeted antibodies that quickly appear in milk. (Immunology; General Principles; Knowledge; Difficulty: 4)

DN-028. The answer is A. Short-gut syndrome does not appear to be related to infant feeding. All of the others are much more common in those who were artificially fed. Pasteurized donor human milk is sometimes used to treat short-gut syndrome. (Immunology; General Principles; Knowledge; Difficulty: 2)

DN-029. The answer is C. Even tuberculosis may be less of a risk in the breastfed infant. The other diseases are strongly associated with artificial feeding. (Immunology; General Principles; Knowledge; Difficulty: 5)

DN-030. The answer is C. No studies have yet reported on a direct correlation between coronary heart disease and infant feeding, although recent studies of adolescents show an increase in serum lipids in those who were artificially fed. A significant relationship to mode of infant feeding has been shown in the other conditions. (Immunology; Preconception; Knowledge; Difficulty: 5)

DN-031. The answer is B. SIgA may be targeted to a specific pathogen, but it does not directly kill bacteria. (Immunology; General Principles; Knowledge; Difficulty: 2)

DN-032. The answer is A. Viral fragments in milk do not appear to actually transmit disease from mother to infant. (Immunology; General Principles; Knowledge; Difficulty: 2)

DN-033. The answer is A. To date, studies have not established a relationship between gross motor performance and infant feeding mode. The other elements are strongly linked to duration and intensity of breastfeeding. (Immunology; General Principles; Knowledge; Difficulty: 5)

DN-034. The answer is B. As of this writing, a link between osteoarthritis and artificial feeding has not been demonstrated in the scientific literature. Eczema is strongly related to allergy, which is related to artificial feeding; ulcerative colitis and respiratory infections are associated with artificial feeding. (Immunology; General Principles; Difficulty: 4)

DN-035. The answer is D. Steroids do not reduce the infant's risk of allergy, and they have other consequences. The other strategies will help postpone the onset of and/or reduce the severity of allergic disease in her child. (Immunology; Prenatal; Application; Difficulty: 2)

DN-036. The answer is D. There is no evidence that the mother will become less ill because she is lactating. Antibodies and white cells that she produces quickly get into her milk and protect the baby. A mother who is sick may be further stressed by the additional work of preparing artificial feeds. (Immunology; 4–6 months; Application; Difficulty: 2)

DN-037. The answer is C. The biochemical, physical, immunological, and neurodevelopmental effects of breastfeeding and lactation forever change the mother and baby. (Immunology; General Principles; Knowledge; Difficulty: 3)

DN-038. The answer is D. White cells in milk do not directly attack dietary allergens. The other answers are true. (Immunology; General Principles; Knowledge; Difficulty: 2)

DN-039. The answer is A. As of this writing, no relationship between breastfeeding and the risk of cervical cancer has been investigated. The risk for all of the others are higher for women who do not breastfeed/lactate. (Immunology; General Principles; Knowledge; Difficulty: 4)

DP-040. The answer is A. The newborn is born sterile. Colonization with the mother's normal gut flora by coming in contact with her feces prevents the newborn from being colonized with harmful bacteria in its environment. Some babies will rotate to a more favorable position for birth in this position, but there is no research (at this date) that directly links mother's position at birth with infant outcomes. (Immunology; Labor/Birth; Knowledge; Difficulty: 4)

DP-041. The answer is B. Facial rashes are a common allergic reaction to cow's milk proteins. Direct exposure from artificial baby milk is the most likely trigger. (Immunology; 1–3 months; Application; Difficulty: 4)

DP-042. The answer is A. The baby is entirely healthy and thriving except for an allergic diaper rash caused by dairy in her mother's diet. The other options are inappropriate and incorrect. There are no signs of fungal infection on the baby in this picture. (Immunology; 15–28 days; Application; Difficulty: 3)

Scoring:

Total number of questions in this section   _____

Number of questions answered correctly   _____

Percent correct (divide number correct by total number)   _____

E. MATERNAL AND INFANT PATHOLOGY

In the 2000 exam blueprint, 19 to 33 questions are dedicated to maternal and infant pathology.

SUBTOPICS INCLUDED IN THIS CATEGORY

1. Infant

   a. Birth-related, including hyperbilirubinemia and hypoglycemia
   b. Genetic, metabolic, and chronic abnormalities
   c. Prematurity
   d. Neurological immaturity or impairment
   e. Physical and structural issues
   f. Oral pathology, including suck problems
   g. Gastrointestinal, digestive
   h. Infectious diseases, including yeast
   i. Failure to thrive

2. Maternal

   a. Pregnancy complications; labor medications; cesarean, placenta problems
   b. Chronic infections and conditions
   c. Genetic, endocrine, and metabolic—e.g., diabetes, cancer
   d. Physical and sensory
   e. Breast and nipple problems, including engorgement and mastitis

3. Impact on lifelong health

   a. Epidemiology of illnesses associated with feeding methods
   b. Impact of maternal or infant illness on breastfeeding

CORE READING

Textbooks

Amir L, Hoover K. *Candidiasis and Breastfeeding*. Schaumburg, IL: La Leche League International; 2002.

Auerbach K, Riordan J. *Clinical Lactation: A Visual Guide*. Sudbury, MA: Jones & Bartlett Publishers; 2000.

Brodribb W, ed. *Breastfeeding Management*. East Malvern, Australia: Australian Breastfeeding Association; 2004.

Cadwell K, Turner-Maffei C. *Breastfeeding A–Z: Terminology and Telephone Triage*. Sudbury, MA: Jones & Bartlett Publishers; 2006.

Cadwell K, Turner-Maffei C. *Case Studies in Breastfeeding: Problem Solving Skills and Strategies*. Sudbury, MA: Jones & Bartlett Publishers; 2006.

Cadwell K, Turner-Maffei C, O'Connor B, et al. *Maternal and Infant Assessment for Breastfeeding and Human Lactation: A Guide for the Practitioner.* 2nd ed. Sudbury, MA: Jones & Bartlett Publishers; 2006.

Dunnewold A, Sanford DG. *Postpartum Survival Guide.* Oakland, CA: New Harbinger Press; 1994.

Good Mojab C. *Congenital Disorders in the Nursling.* Schaumburg, IL: La Leche League International; 2002.

Kendall-Tackett K. *Postpartum Depression and the Breastfeeding Mother.* Schaumburg, IL: La Leche League International; 2004.

Kroeger M, Smith L. *Impact of Birthing Practices on Breastfeeding.* Sudbury, MA: Jones & Bartlett Publishers; 2004.

Lawrence RA, Lawrence RM. *Breastfeeding: A Guide for the Medical Profession.* 6th ed. St. Louis: Elsevier Mosby; 2005.

Merewood A, Phillip B. *Breastfeeding Conditions and Diseases.* Amarillo, TX: Hale Publishing (Pharmasoft Publishing); 2001.

Mohrbacher N, Stock J. *The Breastfeeding Answer Book.* Schaumburg, IL: La Leche League International; 2003.

Popper B. *The Hospitalized Nursing Baby.* Schaumburg, IL: La Leche League International; 2003.

Riordan J. *Breastfeeding and Human Lactation.* 3rd ed. Sudbury, MA: Jones & Bartlett Publishers; 2004.

The Royal College of Midwives, UK. *Successful Breastfeeding.* London: Churchill Livingstone; 2003.

Walker M. *Breastfeeding Management for the Clinician: Using the Evidence.* Sudbury, MA: Jones & Bartlett Publishers; 2006.

Walker M. *Mastitis and the Lactating Woman.* Schaumburg, IL: La Leche League International; 2002.

Wilson-Clay B, Hoover K. *The Breastfeeding Atlas.* 3rd ed. Austin, TX: Lactnews Press; 2005.

Wolf LS, Glass RP. *Feeding and Swallowing Disorders in Infancy: Assessment and Management.* Tucson, AZ: Therapy Skill Builder; 1992.

Key Research Articles

The Academy of Breastfeeding Medicine. *Clinical protocols.* New Rochelle, NY: Academy of Breastfeeding Medicine. Available at: http://www.bfmed.org/?menuID=139&firstlevelmenuID=139. Accessed Oct 1, 2006.

Francis-Morrill J, Heinig MJ, Pappagianis D, Dewey KG. Diagnostic value of signs and symptoms of mammary candidosis among lactating women. *J Hum Lact.* 2004;20(3):288–295.

Heinig MJ, Francis J, Pappagianis D. Mammary candidosis in lactating women. *J Hum Lact.* 1999;15(4):281–288.

Hypoglycaemia of the Newborn: Review of the Literature. Geneva, Switzerland: World Health Organization; 1998.

Morrill JF, Heinig MJ, Pappagianis D, Dewey KG. Risk factors for mammary candidosis among lactating women. *J Obstet Gynecol Neonatal Nurs.* 2005;34(1):37–45.

MATERNAL AND INFANT PATHOLOGY QUESTIONS

Notice on question numbering: E-000 means a basic question, with one correct answer and three wrong answers. EP-000, along with the camera icon, means there is a picture that needs to be viewed to answer the question. The pictures are located on the CD-ROM included with this book and are numbered to correspond with the questions. EN-000, along with the frowning face icon, means the question has a NEGATIVE stem; therefore, read the entire question very carefully to find the one WRONG answer among the choices. EPN-000, with both icons in the margin, means there is a picture associated with the question AND the question has a negative stem. See Appendix A for a fuller explanation of negative stem questions.

E-001. You have been working with a mother who describes excruciating pain every time her baby's mouth touches her breast, even if he does not latch on and breastfeed. You have ruled out injury, infections, and other causes of nipple pain, and her nipples are not reddened or irritated. You should next consider whether the mother has:

a. a history of any kind of abuse.
b. no interest in breastfeeding.
c. a low pain threshold.
d. allergies.

E-002. A breastfeeding mother fractured her pelvis and right leg in a car accident. She is in traction and taking pain medications. Her exclusively breastfed 3-month-old baby has never taken a bottle. The most helpful action to support this family is:

a. get her a breast pump so she does not become engorged.
b. encourage her husband to teach the baby to take milk from a spoon or cup.
c. help her position the baby for nursing in a way that does not disturb her injuries.
d. obtain a prescription for birth control pills to dry up her milk.

E-003. A mother comes to you for help with breastfeeding her 3-week-old baby, stating, "He just doesn't seem to be able to get it right." When you observe the baby breastfeeding, you note that the baby has a highly erratic suck-swallow pattern and that he never develops a good rhythmic suckling action. Which of the following is most likely to explain his sucking behavior?

a. Many babies do not establish effective suckling patterns until 4–6 weeks after birth.
b. The baby's head is still quite molded.
c. The baby was born at 37 weeks' gestation.
d. The baby has cerebral palsy.

E-004. A 16-year-old mother delivered her first baby by cesarean section and sustained significant blood loss requiring a blood transfusion. Four days later, her milk has not yet come in. The most likely reason for delay in onset of copius milk synthesis is:

a. young age.
b. cesarean delivery.
c. first lactation cycle.
d. significant blood loss.

E-005. A mother complains of raw, inflamed skin on both areolas. Her infant is teething, has recently started solid foods, and is taking an antibiotic for strep throat. The most likely cause of this areolar irritation is:

a. an allergic reaction to a food the baby consumed.
b. an allergic reaction to the medication being given to her infant.
c. psoriasis that was exacerbated by the infant's saliva.
d. a bacterial infection of the nipple skin.

E-006. Within the first minute or two of beginning a breastfeed, a 2-week-old infant gulps, coughs, and chokes, then releases the breast. This incident most likely describes:

a. an infant with decreased oral tone.
b. poor coordination of sucking, swallowing, and breathing.
c. strong milk ejection reflex.
d. gastroesophageal reflux.

E-007. Which of the following questions suggests a qualitative research design?

a. What are mothers' experiences of breastfeeding after cesarean birth?
b. How many mothers in Norway gave birth by cesarean section in 2003?
c. Is there a relationship between cesarean birth and infant suck dysfunction?
d. What percent of babies are helped by lactation consultant contact 3 days after a cesarean birth?

E-008. Sudden onset of painless bright red bleeding from the nipple of a mother during the first week postpartum indicates the probable presence of:

a. breast cancer.
b. fibrocystic disease.
c. intraductal papilloma.
d. nipple tissue breakdown.

E-009. A pregnant woman contracted chicken pox a short time ago. The lesions are now completely crusted over, and she is in labor. The most appropriate action to take when she gives birth is:

a. separate her from the baby until she is noninfectious.
b. allow her to hold, but not breastfeed her baby.
c. separate her from the baby but feed her expressed milk to the baby.
d. help her breastfeed immediately after birth with 24-hour rooming-in.

E-010. Lack of eye contact by the mother and little talking or caressing of her infant should alert you to the possibility of:

a. a neurologically impaired infant.
b. a neurologically impaired mother.
c. a developmentally delayed infant.
d. a clinically depressed mother.

E-011. A mother of a fussy, gassy baby has been drinking 10 glasses of cow's milk per day on her doctor's recommendation. Your first action would be:

a. encourage her to follow her doctor's dietary advice.
b. take a thorough history including allergy and food sensitivity in the family.
c. tell her that 6–8 glasses of any liquid is adequate during lactation.
d. tell her that consumption of dairy products is not related to her baby's symptoms.

E-012. Some brands of artificial baby milk produced in the 1980s lacked one essential mineral, causing brain damage and learning disabilities in the children who received this product exclusively. Absence of which of the minerals listed would have that effect?

a. sodium
b. chloride
c. potassium
d. calcium

EN-013. A mother calls you, frustrated, because her 3-week-old baby's preference for nursing at the right breast is so strong that she is unable to get him to nurse on her left side. What is the **LEAST LIKELY** explanation for this baby's nursing behavior?

a. There is a subtle positioning difference in the mother's hold on her left side.
b. The baby has a cephalohematoma on his right side.
c. The mother has an undetected breast cancer in her left breast.
d. The baby's right clavicle is fractured.

EN-014. A mother who is becoming ill with influenza should continue breastfeeding her 5-month-old, exclusively breastfed child for all of the following reasons **EXCEPT**:

a. her milk will quickly obtain specific antibodies to reduce the chance that her child will get this infection.
b. her milk contains white cells that will help her baby fight this infection.
c. lactation speeds up her own production of antibodies so her illness will be less severe.
d. she will recover quicker without the additional burden of preparing artificial feeds.

EN-015. Which component of human milk is **LEAST** important in preventing neonatal septicemia?

a. lysozyme in colostrum
b. secretory IgA antibodies
c. oligosaccharide receptor analogues
d. lactoferrin protein

EP-016. This picture was taken immediately after a feed ended. Which statement most likely describes the preceding feed?

a. The baby had a shallow latch.
b. The baby was deeply latched.
c. The baby effectively transferred milk.
d. The baby fed well and then self-detached.

EP-017. This full-term baby is 36 hours old. The most likely condition requiring this treatment is:

a. exclusive, effective breastfeeding.
b. ABO incompatibility.
c. breast milk jaundice.
d. hypoglycemia.

EP-018. This baby is being breastfed with a silicone nipple shield, jaw support, and a straddle position at breast. The underlying condition that is being helped by these strategies is most likely:

a. hypertonia.
b. hypotonia.
c. ataxia.
d. hypoglycemia.

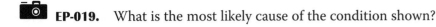 **EP-019.** What is the most likely cause of the condition shown?

a. bacterial infection
b. allergic reaction from laundry soap
c. friction damage from baby's tongue
d. the mother has fair skin

EP-020. The mother of this baby complains of a stinging, burning pain in her nipples. The recommendation most likely to resolve her pain is:

a. breastfeed for frequent, short periods of time.
b. wear nipple shields during breastfeeding for one week.
c. the mother and the baby should be treated with antifungal medication.
d. boil all of the baby's pacifiers.

EP-021. This mother of a 3-month-old began feeling pinpoint pain on her nipple tip 2 days ago. The pain is most likely due to:

a. mastitis.
b. a plugged nipple pore.
c. a bacterial infection.
d. a friction blister.

EP-022. This mother's baby is 8 days old. The most likely cause of the condition pictured is:

a. normal breastfeeding.
b. the baby is tongue-tied.
c. the baby is not latching deeply.
d. the baby is biting during feeds.

EP-023. What could you do to decrease this baby's risk of SIDS?

a. Move the mattress away from the unused fireplace.
b. Put the baby in a crib.
c. Give the baby a pacifier.
d. Roll the baby onto her back.

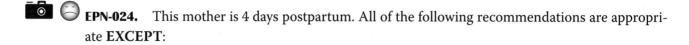

EPN-024. This mother is 4 days postpartum. All of the following recommendations are appropriate **EXCEPT**:

a. apply cool cabbage compresses to the lump in your right armpit.
b. feed your baby at least every 2–3 hours, or more often if he cries.
c. apply hot compresses to help milk flow in your left breast.
d. use cool compresses after feeds if breasts feel full.

EPN-025. After examining this woman's breasts, you would do all of the following actions **EXCEPT**:

a. instruct her on better cleaning procedures for her breast pump.
b. provide her with a nipple shield to wear during feeds.
c. request that the primary care provider culture the baby's mouth.
d. recommend that she wean immediately.

EPN-026. Appropriate treatments for this condition include all of the following **EXCEPT**:

a. cabbage leaf compresses.
b. hot compresses.
c. cold compresses.
d. gentle massage.

EPN-027. Which of the following behaviors is **LEAST LIKELY** to occur in the breastfeeding child of this age?

a. The mother and the child have a code word for breastfeeding.
b. The child can postpone nursing for short periods.
c. Nighttime breastfeeding increases the child's risk of dental caries.
d. The child receives substantial immune protection from breastfeeding.

EPN-028. What is the **LEAST LIKELY** cause of the condition shown?

a. Paget's disease
b. plugged nipple pore
c. persistent wound from baby's tongue thrust
d. nipple thrush (*Candida*)

EPN-029. This breastfeeding mother says that this condition appeared when her baby was about 4 months old. Which is the **LEAST LIKELY** cause of the condition shown?

a. atopic dermatitis
b. fungal infection
c. eczema
d. psoriasis

 EPN-030. All of the following are appropriate actions for this mother's situation **EXCEPT**:

a. advising her to stop breastfeeding on this breast.
b. assisting her to express milk from this breast thoroughly every few hours.
c. encouraging her to rest and continue breastfeeding on the other breast.
d. supporting her in taking any prescribed antibiotics.

E-031. A mother has been feeding her baby on a rigid schedule for several months on the advice of friends. Her child is now underweight, appears anxious, and cries frequently. She strongly desires to continue breastfeeding. Your best recommendation is to:

a. increase the amount of solid food he is getting.
b. pump your milk between feeds to keep up your supply.
c. add artificial milk to his feeds so he can stay on this schedule.
d. feed the baby whenever he is hungry, at least 8 times a day.

E-032. A breastfeeding mother complains of a lump in her breast. Which characteristic of the lump is most likely to be dangerous and require medical evaluation?

a. The lump feels like a soft, fluid-filled sac.
b. The skin over the lump is red and warm.
c. The mother began running a low-grade fever at the same time the lump appeared.
d. The lump does not change size before and after the baby feeds.

E-033. Separating babies from their mothers shortly after birth and caring for them in separate rooms is most likely to result in which of the following?

a. improved sleep-wake patterns in infants
b. increased infant stress hormones
c. more rest for the mother
d. improved infection control practices

E-034.   A woman in the active phase of labor complains of a severe backache. This is most likely due to:

a.   a weak back due to lack of exercise.
b.   a herniated disk in the lumbar spine.
c.   the fetus being in a posterior presentation.
d.   a tetanic contraction of the uterus.

E-035.   A mother experiences a severe hemorrhage postpartum. She is at risk for which of the following conditions?

a.   retained placental fragments
b.   anemia
c.   Sheehan's syndrome
d.   eclampsia

EN-036.   A mother of a 2-week-old baby states that her baby's suck feels weak compared to her first baby's suck. This second baby, she states, "always seems hungry" and has also lost weight since birth. The **LEAST LIKELY** cause of this breastfeeding problem is:

a.   low birthweight.
b.   the baby is lazy.
c.   poor intraoral tone.
d.   shallow attachment at breast.

EN-037.   Allergy in children is associated with all of the following **EXCEPT**:

a.   a strong history of allergy in parents.
b.   over half the visits to pediatric practices in the first year of life.
c.   one third of chronic illnesses in children under age 17.
d.   asthma, which accounts for one third of all lost school days.

EN-038.   A pregnant woman who has insulin-dependent diabetes expresses interest in breastfeeding. Your responses should include all the following **EXCEPT**:

a.   it may be easier to control your insulin if you breastfeed.
b.   breastfeeding will help reduce your baby's risk of being diabetic.
c.   it will be more difficult to control your insulin if you breastfeed.
d.   your colostrum is perfect for your baby especially in adjusting to extrauterine life.

EN-039. A baby born at 32 weeks' gestation was growing normally for 2 weeks, then his growth began slowing. The **LEAST LIKELY** cause of this sudden slowing of weight gain is:

a. exclusive use of human milk.
b. respiratory infection.
c. necrotizing enterocolitis.
d. cardiac anomaly.

EN-040. A breastfeeding woman with multiple sclerosis (MS) should be told all of the following **EXCEPT**:

a. use extra household help whenever you can.
b. many medications used for multiple sclerosis are compatible with breastfeeding.
c. breastfeeding lowers the risk that your baby will develop multiple sclerosis.
d. breastfeeding decreases the likelihood of acute episodes of MS during the early postpartum period.

EN-041. A breastfeeding infant has been diagnosed with oral thrush. You should begin all of the following interventions **EXCEPT**:

a. simultaneously treat the baby and the mother's breasts.
b. unless the mother has signs of infection, treat only the baby's mouth with an antifungal medication.
c. check the mother's nipples for signs or symptoms of infection.
d. assume that the mother's nipples, all infant sucking objects, and possibly other infant areas are infected until proven otherwise.

EN-042. A full-term baby breastfeeds effectively in only one position, and only on one of his mother's breasts. The **LEAST LIKELY** explanation is:

a. the baby has a broken clavicle.
b. one side of the baby's head was injured during birth.
c. the mother has a stronger letdown in one breast.
d. the mother fed him in this position shortly after birth and he doesn't like change.

EN-043. The **LEAST LIKELY** cause for a mother's nipples to be cracked and bleeding on the second postpartum day is:

a. the baby has ankyloglossia.
b. the baby is latching onto the nipple only.
c. the mother has unusually fragile nipple skin.
d. the mother is feeding her baby every 2 hours for 30 minutes each.

🙁 **EN-044.** When a mother is giving birth to twins, the **LEAST LIKELY** reason that the second baby might have a problem initiating breastfeeding is:

a. a higher likelihood of a prolapsed cord.
b. malpresentation causing birth injury.
c. the mother is busy with the first-born twin.
d. the second baby is usually the smaller of the 2.

🙁 **EN-045.** Which is the **LEAST LIKELY** cause of sudden-onset breast pain while nursing an 8- to 10-month-old?

a. baby sliding down onto the nipple tip
b. hormonally induced tenderness due to subsequent pregnancy
c. allergic reaction to family foods that the baby is eating
d. low milk supply due to prolonged lactation

📷 **EP-046.** Any breastfeeding difficulties experienced by this infant are most likely related to:

a. fetal alcohol syndrome.
b. congenital hypothyroidism.
c. Down syndrome.
d. Pierre Robin syndrome.

📷 **EP-047.** This full-term baby is 36 hours old. The most likely condition requiring this treatment is:

a. breast-milk jaundice.
b. ABO incompatibility.
c. exclusive breastfeeding.
d. hypoglycemia.

📷 **EP-048.** The bulge on this mother's breast is most likely :

a. a plugged duct.
b. a galactocele.
c. mastitis.
d. an abscess.

📷 **EP-049.** After assessing this baby, your first suggestion to the mother should be:

a. use a nipple shield during feeds.
b. your baby needs an oral surgery consultation immediately.
c. let's see how your baby does at breast.
d. pump your milk and feed with a bottle today.

📷 **EP-050.** Which of the following sensations is this mother most likely to be experiencing?

a. comfort during and between feeds
b. systemic fever and chills
c. deep, aching breast pain
d. burning, stabbing pain of both nipples/areolas

📷 **EP-051.** The nipple damage shown in this picture is most likely due to:

a. poor positioning at breast.
b. bacterial or fungal infection.
c. tongue-tied baby.
d. overuse of a breast pump.

📷 **EP-052.** This mother had persistent deep breast pain and low grade fever for 2 weeks. What is the most likely reason for the treatment pictured?

a. infectious mastitis
b. breast abscess
c. intraductal papilloma
d. mammary duct ectasia

📷 **EP-053.** This condition is most likely associated with which of the following?

a. delayed or inadequate treatment of mastitis
b. ductal yeast infection
c. transmission of oral bacteria from the baby's mouth
d. bruising or trauma to the breast

📷 **EP-054.** This mother says her nipples started itching and stinging a few days ago. The most likely cause of her symptoms is

a. dry skin.
b. eczema.
c. nipple thrush.
d. positional soreness.

📷 **EP-055.** Which is the most likely cause of the condition pictured?

a. teething baby
b. allergic response to laundry soap used to wash bra
c. suction too high on breast pump
d. bacterial infection of the baby's mouth

EP-056. This mother is 1 week postpartum and experiencing nipple pain. The most likely explanation is

a. an inversion in the center of the tip rubbing on the baby's palate.
b. a large, fibrous nipple being compressed by the baby's mouth.
c. edema of the nipple from the baby's vigorous suck.
d. primary engorgement.

 EP-057. What is the most likely explanation for the condition pictured?

a. milk residue after pumping
b. nipple candidiasis
c. herpes lesions
d. lanolin

 EP-058. This baby just came off the breast. What is this mother most likely feeling?

a. pinching nipple pain
b. aching breast pain
c. relaxation and sleepiness
d. relief that the baby fed well

 EP-059. What is the most likely cause of the dark marks on this mother's areola?

a. herpes lesions
b. tooth marks from the toddler's biting
c. bruise from her baby's off-center latch
d. improper use of a breast pump

 EP-060. This baby prefers this position and has significant difficulty nursing in other positions. What is the most likely cause of this preference?

a. interesting objects on one side of his crib
b. mother feeds only on one breast
c. torticollis
d. ankyloglossia

 EP-061. Which of the following is most associated with this sleep position?

a. increased time in deep sleep
b. less risk of sudden infant death syndrome
c. less chance of aspiration of milk
d. decreased number of awakenings at night

EP-062. What is the most likely reason this mother is experiencing pain in her left axilla?

a. severe postpartum engorgement
b. lactogenesis II in axillary mammary tissue
c. allergic reaction to a new deodorant
d. overuse strain of the pectoral muscles

EP-063. What correlates most closely with the age of the child pictured?

a. will no longer take a pacifier
b. highest risk of SIDS
c. ability to roll over
d. highest risk of otitis media

EPN-064. This breastfeeding mother is being treated for a fungal (*Candida*) infection on her nipples. You should recommend all of the following **EXCEPT**:

a. boil all baby's teething objects including his toothbrush.
b. wash hands before and after contact with baby's mouth or diaper area.
c. wash bras in hot water with a small amount of bleach.
d. use a nipple shield during feeds to prevent transfer to baby.

EPN-065. This child has recently begun solid foods. Based on the condition pictured, she is likely to also have any of the other reactions listed below **EXCEPT**:

a. wheezing.
b. colic.
c. sleepiness.
d. irritability.

EPN-066. This mother's nipple pain has persisted for over 2 weeks. You would check her baby for all of the following conditions **EXCEPT**:

a. micrognathia.
b. short lingual frenulum.
c. tongue thrust movements.
d. cleft of the soft palate.

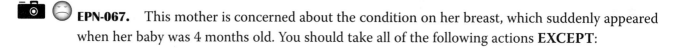

EPN-067.   This mother is concerned about the condition on her breast, which suddenly appeared when her baby was 4 months old. You should take all of the following actions **EXCEPT**:

a. visually examining the baby's mouth and throat.
b. taking a thorough history of the mother and baby.
c. giving her a topical steroid cream to reduce inflammation.
d. recommending that she get a medical evaluation.

EPN-068.   The cause of this toddler's dental condition is **LEAST LIKELY** due to:

a. a high intake of sweetened foods.
b. a lack of tooth brushing.
c. congenital enamel defects.
d. unrestricted breastfeeding at night.

EP-069.   What is the most likely situation leading to this breast condition?

a. The child is over a year and using the mother's breast as a pacifier.
b. The mother did not wash her breasts after each nursing.
c. The child is biting during breastfeeding.
d. The child has an oral infection that was transmitted to the nipple skin.

EP-070.   What is the mother of this baby most likely to be feeling?

a. stinging, burning nipple pain
b. deep, aching pain in her breast
c. comfortable breasts and nipples
d. sharp pain after and between feedings

MATERNAL AND INFANT PATHOLOGY ANSWERS

The parenthetical material at the end of each answer includes the discipline and time period, indicates whether the question pertains to knowledge or application, and specifies the degree of difficulty.

E-001. The answer is A. Extreme nipple pain in the absence of visual symptoms may indicate a deeper problem such as prior history of abuse. (Pathology; 1–2 days; Knowledge; Difficulty: 5)

E-002. The answer is C. The only limiting factor to breastfeeding is the mother's injuries. Compatible pain medications are available. She and her baby still need each other while she recovers. (Pathology; 15–28 days; Application; Difficulty: 4)

E-003. The answer is B. Persistent cranial molding can interfere with nervous system functioning in the early weeks, which can interfere with the suck-swallow pattern. (Pathology; 15–28 days; Application; Difficulty: 3)

E-004. The answer is D. Severe blood loss can cause pituitary shock (Sheehan's syndrome), which blocks prolactin responses needed for lactogenesis III. (Pathology; 3–14 days; Knowledge; Difficulty: 5)

E-005. The answer is D. She was diagnosed with a bacterial infection of the nipple skin, most likely streptococcus transferred from the baby's mouth. The rash is exactly where the baby's mouth had come in contact with the areolar tissue. A and B are possibly correct, but less likely. (Pathology; 4–6 months; Application; Difficulty: 5)

E-006. The answer is B. By 2 weeks, most term infants should be able to handle mother's milk-ejection reflex. If the baby cannot coordinate sucking and swallowing with breathing, he may choke and gasp for breath as the milk releases. Occasionally, a normal baby may still have difficulty handling a mother's strong milk-ejection reflex. (Pathology; 15–28 days; Application; Difficulty: 3)

E-007. The answer is A. Studying experiences of an event is a qualitative research method. The other responses are quantitative designs, B is descriptive, C is correlational, and D is experimental research. (I. Research; General Principles; Knowledge; Difficulty: 4)

E-008. The answer is C. Intraductal papilloma is the most likely cause of painless, bright red bleeding in the early postpartum period. (Pathology; 1–2 days; Knowledge; Difficulty: 4)

E-009. The answer is D. Chicken pox is no longer contagious when all the lesions are completely crusted over. The mother can breastfeed normally. (Pathology; Labor/Birth; Application; Difficulty: 5)

E-010. The answer is D. Lack of eye contact by the mother and little talking or caressing of her infant may be signs of postpartum depression. The lactation consultant should report these signs to the mother's primary care provider immediately. (Pathology; 1–2 days; Knowledge; Difficulty: 4)

E-011. The answer is B. Taking a thorough history is top priority when solving a breastfeeding problem. The baby may be having an allergic reaction to the large amount of milk consumed by the mother. (Pathology; 1–3 months; Application; Difficulty: 3)

E-012. The answer is B. Manufacturers omitted chloride in a mistaken effort to impact adult cardiac disease by changing infant intake of salt. Chloride is an essential nutrient for human brain development. (Pathology; General Principles; Knowledge; Difficulty: 5)

EN-013. The answer is C. Undetected breast cancer is very unlikely this early postbirth. Any birth injury may be painful for the baby. Placing the sore side higher than the normal side may reduce pain, resulting in the baby's strong preference for the more comfortable position. Breasts differ in configuration and flow, and one side may be much easier for the baby to manage in the early weeks. (Pathology; 15–28 days; Application; Difficulty: 2)

EN-014. The answer is C. It is currently unknown whether lactation boosts the mother's own immune system. Antibodies and white cells that she produces quickly get into her milk and protect the baby, and a mother who is sick certainly does not benefit from the additional work of preparing artificial feeds and coping with probable sudden milk stasis. (Pathology; 4–6 months; Application; Difficulty: 2)

EN-015. The answer is A. Lysozyme is probably the least important, even though it may play a role. The other responses are major factors in protecting against neonatal septicemia. (Pathology; Prematurity; Knowledge; Difficulty: 4)

EP-016. The answer is A. The peaked shape with barely visible damage in the center of the nipple tip is most often associated with either a poor (shallow) latch, or a baby with a sucking problem. In this case, the baby was tongue-tied. Rarely would a deeply-latched baby cause this severe nipple distortion. When a baby is poorly latched or has a suck deficit, effective milk transfer and self-detachment are less likely. (Pathology; 4–6 months; Application; Difficulty: 4)

EP-017. The answer is B. ABO incompatibility is a cause of early-onset jaundice. Breast-milk jaundice becomes apparent or continues to rise after the third day, and bilirubin levels may peak at any time from the 7th to the 10th day, or even as late as the 15th day. Effective, exclusive breast-feeding does not result in high enough levels of bilirubin to warrant treatment with light therapy. Hypoglycemia is not treated in this manner. (Pathology; 3–14 days; Application; Difficulty: 4)

EP-018. The answer is B. This baby's hypotonia (low muscle tone) is caused by Prader Willi syndrome. The nipple shield (barely visible), jaw support, and upright straddle position are all techniques that can assist a baby with low tone to maximize milk obtained directly at breast. (Pathology; 1–3 months; Application; Difficulty: 2)

EP-019. The answer is C. This is mechanical (friction) damage from a tongue-tied baby. A and B do not cause open wounds. D is an old myth, not consistent with current knowledge and research evidence. (Pathology; 1–2 days; Application; Difficulty: 2)

EP-020. The answer is C. The baby's mouth is infected with thrush (*Candida*), which is a fungus. The mother and the baby need to be treated simultaneously with an antifungal agent. (Pathology; 3–14 days; Application; Difficulty: 5)

EP-021. The answer is B. This is a plugged nipple pore, also known as a "bleb" or "white spot." These are thought to be due to plugs of milk that solidify at the opening of a milk duct on the nipple skin. (Pathology; 1–3 months; Application; Difficulty: 3)

EP-022. The answer is B. This nipple wound was caused by a baby with tongue-tie (short and/or tight lingual frenulum). Normal breastfeeding does not cause this kind of wound; shallow latch is unlikely to cause this much damage in just 8 days, and an 8-day-old is unlikely to be biting during feeds. (Pathology; 3–14 days; Knowledge; Difficulty: 3)

EP-023. The answer is D. Supine sleeping is the safest position for sleeping, especially if the baby is sleeping alone. This firm, flat mattress on the floor is not a risk, nor is the proximity of the unused fireplace. The child is sleeping in proximity to her mother, who is not shown working in the same room. Pacifier use to prevent SIDS is a controversial recommendation that is not fully supported by research, and often interferes with breastfeeding. (Pathology; 1–3 months; Application; Difficulty: 4)

EPN-024.   The answer is C. There is no research supporting the use of hot compresses to relieve milk stasis or edema. This woman's chief complaint is the accessory breast tissue in her armpit; her breasts are neither overfull nor swollen, and the baby is nursing well. (Pathology; 3–14 days; Application; Difficulty: 2)

EPN-025.   The answer is D. This was diagnosed as a bacterial infection of the nipple skin. Immediate weaning is not appropriate, because the baby has already been exposed and may even have caused the infection. A nipple shield may provide some comfort, providing it is thoroughly cleaned between uses. Choices A and C are also appropriate. (Pathology; 15–28 days; Application; Difficulty: 3)

EPN-026.   The answer is B. This mother's breast is engorged—a combination of edema and milk stasis. Hot compresses can make edema worse and have no documented advantage in correcting milk stasis. (Pathology; 3–14 days; Application; Difficulty: 5)

EPN-027.   The answer is C. There is no evidence of increased dental caries from nighttime breast-feeding in the second year of life. The child who nurses past 12 months of age receives substantial immune protection, nutrition, and psychological benefits from breastfeeding. (Pathology; >12 months; Application; Difficulty: 3)

EPN-028.   The answer is A. Paget's disease is a type of nipple cancer and the least likely cause of the small wound shown. The lesion is an unhealed sore caused by the baby's poor suck due to a short frenulum that persisted for 2 months. (Pathology; 1–3 months; Knowledge; Difficulty: 5)

EPN-029.   The answer is B. Fungal infections on the lactating breast are typically not localized to one small area. The other conditions are more likely, and the lactation consultant should be collaborating with her medical care provider for a thorough diagnosis. (Pathology; 4–6 months; Knowledge; Difficulty: 3)

EPN-030.   The answer is A. Weaning from the affected breast following abscess formation or treatment is rarely necessary. All the other actions are appropriate. (Pathology; 1–3 months; Application; Difficulty: 2)

E-031.   The answer is D. Scheduled feeds are inappropriate and can result in underfeeding and failure to thrive. Feeding on cue is appropriate regardless of the baby's age. (Pathology; 1–3 months; Application; Difficulty: 3)

E-032. The answer is D. Lumps that do not change size related to milk flow are considered ominous. The mother should be evaluated by a physician immediately. The other characteristics are fairly common during lactation. (Pathology; 15–28 days; Application; Difficulty: 2)

E-033. The answer is B. Research shows that babies separated from their mothers are in a state of higher stress, as measured by salivary cortisol levels and other physiological markers. (Pathology; Labor/Birth; Knowledge; Difficulty: 4)

E-034. The answer is C. Backache in active labor is most likely due to the baby/fetus being in a posterior presentation. This is relevant to breastfeeding because difficult labors, including posterior presentation, may affect the baby's ability to breastfeed. Back pain in labor may also slow labor progress and result in even more drugs for pain relief and other interventions, further affecting the baby's ability to breastfeed. (Pathology; Labor/birth; Knowledge; Difficulty: 4)

E-035. The answer is C. Hemorrhage postbirth may trigger Sheehan's syndrome, or necrosis of all or part of the pituitary gland. Sheehan's syndrome may reduce prolactin levels beyond that needed for lactogenesis, thus causing primary lactation failure. (Pathology; Labor/birth; Knowledge; Difficulty: 4)

EN-036. The answer is B. Babies are not lazy. Labeling babies in this manner prevents looking for, finding, and resolving the cause of the problem. All of the other choices are possible causes of poor milk transfer and low weight gain in a newborn. (Pathology; 15–28 days; Application; Difficulty: 5)

EN-037. The answer is B. Allergic disease is responsible for a third of pediatric office visits in the United States. The other statements are true. (Pathology; General Principles; Knowledge; Difficulty: 2)

EN-038. The answer is C. Mothers with diabetes may need less insulin during lactation. Careful monitoring is essential. (Pathology; Prenatal; Application; Difficulty: 2)

EN-039. The answer is A. Effective, exclusive breastfeeding does not result in growth faltering. (Pathology; 4–6 months; Application; Difficulty: 2)

EN-040. The answer is D. Whether or not she is breastfeeding, a new mother with MS is likely to experience an increase in acute episodes during the postpartum period. Often, breastfeeding is wrongly blamed for this phenomenon. (Pathology; 1–2 days; Knowledge; Difficulty: 3)

EN-041. The answer is B. Mother–baby cross-infection is likely when the baby has an oral infection. Assume that the mother's nipples are also infected with the same organism, as well as other infant body parts and any/all sucking objects. (Pathology; 15–28 days; Application; Difficulty: 3)

EN-042. The answer is D. Normal babies without injury can nearly always feed in various positions on either breast. A baby who has sustained a birth injury may only have one position where breastfeeding is comfortable and successful. Over time as the injuries heal, he should be able to feed in a variety of positions. (Pathology; Labor/birth; Knowledge; Difficulty: 5)

EN-043. The answer is D. The length and/or frequency of breastfeeds are far less important causes of nipple damage than maternal skin conditions or the baby's ability to suck correctly. Most early cracked nipples are cause by poor breastfeeding technique and/or sucking problems. (Pathology; 1–2 days; Knowledge; Difficulty: 5)

EN-044. The answer is C. The mother's activity is the least likely to cause a problem with initiation of breastfeeding in the second-born twin. (Pathology; Labor/birth; Application; Difficulty: 3)

EN-045. The answer is D. Low milk supply is not a given in the second 6 months of lactation, and toddlers often wake several times at night during this age. Sloppy positioning, subsequent pregnancy, and allergic reactions are all possible causes of sudden breast pain at this stage. (Pathology; 7–12 months; Application; Difficulty: 5)

EP-046. The answer is C. This baby has Down syndrome (Trisomy 21). However, not all babies with Down syndrome have problems with breastfeeding. (Pathology; 15–28 days; Application; Difficulty: 3)

EP-047. The answer is B. The baby is being treated for hyperbilirubinemia. If this appears in the first 24–48 hours, the most likely cause is ABO incompatibility. (Pathology; 1–2 days; Knowledge; Difficulty: 2)

EP-048. The answer is B. The bulge is a galactocele. Plugged ducts are rarely visible on the breast surface. Inflammation is characteristic of both mastitis and abscess. (Pathology; 3–14 days; Knowledge; Difficulty: 5)

EP-049. The answer is C. The baby has a short, tight frenulum, which might interfere with effective breastfeeding. However, direct breastfeeding is the ultimate goal and the normative behavior to reinforce. Not all babies with tight frenula will have a problem breastfeeding. If direct breastfeeding is ineffective or painful, options A, B, or D could be considered. (Pathology; 1–2 days; Application; Difficulty: 4)

EP-050. The answer is D. The reddened areola and nipple area indicate the probable presence of nipple thrush (*Candida*) infection, which is commonly accompanied by burning, stinging, or itching. Fever and chills and deep, aching breast pain are more likely to be caused by a bacterial breast infection. A few mothers will feel no discomfort even with this amount of nipple thrush. (Pathology; 15–28 days; Application; Difficulty: 3)

EP-051. The answer is B. The damage shown is infectious in origin, not mechanical. The shape of the nipple is normal, suggesting pressure is not the cause of the damage. (Pathology; > 12 months; Application; Difficulty: 4)

EP-052. The answer is B. This surgery (incision and drainage) was performed to treat a breast abscess. The location of the incision may have long-term consequences on lactation in this breast. (Pathology; 1–3 months; Application; Difficulty: 3)

EP-053. The answer is A. Breast abscesses are usually the result of delayed or inadequate treatment for mastitis. Rarely, physical trauma may precipitate abscess formation. The baby's oral bacteria are not implicated in abscess formation in the lactating breast. (Pathology; 1–3 months; Application; Difficulty: 4)

EP-054. The answer is C. Nipple thrush often has few visible signs—identification is based on clinical symptoms of itching, stinging, and/or burning. The slightly pink color of her nipples, combined with the sensations reported, is highly suggestive of nipple thrush (*Candida*). (Pathology; 15–28 days; Application; Difficulty: 5)

EP-055. The answer is D. This is a bacterial infection of the nipple skin. The baby had just begun treatment for an oral staph infection that was acquired at daycare. (Pathology; 15–28 days; Application; Difficulty: 4)

EP-056. The answer is B. This mother's large, fibrous nipple was being compressed by her baby's small mouth and shallow palate. (Pathology; 3–14 days; Application; Difficulty: 2)

EP-057. The answer is A. This is milk residue. The mother had just finished pumping her milk. (Pathology; 3–14 days; Application; Difficulty: 4)

EP-058. The answer is A. The flattened nipple is most likely causing a pinching nipple pain. This type of postfeed distortion is an indication that the baby did not feed well. (Pathology; 3–14 days; Application; Difficulty: 4)

EP-059. The answer is C. The dark marks are bruises from her baby's off-center latch. The photo was taken on day 3. (Pathology; 3–14 days; Application; Difficulty: 4)

EP-060. The answer is C. Torticollis is the most likely reason that this baby prefers to turn his head right. Torticollis is an abnormal condition of the neck muscles, especially the sternocleido mastoid. (Pathology; 15–28 days; Knowledge; Difficulty: 3)

EP-061. The answer is B. Supine sleeping is strongly associated with a lower risk of sudden infant death syndrome (SIDS). This position also makes breastfeeding at night easier. (Pathology; 3–14 days; Knowledge; Difficulty: 3)

EP-062. The answer is B. This mother has axillary mammary tissue that has no outlet, and the photo was taken 4 days postbirth. Lactogenesis II is causing milk secretion in the axillary mammary tissue. (Pathology; 3–14 days; Knowledge; Difficulty: 3)

EP-063. The answer is B. The highest risk for SIDS is 2 to 4 months of age; the baby pictured is 3 months old. (Pathology; 7–12 months; Application; Difficulty: 5)

EPN-064. The answer is D. Using a nipple shield is unlikely to reduce cross-infection, and this age child will likely vigorously object to introduction of this device. (Pathology; 7–12 months; Application; Difficulty: 2)

EPN-065.   The answer is C. Hypersensitivity reactions to ingested substances rarely include sleepiness. Skin rashes, wheezing, colic, and irritability are all common hypersensitivity reactions. (Pathology; 4–6 months; Difficulty: 3)

EPN-066.   The answer is D. A cleft palate is unlikely to cause the horizontal crack in this mother's nipples. This mother's baby was thrusting his tongue forward to control the mother's oversupply of milk and strong milk-ejection reflex. The picture was taken at 2 weeks postbirth. (Pathology; 15–28 days; Application; Difficulty: 3)

EPN-067.   The answer is C. Providing medications is not within the current scope of practice of the lactation consultant. The other actions are appropriate. (Pathology; 4–6 months; Application; Difficulty: 4)

EPN-068.   The answer is D. There is no research or epidemiological evidence that unrestricted breastfeeding at night is a cause of baby-bottle tooth decay or nursing caries. The other choices are associated with rampant caries in young children. (Pathology; > 12 months; Application; Difficulty: 3)

EP-069.   The answer is D. The child was diagnosed with strep throat, which caused a strep infection of the nipple and the damage shown in this picture. Ordinary breastfeeding does not cause nipple damage. Washing the breasts after every feed is impractical and unnecessary. Biting rarely causes a lesion on the areola and crack at the nipple base. (Pathology; 4–6 months; Application; Difficulty: 4)

EP-070.   The answer is A. This baby's diaper-area rash was caused by *Candida* (thrush) infection, which was also present in his mouth and on the mother's nipples. The mother was experiencing itching, stinging, burning nipple pain consistent with thrush infection of the nipples. (Pathology; 7.15–28 days; Application; Difficulty: 4)

Scoring:

Total number of questions in this section   _____

Number of questions answered correctly   _____

Percent correct (divide number correct by total number)   _____

F. MATERNAL AND INFANT PHARMACOLOGY AND TOXICOLOGY

In the 2000 exam blueprint, 10 to 16 questions are dedicated to maternal and infant pharmacology and toxicology.

SUBTOPICS INCLUDED IN THIS CATEGORY

1. Principles of pharmacokinetics

2. Maternal use of medications

   a. Prescription drugs
   b. Herbs and homeopathic substances
   c. Over-the-counter drugs; alcohol and tobacco; dietary drugs
   d. Social or recreational drugs, including drugs of abuse
   e. Pesticide residues; environmental contaminants
   f. Complementary therapies

3. Compounds that affect milk supply

   a. Effect on the infant, on milk composition, and on lactation
   b. Galactagogues and suppressants
   c. Medications used in labor and birth
   d. Medications that alter fertility

4. Lactation consultant's role and resources

CORE READING

Textbooks

Hale T. *Medications and Mothers' Milk 2006.* Amarillo, TX: Hale Publishing (Pharmasoft Publishing); 2006.

Hale T, Berens P. *Clinical Therapy in Breastfeeding Patients.* 2nd ed. Amarillo, TX: Hale Publishing (Pharmasoft Publishing); 2002.

Hale T, Ilett K. *Drug Therapy and Breastfeeding.* Amarillo, TX: Hale Publishing (Pharmasoft Publishing); 2002.

Humphrey S. *The Nursing Mother's Herbal.* Minneapolis, MN: Fairview Press; 2003.

Kroeger M, Smith L. *Impact of Birthing Practices on Breastfeeding.* Sudbury, MA: Jones & Bartlett Publishers; 2004.

Lawrence RA, Lawrence RM. *Breastfeeding: A Guide for the Medical Profession.* 6th ed. St. Louis: Elsevier Mosby; 2005.

Riordan J. *Breastfeeding and Human Lactation*. 3rd ed. Sudbury, MA: Jones & Bartlett Publishers; 2004.
US National Library of Medicine Drugs and Lactation Database <http://toxnet.nlm.nih.gov/cgi-bin/sis/htmlgen?LACT> (accessed 10/6/2006)

Key Research Articles

Aljazaf K, Hale TW, Ilett KF, et al. Pseudoephedrine: effects on milk production in women and estimation of infant exposure via breastmilk. *Br J Clin Pharmacol.* 2003;56(1):18–24.
Hale TW. Anesthetic medications in breastfeeding mothers. *J Hum Lact.* 1999;15(3):185–194.
Hale TW. Maternal medications during breastfeeding. *Clin Obstet Gynecol.* 2004;47(3):696–711.
Hale TW. Medications in breastfeeding mothers of preterm infants. *Pediatr Ann.* 2003;32(5):337–347.
Hale TW, McDonald R, Boger J. Transfer of celecoxib into human milk. *J Hum Lact.* 2004;20(4):397–403.
Ilett KF, Hale TW, Page-Sharp M, Kristensen JH, Kohan R, Hackett LP. Use of nicotine patches in breast-feeding mothers: Transfer of nicotine and cotinine into human milk. *Clin Pharmacol Ther.* 2003;74(6):516–524.

MATERNAL AND INFANT PHARMACOLOGY AND TOXICOLOGY QUESTIONS

Notice on question numbering: F-000 means a basic question, with one correct answer and three wrong answers. FP-000, along with the camera icon, means there is a picture that needs to be viewed to answer the question. The pictures are located on the CD-ROM incuded with this book and are numbered to correspond with the questions. FN-000, along with the frowning face icon, means the question has a NEGATIVE stem; therefore, read the entire question very carefully to find the one WRONG answer among the choices. FPN-000, with both icons in the margin, means there is a picture associated with the question AND the question has a negative stem. See Appendix A for a fuller explanation of negative stem questions.

F-001. Which drug property is most likely to permit high passage of the drug into milk?

a. high lipid solubility
b. high pH
c. large molecular weight
d. high protein binding

F-002. Which category of drug administered to the mother is usually contraindicated during breastfeeding?

a. antimicrobial
b. antihypertensive
c. antineoplastic
d. antidepressant

F-003. When would a drug given to the mother most readily pass into the milk?

a. when the mother is collecting milk for a premature baby
b. in the first 4 days postbirth
c. when the mother has a breast infection
d. when the drug is given transdermally

F-004. What is the average percentage of a drug administered to a lactating woman that actually reaches the breastfeeding baby?

a. 0.01%
b. 0.1%
c. 1.0%
d. 10%

F-005. Which property of maternal medications increases the amount of the drug that gets to the breastfeeding baby via breast milk?

a. short half-life
b. no active metabolites
c. high oral absorption
d. high gut destruction

F-006. A breastfeeding mother has been diagnosed with postpartum depression. Her physician contacts you to discuss whether or not she should continue to breastfeed during drug treatment. Your best response is:

a. there are several antidepressant medications that are considered compatible with breastfeeding.
b. all medications used to treat mental illness are contraindicated during breastfeeding.
c. her baby is in great danger and should be kept away from her at all costs.
d. the hormones of breastfeeding will exacerbate her illness.

F-007. A mother was given high doses of pain-relieving drugs during labor. When the baby's cord blood is tested for the presence of drugs, none is found. The most likely explanation is:

a. Pain-relieving drugs are lipid-soluble and concentrate in the infant's brain.
b. Pain-relieving drugs do not cross the placenta.
c. The mother's body metabolizes most drugs before birth.
d. Pain-relieving drugs have a very short half-life.

F-008. A mother is concerned because her 3-week-old, exclusively breastfed baby suddenly became very fussy in the evenings. Her breastfeeding pattern did not change, and the baby is otherwise healthy. Which recently added item in her diet is most likely to be related to her baby's reaction?

a. lemonade
b. herbal tea
c. green vegetables
d. vitamin supplements

F-009. Which mother would have the highest risk of drug passage into milk?

a. Sue, whose baby was born at 26 weeks' gestation and is now 3 weeks old
b. Mary, who breastfeeds 5 times a day and supplements with infant formula
c. Irene, who had a cesarean birth 2 days ago
d. Claudia, whose 5-month-old twins are exclusively breastfed

F-010. A mother was given 40 mg of a drug with a half-life of 4 hours. How much of the drug is left in her system after 4 half-lives have elapsed?

a. 20 mg
b. 10 mg
c. 5 mg
d. 2.5 mg

F-011. Which drug property results in more transfer of the drug into the mother's milk?

a. milk-plasma ratio < 1.0
b. molecular weight > 500
c. high protein binding
d. lipid solubility

FN-012. A newborn baby, 6 hours old, is awake and alert but having trouble breastfeeding. Which of the following is the **LEAST LIKELY** cause of his difficulty?

a. His mother received antibiotic treatment for Group B streptococcus during labor.
b. His mother was given epidural anesthesia 4 hours before delivery.
c. His mother received narcotic analgesia immediately prior to delivery.
d. His mother's labor was stimulated by Pitocin (oxytocin) given intravenously.

FN-013. A pregnant woman has heard that letting epidural anesthesia wear off prior to delivery will avoid anesthesia-related breastfeeding problems. You should tell her all of the following **EXCEPT**:

a. drugs can take much longer to clear the baby's system, so there is still possible breastfeeding risk with this approach.

b. the combination of drugs used in epidural anesthesia makes it difficult to determine which medications cause breastfeeding problems.

c. epidural anesthesia has minimal or no effect on the baby regardless of how long before delivery it is administered.

d. epidural anesthesia increases the likelihood of other birth interventions that can affect breast-feeding.

FN-014. A student in your prenatal class asks about the impact of labor pain-relieving medications on the baby. Your responses should include all of the following **EXCEPT**:

a. narcotic analgesics can depress the baby's breathing and sucking.

b. epidural anesthesia has no effect on the baby.

c. the effect of labor drugs on the baby is dose-related.

d. tranquilizers potentiate the action of other drugs.

F-015. A woman who received intravenous magnesium sulfate during labor to control her blood pressure is having trouble initiating breastfeeding. The most likely explanation for this is:

a. this medication can cause maternal lethargy, confusion, and muscle relaxation.

b. the medication affected the baby's ability to suck.

c. her milk tastes unpleasant because of the medication.

d. the drug reduced the amount of colostrum available, and the baby is frustrated.

F-016. A woman with a 5-month-old, exclusively breastfed baby is prescribed amoxicillin for her breast infection. The most likely possible consequence for the infant is:

a. interference with bilirubin binding.

b. vomiting and dehydration.

c. none.

d. diarrhea or loose stools.

FN-017. Epidural narcotic drugs given to the laboring woman may have all of the following effects **EXCEPT**:

a. improved neonatal neuromuscular coordination.
b. longer second stage of labor.
c. increased risk of cesarean birth.
d. increased risk for forceps or vacuum-assisted birth.

FN-018. A breastfeeding mother is prescribed fluconazole to treat a vaginal infection. She asks the lactation consultant whether it is safe to take this drug while breastfeeding. All of the following are appropriate responses by the lactation consultant **EXCEPT**:

a. yes, it's safe to take fluconazole while breastfeeding.
b. what has the baby's pediatrician said?
c. I would be glad to look it up in reference books.
d. what are your baby's age and health status?

FN-019. A mother complains of sudden-onset sore nipple when her baby is 10 months old. To identify the cause, you would ask all of the following questions **EXCEPT**:

a. did you recently begin taking oral contraceptive pills?
b. is your baby taking any solid foods or artificial baby milk?
c. have you or your baby taken an antibiotic recently?
d. has anyone in the family been sick with an infection?

FN-020. Local perineal injection of an anesthetic drug prior to performing an episiotomy may have all the following consequences **EXCEPT**:

a. the mother's discomfort sitting up to feed.
b. infant bradycardia due to the medication used.
c. increased risk of perineal infection.
d. tissue damage from the procedure.

MATERNAL AND INFANT PHARMACOLOGY AND TOXICOLOGY ANSWERS

The parenthetical material at the end of each answer includes the discipline and time period, indicates whether the question pertains to knowledge or application, and specifies the degree of difficulty.

F-001. The answer is A. High lipid solubility would increase drug transfer into milk. The other factors would inhibit passage into milk. (Pharmacology; General Principles; Application; Difficulty: 2)

F-002. The answer is C. Antineoplastics, often called chemotherapy agents, are used in treating malignant tumors. Breastfeeding is usually contraindicated because of the potential risk to the infant. (Pharmacology; General Principles; Knowledge; Difficulty: 4)

F-003. The answer is B. Drugs more readily pass into milk in the first few days postbirth because the junctures between mammary secretory cells are open at this point, permitting passage of medications and other substances into the alveolar lumen. (Pharmacology; 1–2 days; Knowledge; Difficulty: 4)

F-004. The answer is C. About 1% of most medications given to a lactating woman actually gets to her breastfed baby. (Pharmacology; General Principles; Knowledge; Difficulty: 3)

F-005. The answer is C. Drugs that are highly absorbable via oral ingestion more easily transfer to breast milk. The other properties reduce the amount that may get to the baby. (Pharmacology; General Principles; Knowledge; Difficulty: 2)

F-006. The answer is A. There are several antidepressant medications considered compatible with breastfeeding. Continuing to breastfeed may help her recover from her illness. (Pharmacology; 1–2 days; Application; Difficulty: 4)

F-007. The answer is A. Pain-relieving drugs work on the central nervous system and therefore are highly lipid-soluble and sequester in the infant's brain. The other answers are incorrect. (Pharmacology; Labor/Birth; Application; Difficulty: 3)

F-008. The answer is B. Herbal teas may contain substances that exert a pharmacological effect on the baby. (Pharmacology; 15–28 days; Application; Difficulty: 4)

F-009.   The answer is C. The risk of drug passage into milk is highest in the early postpartum period when the junctures between the mammary secretory epithelial cells (lactocytes) are open. After the first week or so, the tight junctures between cells inhibit most drugs from passing into milk. (Pharmacology; 1–2 days; Application; Difficulty: 4)

F-010.   The answer is D. One half-life is the time it takes for half of the drug to be metabolized. In the first half-life, 20 mg would be metabolized, leaving 20 mg. After the second half-life, half of the remaining 20 mg would be metabolized, leaving 10 mg. After the third half-life, 5 mg would be left. After 4 half-lives, 2.5 mg of the drug would remain. (Pharmacology; General Principles; Application; Difficulty: 4)

F-011.   The answer is D. Lipid solubility facilitates transfer of drugs into a mother's milk. The other factors inhibit drug transfer to milk. (Pharmacology; General Principles; Knowledge; Difficulty: 4)

FN-012.   The answer is A. Antibiotic drugs have no documented effect on the fetus's or newborn's ability to breastfeed. The other choices are more likely to contribute to breastfeeding difficulties. (Pharmacology; General Principles; Application; Difficulty: 2)

FN-013.   The answer is C. All labor drugs cross the placenta, including those administered in the epidural space. The effect on the baby's ability to breastfeed appears to be dose-related. (Pharmacology; Labor/Birth; Application; Difficulty: 5)

FN-014.   The answer is B. Epidural analgesia and narcotics cross the placenta and have documented effects on the baby's motor and neurobehavioral scores. (Pharmacology; Labor/Birth; Application; Difficulty: 2)

F-015.   The answer is A. Magnesium sulfate can cause maternal drowsiness and lethargy. The American Academy of Pediatrics considers this medication compatible with breastfeeding. (Pharmacology; 1–2 days; Knowledge; Difficulty: 5)

F-016.   The answer is D. Even though amoxicillin is considered compatible with breastfeeding, the infant may develop diarrhea or loose stools. (Pharmacology; 4–6 months; Knowledge; Difficulty: 4)

FN-017.   The answer is A. Epidural narcotic or anesthetic drugs cross the placenta and appear in cord blood. Epidurals are documented to lengthen the second stage of labor and increase the likelihood of operative birth. (Pharmacology; Labor/Birth; Application; Difficulty: 2)

FN-018.   The answer is A. Determining the safety of maternal medications is reserved for appropriately licensed health care providers. The other three responses are appropriate for the lactation consultant. (Pharmacology; General Principles; Application; Difficulty: 5)

FN-019.   The answer is A. Taking oral contraceptives is not likely to have caused sudden-onset sore nipples. Hoever, if she stopped taking oral contraceptives, she could be pregnant, which could cause sudden-onset nipple pain. The other questions are appropriate. (Pharmacology; 7–12 months; Application; Difficulty: 2)

FN-020.   The answer is B. Perineally injected medications transfer to the infant poorly. Pudendal block does affect the newborn's motor skills immediately postbirth. (Pharmacology; Labor/Birth; Application; Difficulty: 5)

Scoring:

Total number of questions in this section   _____

Number of questions answered correctly   _____

Percent correct (divide number correct by total number)   _____

G. PSYCHOLOGY, SOCIOLOGY, AND ANTHROPOLOGY

In the 2000 exam blueprint, 10 to 16 questions are dedicated to psychology, sociology, and anthropology.

SUBTOPICS INCLUDED IN THIS CATEGORY

1. Counseling and adult education skills

2. Grief, postnatal depression, and psychosis

3. Effect of socioeconomic, lifestyle, and employment issues on breastfeeding

4. Maternal role adaptation and maternal–infant relationship

   a. Parenting skills
   b. Sleep patterns
   c. Cultural beliefs and practices
   d. Family and support systems
   e. Multiple infants

5. Mothers with special needs, including adolescents and migrants

6. Domestic violence and abuse

CORE READING

Textbooks

Brodribb W, ed. *Breastfeeding Management.* Melbourne: Australian Breastfeeding Association; 2004.

Gromada KK. *Mothering Multiples.* Schaumburg, IL: La Leche League International; 2001.

Kendall-Tackett KA. *The Hidden Feelings of Motherhood: Coping with Mothering Stress, Depression and Burnout.* Oakland, CA: New Harbinger; 2001.

Kendall-Tackett KA. *Breastfeeding and the Sexual Abuse Survivor.* Schaumburg, IL: La Leche League International; 2004. *Lactation Consultant* Series 2, Unit 9.

Kendall-Tackett KA. *Depression in New Mothers: Causes, Consequences, and Treatment Options.* Binghamton, NY: Haworth; 2005.

Kendall-Tackett KA. *Handbook of Women, Stress and Trauma.* NY: Taylor & Francis; 2005. Figley C, ed. *Stress and Trauma.*

Lauwers J, Swisher A. *Counseling the Nursing Mother.* 4th ed. Sudbury, MA: Jones & Bartlett; 2003.

Lawrence RA, Lawrence RM. *Breastfeeding: A Guide for the Medical Profession*. 6th ed. St. Louis: Elsevier Mosby; 2005.

Mohrbacher N, Kendall-Tackett KA. *Breastfeeding Made Simple: Seven Natural Laws for Nursing Mothers*. Oakland, CA: New Harbinger; 2005.

Montagu A. *Touching: The Human Significance of the Skin*. Third Edition. New York: Harper and Row; 1986.

Riordan J. *Breastfeeding and Human Lactation*. 3rd ed. Sudbury, MA: Jones & Bartlett Publishers; 2004.

Small MF. In: *Our Babies, Ourselves: How Biology and Culture Shape the Way We Parent*. New York: Random House; 1998:109–137.

Smith LJ. *Coach's Notebook: Games and Strategies for Lactation Education*. Sudbury, MA: Jones & Bartlett Publishers; 2002.

Stuart-Macadam P, Dettwyler KA. *Breastfeeding: Biocultural Perspectives*. New York: Aldine De Gruyter; 1995.

The Royal College of Midwives, UK. *Successful Breastfeeding*. London: Churchill Livingstone; 2003.

Trevathan W, Smith EO, McKenna J, eds. In: *Evolutionary Medicine*. Oxford University Press: Oxford; 1999:53–74.

INTERNET RESOURCES

The Cochrane Collection. Available at www.cochrane.org. Accessed Oct. 1, 2006.

Core Library for Evidence-Based Practice. Available at www.shef.ac.uk/scharr/ir/core.html. Accessed Oct. 1, 2006.

National Library of Medicine and National Institutes of Health. PubMed website. Available at www.ncbi.nlm.nih.gov/PubMed. Accessed Oct. 1, 2006.

Key Research Articles

Kendall-Tackett KA, Sugarman M. The social consequences of long-term breastfeeding. *J Hum Lact.* 1995;11:179–183.

McKenna JJ, McDade T. Why babies should never sleep alone: A review of the co-sleeping controversy in relation to SIDS, bedsharing and breast feeding. *Paediatr Respir Rev.* 2005;6(2):134–152.

Pugh LC, Milligan RA, Frick KD, Spatz D, Bronner Y. Breastfeeding duration, costs, and benefits of a support program for low-income breastfeeding women. *Birth.* 2002;29(2):95–100.

PSYCHOLOGY, SOCIOLOGY, AND ANTHROPOLOGY QUESTIONS

Notice on question numbering: G-000 means a basic question, with one correct answer and three wrong answers. GP-000, along with the camera icon, means there is a picture that needs to be viewed to answer the question. The pictures are located on the CD-ROM included with this book and are numbered to correspond with the questions. GN-000, along with the frowning face icon, means the question has a NEGATIVE stem; therefore, read the entire question very carefully to find the one WRONG answer among the choices. GPN-000, with both icons in the margin, means there is a picture associated with the question AND the question has a negative stem. See Appendix A for a fuller explanation of negative stem questions.

G-001. A mother of 10-week-old twins calls. She says that all she does all day is feed babies and she can't take it anymore. She asks how she can introduce some artificial baby milk or infant cereal without weaning her babies from the breast. The first thing you should do is:

a. suggest she feed her infants simultaneously in order to save time.
b. tell her that offering other foods will decrease milk production.
c. ask if she has any help with household chores.
d. actively listen, and praise her for breastfeeding 2 babies.

G-002. A mother of newborn twins asks whether to feed her babies separately or together. Your best response is:

a. let's see which works best for you.
b. separately is better so you can focus on one at a time.
c. together is better to save you time.
d. feed them together to get their feeding patterns synchronized.

G-003. Which of the following approaches will be most helpful to assisting a breastfeeding mother who has a hearing impairment?

a. Speak to her more slowly.
b. Talk directly to her interpreter.
c. Make frequent eye contact with her.
d. Help her observe the baby's visual cues.

G-004. A cultural attitude that emphasizes the sexual nature of breasts is most likely associated with:

a. harassment for breastfeeding in public.
b. increased breast augmentation surgery.
c. mothers enjoying the attention created by larger breasts during lactation.
d. conflicts in custody disputes involving breastfeeding babies.

G-005. A mother with a 5-day-old infant repeatedly requests rules for how many times a day she should feed her baby. This behavior is typical of which stage of maternal role acquisition?

a. anticipatory
b. formal
c. informal
d. personal

G-006. A breastfeeding mother 6 weeks postbirth tells you, "None of your suggestions have worked, and I'm at the end of my rope. I'm a complete failure as a mom!" Which is the most likely condition affecting the mother?

a. bipolar disorder
b. anxiety disorder
c. postpartum depression
d. Asperger's syndrome

GN-007. Which is the **LEAST LIKELY** reason a 1-month-old child breastfeeds 4–8 times every day, including 1–2 times at night?

a. The mother is pressuring the child to gratify her own desires.
b. The child is recovering from gastroenteritis.
c. The child is allergic to many foods.
d. The mother is recovering from a hospital stay where the child could not visit.

GN-008. Separating mothers and babies shortly after birth has all of the following consequences **EXCEPT**:

a. increased rates of infection.
b. improved rest for mother.
c. increase in infant stress hormones.
d. difficulty initiating breastfeeding.

GN-009. A mother asks you to help her write a birth plan that will optimize her success with breastfeeding. Her plan should include all of the following **EXCEPT**:

a. the place of birth where she feels safest.
b. her choice of companions and family members.
c. access to furniture, hot tub, equipment that encourages motion, and posture changes.
d. a professional attendant who will direct her actions during labor.

GP-010. This child's imitative behavior suggests which of the following?

a. latent homosexuality
b. normal behavior modeling
c. deviant behavior
d. precocious sexuality

GP-011.   You are caring for this mother and baby. The baby is 4 hours old and has breastfed well shortly after birth. Upon entering this mother's room, the first thing you should do is:

a.   attempt to wake the baby for another feeding.
b.   check the baby's blood glucose by doing a heel stick.
c.   quietly observe the mother and baby but do not intervene.
d.   have the mother put the baby in a crib next to the bed.

GP-012.   This pregnant mother calls and complains of tender nipples and lower milk supply. Your best response is:

a.   it's best if you start weaning your daughter; she's nursed long enough already.
b.   see your doctor about the sudden-onset nipple pain—it might be thrush.
c.   drink fenugreek tea to increase your milk supply.
d.   what you're experiencing is common for women who are pregnant and still breastfeeding. How do you feel about continuing to breastfeed?

GP-013.   This baby was born about 10 minutes ago. What is the first thing you would say to this mother?

a.   You and your baby look so comfortable and happy!
b.   When she's ready, I can help you get started with breastfeeding.
c.   We'll give the baby a bath before you try breastfeeding.
d.   Aren't you going to let your partner hold the baby, too?

GP-014.   A woman requests information on allowing her children to nap together. Your best response is

a.   the children look very cute when they are asleep.
b.   the infant is at some danger from overlying, so make sure they sleep where you can observe them.
c.   children should learn to sleep in their own beds. The toddler certainly belongs in a crib.
d.   siblings sleeping together is common around the world. There is no risk to this practice.

GPN-015.   This exclusively breastfed baby suddenly begins nursing every 1–2 hours around the clock. The mother is worried that her milk supply has dried up. Your responses would include all of the following **EXCEPT**:

a.   milk supply often dips at this age, so you should begin supplementing.
b.   this sounds like a typical growth spurt, which is common at this age.
c.   babies often nurse in that pattern even when they nurse as well as your baby does.
d.   it's reassuring to see your baby gaining weight even when he seems to need to nurse that often.

GPN-016.   What is the **LEAST LIKELY** reason this grandmother would engage in the behavior shown?

a.   She is in competition with the baby's mother.
b.   She is trying to soothe the baby while the mother finishes a nap.
c.   The baby has a medical condition that requires upright posture.
d.   She is showing genuine affection for her grandchild.

G-017.   Which of the following behaviors suggests a woman is having difficulty moving through the normal developmental tasks of pregnancy?

a.   wearing maternity clothing in her second trimester
b.   choosing possible baby names
c.   discontinuing smoking and consumption of alcohol
d.   waiting until the third trimester to tell family members of her pregnancy

G-018.   Which practice is most likely to suggest that a healthcare provider is unsupportive of breastfeeding?

a.   breastfeeding texts on office shelves
b.   providing gift packs that include formula samples
c.   lactation consultant on staff
d.   list of mother support groups provided to all clients

G-019.   You have been collaborating with a physician regarding a breastfeeding mother who experienced a psychotic episode. The question is whether or not she should continue to breastfeed during drug treatment. The drug prescribed is considered compatible with breastfeeding. Your best response is:

a.   Breastfeeding may be healing for her under carefully controlled conditions.
b.   Breastfeeding is contraindicated for mothers with mental illnesses.
c.   Her baby is in great danger and should be kept away from her at all costs.
d.   The hormones of breastfeeding will exacerbate her illness.

G-020.   A mother tells you, "Breastfeeding has been so wonderful! Now I want to talk to every pregnant woman and tell her to breastfeed!" This statement is an example of:

a.   overenthusiasm.
b.   empowerment.
c.   delusion of grandeur.
d.   self-actualization.

G-021. A mother in Western industrialized cultures is most likely to continue breastfeeding past 1 year if which of the following people support this idea?

a. her male partner
b. her father
c. her doctor
d. her sister

G-022. A mother's psychological and emotional reactions to birth are most likely to be affected by:

a. her age.
b. whether her pregnancy was planned.
c. how she was treated and nurtured during labor.
d. the temperament and health of her baby.

G-023. A healthcare provider wants to encourage pregnant women to choose breastfeeding. Which question is most supportive of breastfeeding?

a. Are you considering breastfeeding?
b. What have you heard about breastfeeding?
c. Are you going to breastfeed or bottle-feed?
d. You aren't thinking about breastfeeding, are you?

G-024. A mother calls in a panic on day 3 postbirth. She has been crying all morning, her breasts hurt, and her baby is having a hard time feeding. Your first response to her should be:

a. How many times did your baby produce stool today?
b. Things sure are overwhelming for you today!
c. Have you been pumping your breasts?
d. You'll be fine—lots of mothers have problems on day 3.

G-025. Breastfeeding care in the modern industrialized healthcare system is impeded most by its:

a. heightened emphasis on the baby at the expense of the mother.
b. heightened emphasis on the mother at the expense of the baby.
c. failure to consider the breastfeeding dyad as a unique biological unit.
d. failure to consider the role of the father in solving breastfeeding problems.

G-026. Which feature of a mother's birth plan is most likely to optimize breastfeeding success?

a. The birth takes place in a major hospital.
b. The mother has a supportive companion of her choice.
c. The mother may move around freely during the first stage of labor.
d. Medication for pain relief is available early in labor.

GN-027. Employers with breastfeeding support programs for employees are likely to experience all of the following **EXCEPT**:

a. reduced employee absenteeism.
b. reduced employee productivity.
c. increased retention of employees.
d. increased employee morale.

GN-028. A mother is planning to go back to work after her baby is born. You can best support her breastfeeding by encouraging her to do all of the following strategies **EXCEPT**:

a. using the maximum amount of maternity leave to which she is entitled.
b. discussing part-time or flexible schedules with her supervisor.
c. planning to bottle-feed with formula while at work and continue breastfeeding during off-duty hours.
d. investigating child care at her work site or nearby.

GN-029. A mother asks for your help with weaning her toddler. Your responses should include all of the following **EXCEPT**:

a. For both you and him, it is best to wean gradually.
b. Put some bitter substance on your nipples to discourage him.
c. Let's look for other ways to meet his needs for closeness.
d. Be aware that your fertility will likely return in a few weeks.

GN-030. Breastfeeding mothers are **LEAST LIKELY** to experience which of the following psychosocial effects?

a. calming effect of lactational hormones
b. enhanced fulfillment of their maternal role
c. less work time lost because of children's illness
d. higher blood pressure because of the metabolic demands of breastfeeding

GN-031. Of the following options for mothers returning to work, which is the **LEAST** protective of the breastfeeding relationship?

a. on-site child care
b. extended paid maternity leave
c. flexible working hours
d. facilities for collecting and storing milk

📷 **GP-032.** The likelihood that this mother and baby will enjoy a successful start to breastfeeding is:

a. decreased, because new mothers prefer to do for themselves.
b. decreased, because the mother is likely to be confused by so many different people.
c. increased, because many people are supporting her.
d. increased, because family members can take over night feedings while she rests.

📷 **GP-033.** This mother is uncomfortable in this situation. Your best response to her is:

a. You'll get used to it—many mothers breastfeed in public.
b. You could always try the ladies' room.
c. It won't hurt to give the baby a bottle when you're out shopping.
d. It can be embarrassing the first few times you breastfeed away from home.

📷 **GP-034.** In this situation, which aspect of maternal–infant bonding is most likely to occur first?

a. The mother bonds with the unit.
b. The mother bonds with the firstborn.
c. The mother bonds with the last-born.
d. The mother has delayed bonding with all.

📷 **GP-035.** This baby's weight gain and development are normal. What is the first question you would ask the mother?

a. Do you use this position at all feeds?
b. Is your baby sleeping through the night yet?
c. How is breastfeeding going for you?
d. Have your menstrual periods returned?

📷 **GP-036.** On day 6 (as pictured), this mother says she is enjoying breastfeeding. Your first response should be:

a. your baby looks a bit jaundiced—has he seen the doctor?
b. how many times has your baby nursed in the past 24 hours?
c. how many wet diapers have you changed so far today?
d. wonderful! You were ambivalent, and now you look so confident. How are things going?

GPN-037. This mother has been warned that she is spoiling her baby by using the device in the picture. Which of the following statements about this practice is **FALSE**?

a. Continuous body contact helps the baby maintain body temperature.
b. Carrying the baby in a sling allows the baby easy access to breastfeeding.
c. Carrying the baby reduces infant crying.
d. Carrying the baby prolongs dependency of the baby on its mother.

GPN-038. This practice provides all of the following benefits **EXCEPT**:

a. more rest for the mother, because the baby nurses less frequently.
b. decreased apnea spells in the infant.
c. more rest for the mother, because she does not have to wake fully to nurse.
d. delayed return of fertility for the mother.

GPN-039. Which of the following statements about this practice is **FALSE**?

a. It helps the baby maintain body temperature.
b. It allows the baby easy access to breastfeeding.
c. It reduces infant crying.
d. It prolongs dependency on the mother.

PSYCHOLOGY, SOCIOLOGY, AND ANTHROPOLOGY ANSWERS

The parenthetical material at the end of each answer includes the discipline and time period, specifies whether the question pertains to knowledge or application, and indicates the degree of difficulty.

G-001. The answer is D. Active listening is the first action because the mother is obviously emotionally upset. Understanding, addressing, and exploring feelings are key to counseling the breastfeeding mother. (Psychology; 1–3 months; Application; Difficulty: 4)

G-002. The answer is A. Each mother–baby system will develop unique feeding patterns. The lactation consultant supports any and all patterns that meet the mothers' and babies' needs. (Psychology; 1–2 days; Application; Difficulty: 5)

G-003. The answer is D. Mothers with hearing (auditory) impairments are generally very familiar with visual and tactile communication. Breastfeeding may be easier for her than artificial feeding. (Psychology; 1–2 days; Application; Difficulty: 4)

G-004. The answer is A. Cultures that sexualize the breast are often the most resistant to women using their breasts to feed their infants anywhere and everywhere. (Psychology; General Principles; Knowledge; Difficulty: 5)

G-005. The answer is B. During the formal stage, mothers seek consistent, concrete rules to govern their actions. (Psychology; 3–14 days; Knowledge; Difficulty: 4)

G-006. The answer is C. Unresolved stress from the birth can trigger or exacerbate postpartum depression. She needs to see her primary care provider immediately for thorough evaluation, diagnosis, and treatment. (Psychology; 1–3 months; Knowledge; Difficulty: 4)

GN-007. The answer is A. Breastfeeding cannot be forced on a child at any age. The child who does not want to breastfeed will either bite or refuse to latch on. The other reasons are all common reasons for continued breastfeeding well into the second year of the child's life. (Psychology; > 12 months; Application; Difficulty: 2)

GN-008. The answer is B. Research shows mothers rest better when mothers and babies are kept together following birth. (Psychology; 1–2 days; Knowledge; Difficulty: 2)

GN-009. The answer is D. The laboring woman is disempowered when others direct her actions during labor. All of the other items increase her empowerment. The take-charge attitude of the attendant puts her into a passive role, which has been shown to interfere with breastfeeding. (Psychology; Prenatal; Application; Difficulty: 2)

GP-010. The answer is B. Young children imitating breastfeeding with a doll is a common and normal occurrence in most cultures worldwide. (Psychology; Preconception; Application; Difficulty: 2)

GP-011. The answer is C. This mother and baby are content, safe, and warm. Keeping the mother and baby in skin-to-skin contact is ideal for stabilizing the baby's systems. Preserving the mother–baby relationship is a primary responsibility of the lactation consultant. Continue observing the dyad; the baby will likely wake to feed soon. (Psychology; Labor/Birth; Application; Difficulty: 2)

GP-012. The answer is D. The lactation consultant should help the mother clarify her feelings about continuing to breastfeed and support her decision. The other responses are not appropriate. (Psychology; 15–28 days; Application; Difficulty: 3)

GP-013. The answer is A. Supporting the mother is always the first response, especially when she is as happy as the mother in the photo. Choice B would be appropriate after you've complimented the mother. The other two responses are not appropriate. (Psychology; Labor/Birth; Application; Difficulty: 3)

GP-014. The answer is B. Although siblings sleeping together is a practice found in many cultures, new research on sudden unexpected deaths in infancy (SUDI) suggests that infants under 6 months are at some risk of suffocation from bed partners who are relatively unaware of the infant's presence, such as young siblings. Babies should sleep in proximity to an attentive adult. (Psychology; 1–3 months; Application; Difficulty: 4)

GPN-015. The answer is A. This child is about 8 months old, an age at which children go through a period of separation anxiety and may want to breastfeed much more frequently. Other babies normally and naturally nurse in that pattern. It is very unlikely that this mother's supply is reduced, because the baby in the photo is obviously thriving. (Psychology; 7–12 months; Application; Difficulty: 2)

GPN-016. The answer is A. Competition with the baby's own mother is highly unlikely. This picture shows the author carrying her perfectly normal, wonderful, gorgeous, and brilliant granddaughter at about 4 weeks of age. (Psychology; 15–28 days; Knowledge; Difficulty: 2)

G-017. The answer is D. Telling others of her pregnancy is an early developmental task. Failure to reveal her pregnancy suggests lack of acceptance of the fetus. (Psychology; Prenatal; Knowledge; Difficulty: 2)

G-018. The answer is B. Giving formula samples sends the message that the mother will need formula, thereby undermining breastfeeding. (Psychology; General Principles; Knowledge; Difficulty: 2)

G-019. The answer is A. Closely supervised breastfeeding may help her. The key is close supervision to protect her and her baby. (Psychology; General Principles; Knowledge; Difficulty: 2)

G-020. The answer is B. Mothers who breastfeed often want to tell the world, which is a strong theme of empowerment. (Psychology; General Principles; Knowledge; Difficulty: 3)

G-021. The answer is A. Support from her male partner is the most important of the options listed, although any support will increase the likelihood of her continuing to breastfeed. (Psychology; General Principles; Knowledge; Difficulty: 4)

G-022. The answer is C. The mother's treatment during labor strongly affects her sense of accomplishment and self-esteem. The mother's age and other factors are less significant to her experience. (Psychology; Labor/Birth; Knowledge; Difficulty: 3)

G-023. The answer is B. This is the most supportive question because it is an open-ended question designed to explore the mother's preconceived ideas about breastfeeding. (Psychology; Prenatal; Application; Difficulty: 3)

G-024. The answer is B. Beginning your interaction with an empathetic response such as B helps validate the mother's emotions, helps her integrate her experience, and moves her into problem solving. (Psychology; 3–14 days; Application; Difficulty: 4)

G-025. The answer is C. The breastfeeding dyad is a unique biological and psychological entity. (Psychology; General Principles; Knowledge; Difficulty: 5)

G-026. The answer is B. A supportive companion is the most likely (of these options) to optimize breastfeeding success. Medications to relieve labor pain can significantly interfere with breastfeeding and bonding. Freedom to move about will enhance her comfort. (Psychology; Labor/Birth; Application; Difficulty: 3)

GN-027. The answer is B. Employee productivity is actually increased when mothers are enabled to continue breastfeeding their babies. (Psychology; General Principles; Knowledge; Difficulty: 2)

GN-028. The answer is C. While partial breastfeeding is better than none, the other options should be pursued first. (Psychology; General Principles; Knowledge; Difficulty: 5)

GN-029. The answer is B. Application of noxious substances to the nipples to discourage breastfeeding can disrupt the trust relationship that has been carefully established via breastfeeding. The other suggestions are appropriate. (Psychology; > 12 months; Application; Difficulty: 2)

GN-030. The answer is D. Breastfeeding has little known effect on blood pressure. Any significant effect would be likely to lower blood pressure because of the calming effects of lactational hormones. (Psychology; General Principles; Knowledge; Difficulty: 2)

GN-031. The answer is D. Facilitating continued direct breastfeeding is better for the breastfeeding relationship. However, even just having facilities for collecting milk is a positive support for breastfeeding. (Psychology; General Principles; Knowledge; Difficulty: 2)

GP-032. The answer is C. Social support increases the likelihood of successful breastfeeding. (Psychology; Labor/Birth; Application; Difficulty: 3)

GP-033. The answer is D. Identifying with the mother's feelings rather than offering solutions allows her to think about her options. (Psychology; 15–28 days; Application; Difficulty: 2)

GP-034. The answer is A. Mothers of multiples often attach to the unit before the individual baby or babies. (Psychology; 7–12 months; Knowledge; Difficulty: 3)

GP-035. The answer is C. It is always appropriate to begin a counseling session with an open-ended, general, supportive question. Option B is inappropriate at 2 months, the age of the baby pictured. Option A would be a reasonable question, especially if nipple soreness is a problem. Option D might be asked on a routine screening form. (Psychology; 1–3 months; Application; Difficulty: 4)

GP-036. The answer is D. Reinforcing the mother is the first strategy to support her decision and build confidence. After rapport is established, attending to the baby's possible jaundice and breast-feeding management questions are appropriate. (Psychology; 3–14 days; Application; Difficulty: 4)

GPN-037. The answer is D. Breastfeeding frequently on cue and continuous/frequent carrying fosters all aspects of infant mental and physical development. (Psychology; > 12 months; Application; Difficulty: 2)

GPN-038. The answer is A. The baby nurses more frequently during safe bedsharing. (Psychology; 1–3 months; Knowledge; Difficulty: 3)

GPN-039. The answer is D. Continuous/frequent carrying with unrestricted breastfeeding fosters all aspects of infant mental and physical development. (Psychology; 1–3 months; Knowledge; Difficulty: 2)

Scoring:

Total number of questions in this section   _____

Number of questions answered correctly   _____

Percent correct (divide number correct by total number)   _____

H. GROWTH PARAMETERS AND DEVELOPMENTAL MILESTONES

In the 2000 exam blueprint, 10 to 16 questions are dedicated to growth parameters and developmental milestones.

SUBTOPICS INCLUDED IN THIS CATEGORY

1. Fetal and preterm growth patterns

2. Breastfed and artificially fed growth patterns

3. Normal and delayed physical, psychological, and cognitive developmental milestones

4. Normal breastfeeding behaviors to and beyond 12 months

5. Weaning

CORE READING

Textbooks

Baumgarner NJ. *Mothering Your Nursing Toddler*. Schaumburg, IL: La Leche League International; 2002.

Bengson D. *How Weaning Happens*. Schaumburg, IL: La Leche League International; 2000.

Global Strategy for Infant and Young Child Feeding. Geneva, Switzerland: World Health Organization; 2004.

Global Strategy for Infant and Young Child Feeding: A Joint WHO/UNICEF Statement. Geneva, Switzerland: World Health Organization; 2003.

Guiding Principles for Complementary Feeding of the Breastfed Child. Washington, DC: Pan American Health Organization; 2003.

Flower, H. *Adventures in Tandem Nursing*. Schaumburg, IL: La Leche League International, 2003.

Lauwers J, Swisher A. *Counseling the Nursing Mother*. 4th ed. Sudbury, MA: Jones & Bartlett; 2003.

Lawrence RA, Lawrence RM. *Breastfeeding: A Guide for the Medical Profession*. 6th ed. St. Louis: Elsevier Mosby; 2005.

Nutrient Adequacy of Exclusive Breastfeeding for the Term Infant During the First Six Months of Life. Geneva, Switzerland: World Health Organization; 2002.

Riordan J. *Breastfeeding and Human Lactation*. 3rd ed. Sudbury, MA: Jones & Bartlett Publishers; 2004.

Small MF. *Our Babies, Ourselves: How Biology and Culture Shape the Way We Parent*. New York: Random House; 1998.

Stuart-Macadam P, Dettwyler KA. *Breastfeeding: Biocultural Perspectives*. New York: Aldine De Gruyter; 1995.

WHO Child Growth Standards. Geneva: World Health Organization; 2006. Accessed Oct 1, 2006. Available at www.who.int/childgrowth/en/

Key Research Articles

Borghi E, de Onis M, Garza C, et al. Construction of the World Health Organization child growth standards: Selection of methods for attained growth curves. *Stat Med.* 2006;25(2):247–265.

Kramer MS, Chalmers B, Hodnett ED, et al. Promotion of breastfeeding intervention trial (PROBIT): A randomized trial in the Republic of Belarus. *JAMA.* 2001;285(4):413–420.

Kramer MS, Guo T, Platt RW, et al. Breastfeeding and infant growth: Biology or bias? *Pediatrics.* 2002;110(2 pt 1):343–347.

Kramer MS, Kakuma R. The optimal duration of exclusive breastfeeding: A systematic review. *Adv Exp Med Biol.* 2004;554:63–77.

Kramer MS, Kakuma R. Optimal duration of exclusive breastfeeding. *Cochrane Database Syst Rev.* 2002(1):CD003517.

Kramer MS, Chalmers B, Hodnett ED, et al. Promotion of breastfeeding intervention trial (PROBIT): A cluster-randomized trial in the Republic of Belarus; design, follow-up, and data validation. *Adv Exp Med Biol.* 2000;478:327–345.

GROWTH PARAMETERS AND DEVELOPMENTAL MILESTONES QUESTIONS

Notice on question numbering: H-000 means a basic question, with one correct answer and three wrong answers. HP-000, along with the camera icon, means there is a picture that needs to be viewed to answer the question. The pictures are located on the CD-ROM included with this book and are numbered to correspond with the questions. HN-000, along with the frowning face icon, means the question has a NEGATIVE stem; therefore, read the entire question very carefully to find the one WRONG answer among the choices. HPN-000, with both icons in the margin, means there is a picture associated with the question AND the question has a negative stem. See Appendix A for a fuller explanation of negative stem questions.

H-001. At what developmental age is self-feeding most likely to begin?

a. 3–4 months
b. 6–7 months
c. 9–10 months
d. 12+ months

H-002. The mother of a 5-month-old breastfeeding baby is most likely to observe that the baby:

a. plays with her mother's other nipple while breastfeeding.
b. closes her eyes during breastfeeding.
c. is easily distracted while nursing.
d. does not awaken to breastfeed at night.

H-003. At what gestational age does the swallowing reflex first appear?

a. 16 weeks
b. 22 weeks
c. 28 weeks
d. 32 weeks

HN-004. Which of the following is **NOT** an example of mutual interdependency during breast-feeding?

a. The baby's gut closure occurs around the time he is ready for solid foods.
b. The mother's milk contains environmental chemicals, triggering baby's immune system.
c. Skin contact during breastfeeding helps regulate baby's temperature.
d. Sucking at breast triggers release of gut hormones in mother and baby.

HN-005. Breastfeeding as an oral function of the baby involves all of the following **EXCEPT**:

a. a sense of taste and smell of milk
b. oral gratification and comfort
c. tactile sensation of the breast filling the infant's mouth
d. an inability of the infant to control the shape of the breast

HP-006. A child of the age shown is most likely to be developmentally ready to:

a. crawl and attempt to stand alone.
b. wean from the breast.
c. sleep through the night alone.
d. separate easily from mother.

HP-007. Which behavioral state is illustrated by the infant in this picture?

a. active alert
b. quiet alert
c. light sleep
d. drowsy

HP-008. Which statement best describes the reason this baby would begin reaching for table (family) food?

a. The baby is developmentally ready for solid (family) food.
b. The mother's milk supply is no longer adequate.
c. The baby is just imitating and will not be ready for family foods for some time.
d. The baby is jealous because everyone else is eating "real" food.

HP-009. At which age is this breastfeeding behavior most likely to occur?

a. 5–6 months
b. 7–12 months
c. 12–18 months
d. 18–24 months

HP-010. Which of the following is the most common breastfeeding behavior of a child at this age?

a. biting at the end of feeds
b. nursing strike
c. easily distracted while nursing
d. playfulness and vocalization during feeds

HP-011. This mother is getting irritated with her child's nursing habits. The child is afraid of strangers, cries when left with a caregiver, and wakes several times at night. The most likely reason for this behavior pattern is:

a. delayed development of autonomy caused by breastfeeding.
b. the mother clinging to her child and discouraging autonomy.
c. common and normal behavior in the second 6 months of life.
d. the mother's inability to set limits for the child's behavior.

HPN-012. Of the following conditions, which is **LEAST LIKELY** to result in this pattern of growth?

a. Down syndrome
b. exclusive breastfeeding
c. tongue-tied baby
d. cystic fibrosis

HPN-013. The behavior shown in this picture is **LEAST LIKELY** to be:

a. distress at separation from mother.
b. an indication of pain.
c. the infant's attempt to manipulate its mother.
d. stressful to the baby's physiology.

HPN-014. Common breastfeeding behaviors of babies at this age include all of the following **EXCEPT**:

a. smiling up at the mom during feeds.
b. biting or clamping down at the end of a feed.
c. distractibility.
d. feeding mostly with the eyes closed.

H-015. A 6-month-old baby, sitting at the family dinner table, begins reaching for food. Which statement best describes the reason for this behavior?

a. The baby is developmentally ready for solid (family) foods.
b. The mother's milk supply is no longer adequate.
c. The baby is imitating and will not be ready for family foods for some time.
d. The baby is jealous because everyone else is eating "real" food.

H-016. A thriving, exclusively breastfed 3-month-old baby suddenly begins nursing much more frequently, around the clock. Her mother calls you, worried that something has happened to her milk. Your best response to her is:

a. Has the baby been exposed to illness lately?
b. Babies usually nurse more frequently beginning at 3 months of age.
c. This is probably a growth spurt; her usual pattern will probably resume soon.
d. Your milk is higher in casein now, making her fussier.

H-017. The mother of a 4-month-old, exclusively breastfed baby wonders when her baby will sleep through the night without waking to feed. Your best response is:

a. by the time he is 6 months old.
b. when he has doubled his birth weight.
c. when you stop nursing him as soon as he cries.
d. when he is physiologically ready.

H-018. At which ages/stages are babies most likely to self-wean?

a. under 12 months
b. 12–18 months
c. 2–2½ years
d. 3–4 years

H-019.   What window (age) period most likely represents a biologic end of breastfeeding for human infants?

a.   9–15 months
b.   around 18 months
c.   around 24 months
d.   2½ to 7 years

H-020.   A mother asks about a book she has read that recommends letting a baby cry it out to teach him to sleep all night by 3 months of age. The authors claim that responding immediately to the baby's cries will teach the baby to be manipulative. Based on Erickson and Piaget's work regarding the development of trust, your best response to her is:

a.   Three-month-old babies are learning trust. Not responding to him teaches him that he can't trust you.
b.   The book is correct. Babies can learn to self-soothe at that age.
c.   Babies learn to manipulate parents at an early age. You can learn to differentiate his cries of real distress.
d.   By 3 months, his ability to trust you is already developed, and crying it out won't hurt him.

H-021.   The normal and safest nighttime sleep and breastfeeding pattern for the 3-month-old, exclusively breastfed baby is:

a.   The mother and the baby share a bed and the baby feeds several times at night.
b.   The baby sleeps in a room away from his parents.
c.   The baby is put to bed at a regular time and allowed to self-comfort to go to sleep.
d.   The baby is nursed to sleep, then put down with a pacifier in a crib.

H-022.   In order to breastfeed successfully, it is most important for a mother of twins to:

a.   get at least 6 straight hours of sleep each night.
b.   learn to feed her babies simultaneously.
c.   use a nursing pillow.
d.   follow her babies' cues.

H-023. The mother of a 9-month-old is concerned that her baby has suddenly begun waking several times at night to breastfeed. She works at a local factory 4 hours a day, leaving her child in the on-site day care center. Your first response should be:

a. your milk supply is faltering, so increase the amount of family foods you offer to your child.
b. stop into the day care center unannounced to see if any abuse is taking place.
c. express or pump your milk several times a day while you're at work, and feed your child that milk at night.
d. increased nighttime breastfeeding is common at this age. Do continue to breastfeed him on cue, and this phase will pass.

H-024. Which is the latest feeding cue that an infant exhibits?

a. crying
b. hand-to-face or hand-to-mouth
c. grope or mouthing motions
d. moving into feeding position

HN-025. Benefits to a mother and/or her baby of breastfeeding past 12 months include all of the following **EXCEPT**:

a. a continued source of most calories in the baby's diet
b. continued immune protection for the baby
c. mutual pleasure in the relationship
d. reassurance of the mother's permanence

HN-026. Which is the **LEAST LIKELY** feature of a "nursing strike"?

a. It may occur between 6 and 9 months of age.
b. It may coincide with infant illness.
c. With careful attention, the baby will usually go back to the breast.
d. The baby is indicating readiness to wean.

HN-027. A nursing strike by a 7- to 9-month-old child is likely to be precipitated by any of the following **EXCEPT**:

a. illness in the infant.
b. the mother's reaction to baby biting during feeds.
c. a change in the mother's soap, perfume, or deodorant.
d. the infant's readiness to wean.

HN-028. A mother and her breastfeeding toddler twins are likely to experience all of the following **EXCEPT**:

a. mutual enjoyment of breastfeeding
b. sibling rivalry for the breast
c. playfulness between children during feeds
d. higher risk of milk stasis

HP-029. This child's nursing behavior is:

a. highly unusual at this age.
b. indicative of attachment disorder.
c. normal for a child this age.
d. likely to cause dental caries.

HP-030. If her mother moves the dog's water dish out of her sight, this child will probably:

a. crawl straight to it.
b. forget it was there.
c. become confused.
d. search for it without knowing where to look.

HP-031. Which of the following breastfeeding-related behaviors is this baby most likely to exhibit?

a. gazes up and smiles at his mother
b. hands relax as he obtains milk
c. reaches for his mother's face
d. cues to feed by crying

HP-032. This mother has been told that her baby should no longer feed at night. Your best response to her is:

a. It's time to begin solid foods.
b. Try to get him to nurse more in the daytime.
c. Use a pacifier during the night.
d. Feeding at night is normal behavior.

HP-033. Which statement are you most likely going to hear from the mother of this child?

a. My baby has been weaning herself—she's down to 3 nursings a day.
b. She just started sleeping through the night without nursing.
c. She's been so clingy lately—I can't even leave her for a moment!
d. I'm changing diapers all day—she still stools as often as she did as a newborn.

HP-034. Which of the following reflexes is most likely to have faded (integrated) in this baby?

a. gag reflex
b. sucking reflex
c. extrusion reflex
d. stepping reflex

HP-035. What is the most likely age of this baby?

a. 4 months
b. 6 months
c. 8 months
d. 10 months

HPN-036. The likely consequences of this behavior include all of the following **EXCEPT**:

a. the baby receives up to 30% of calories at night.
b. increased risk of baby's smothering.
c. reduced risk of early weaning.
d. reduced risk of pregnancy.

HPN-037. This baby's mother complains that her baby has increased her night feeds. The **LEAST** appropriate suggestion is:

a. This is normal behavior at this age.
b. Try going to a quieter, darker place.
c. You can try feeding more family foods during the day.
d. Night feeds are important to your baby at this age.

HPN-038. A baby of this age is likely to show all of the following behaviors **EXCEPT**:

a. hands are frequently open.
b. can follow light to midline.
c. able to reach for an object.
d. has differentiated cries and sounds.

HPN-039. Common breastfeeding behaviors of babies at this age include all of the following **EXCEPT**:

a. playing with their toes while nursing.
b. increased breastfeeding at night.
c. handling the mother's other breast.
d. lifting the mother's shirt/blouse.

HPN-040. Breastfeeding behaviors common to a child of this age include all of the following **EXCEPT**:

a. playfulness at the breast.
b. ability to breastfeed while the mother is engaging in other activities.
c. persistent biting.
d. breastfeeding at night.

HPN-041. Which behavior is **LEAST LIKELY** to occur in the breastfeeding child shown in this picture?

a. breastfeeding 8–12 times per 24 hours
b. sleeping through the night
c. separation anxiety
d. self-feeding of family foods

HPN-042. Common breastfeeding behaviors of babies at this age include all of the following **EXCEPT**:

a. The mother and baby develop a code word for nursing.
b. The baby takes family foods well.
c. The baby has an increased ability to postpone feeds.
d. The baby passes stool during most feeds.

HPN-043. Which of the following events is **LEAST LIKELY** to be associated with a baby of this age?

a. breastfeeds 7–17 times per 24 hours
b. sleeps 8–9 hours at night
c. looks to locate interesting sounds
d. recognizes mother and smiles

GROWTH PARAMETERS AND DEVELOPMENTAL MILESTONES ANSWERS

The parenthetical material at the end of each answer includes the discipline and time period, indicates whether the question pertains to knowledge or application, and specifies the degree of difficulty.

H-001.   The answer is B. Babies start being able to self-feed around 6 months. Offering a variety of family foods that the child can pick up and explore is appropriate. (Growth; 4–6 months; Knowledge; Difficulty: 4)

H-002.   The answer is C. Distractibility is a common behavioral characteristic in the 4- to 6-month age range. (Growth; 4–6 months; Knowledge; Difficulty: 3)

H-003.   The answer is A. The infant is able to swallow from about 16 weeks and develops an immature suck pattern at around 26 weeks gestational age. (Growth; Prematurity; Knowledge; Difficulty: 4)

HN-004.   The answer is B. Environmental chemicals that may appear in the mother's milk have no documented effect on the baby or its immune system. Mother's milk helps build the baby's immune system. The other choices are true. (Growth; General Principles; Knowledge; Difficulty: 2)

HN-005.   The answer is D. The oral experience of breastfeeding is pleasurable and normal. The infant controls and molds the shape of the breast in its mouth. (Growth; General Principles; Application; Difficulty: 2)

HP-006.   The answer is A. The developmental milestones characteristic of the 7- to 12-month age group include separation anxiety; sleep changes, especially increased night waking; and decreased (not increased) likelihood of self-weaning. (Growth; 7–12 months; Application; Difficulty: 4)

HP-007.   The answer is B. In the quiet alert state, the baby's eyes are open, arms extended and relaxed, hands loosely open. The baby's expression is calm and relaxed. (Growth; 15–28 days; Knowledge; Difficulty: 4)

HP-008.   The answer is A. Many babies show signs of developmental readiness around 6 months of age, such as reaching for family foods. Exclusive breastfeeding is recommended for 6 months. (Growth; 7–12 months; Application; Difficulty: 4)

HP-009. The answer is B. "Gymnastic" nursing, pincer grasp and self-feeding, and increased mobility are typical of the 7- to 12-month-old baby. (Growth; 7–12 months; Knowledge; Difficulty: 5)

HP-010. The answer is D. The over-1-year-old nursing child often plays and explores his mother's body during breastfeeding sessions. (Growth; > 12 months; Application; Difficulty: 5)

HP-011. The answer is C. These are typical and normal behaviors of breastfeeding children in the 7- to 12-month period. (Growth; 7–12 months; Application; Difficulty: 3)

HPN-012. The answer is B. Appropriate exclusive breastfeeding is unlikely to cause this pattern. The other conditions could result in growth compromise as charted. (Growth; 7–12 months; Knowledge; Difficulty: 5)

HPN-013. The answer is C. Babies cue or signal for their needs to be met. Crying is a LATE sign of hunger and also a sign that the baby has exhausted all other resources in getting his needs met. (Growth; 3–14 days; Application; Difficulty: 2)

HPN-014. The answer is D. Four- to six-month-old babies are very interactive with their mothers during breastfeeding, including making intense eye contact. (Growth; 4–6 months; Application; Difficulty: 2)

H-015. The answer is A. Exclusive breastfeeding is recommended for at least 6 months. Many babies show signs of readiness for solid food at that point, such as reaching for family foods. (Growth; 4–6 months; Application; Difficulty: 3)

H-016. The answer is C. Growth occurs in spurts that may parallel changes in breastfeeding frequency, which may occur around 3 months of age. (Growth; 1–3 months; Application; Difficulty: 4)

H-017. The answer is D. Babies have individual needs that are best met by feedings on cue, day and night. They eventually outgrow these needs. About 2/3 of babies breastfeed at night during the first 6 months. (Growth; 4–6 months; Application; Difficulty: 3)

H-018. The answer is D. This is a period of equilibrium, and many believe that babies are more likely to wean at stable ages. (Growth; > 12 months; Knowledge; Difficulty: 4)

H-019. The answer is D. Anthropological evidence suggests the human infant was "designed" to breastfeed for more than 2 years. (Growth; > 12 months; Knowledge; Difficulty: 4)

H-020. The answer is A. Forcing a baby to cry it out destroys the baby's growing sense of trust. Once broken, trust is difficult to repair. A baby's trust develops by consistently and promptly responding to his needs. Over time, his needs diminish and he can tolerate delays in his mother's response. (Growth; 1–3 months; Application; Difficulty: 4)

H-021. The answer is A. This is the biological norm and most common nighttime arrangement worldwide. Separate sleeping is associated with higher risk of SIDS (sudden infant death syndrome). Self-comforting is distressful for many babies. Pacifiers can compromise breastfeeding. (Growth; 1–3 months; Application; Difficulty: 3)

H-022. The answer is D. Most mothers will produce plenty of milk for several breastfed babies, despite higher risk of early birth-related problems. (Growth; 7–12 months; Application; Difficulty: 3)

H-023. The answer is D. Babies breastfeed at this age to reconnect with mother as much as for the milk, and giving bottles is likely to shorten the duration of breastfeeding. An empathetic response, plus factual information on breastfeeding during separation anxiety stage, is the best response. Milk supply rarely falters in the second 6 months. While abuse is a possibility, it is less likely a cause of night waking than the other responses. (Growth; 7–12 months; Application; Difficulty: 4)

H-024. The answer is A. Crying is a late sign of hunger and occurs after all other cues have been ignored. Babies should be fed when they exhibit early feeding cues. (Growth; 1–2 days; Application; Difficulty: 2)

HN-025. The answer is A. The older child is usually nursing for far more than food. Breastfeeding the older child is mutually pleasurable even when the majority of the child's calories come from other sources. (Growth; > 12 months; Knowledge; Difficulty: 2)

HN-026. The answer is D. Self-weaning is developmentally unusual and unlikely to occur before one year of age, at a minimum. Babies may suddenly refuse the breast if they are ill and/or breast-feeding is painful, and will usually begin again when the crisis has resolved. (Growth; 7–12 months; Application; Difficulty: 2)

HN-027. The answer is D. Nursing strikes are indications that the baby is having some difficulty with breastfeeding or the mother–baby breastfeeding relationship. Self-weaning before 12 months of age is unusual. (Growth; 7–12 months; Knowledge; Difficulty: 2)

HN-028. The answer is B. Breastfed twins are often best friends and copy each other's breastfeed-ing behaviors. High milk volume may increase mother's susceptibility to milk stasis. (Growth; > 12 months; Knowledge; Difficulty: 3)

HP-029. The answer is C. This 13-month-old's nursing pattern is entirely normal. (Growth; > 12 months; Knowledge; Difficulty: 3)

HP-030. The answer is A. Object permanence emerges in the 4- to 8-month-old period. The child can remember her intention even when the object is moved out of visual range. (Growth; 7–12 months; Application; Difficulty: 3)

HP-031. The answer is B. In the early weeks, babies often feed with closed fists that open and relax as the baby becomes satiated at breast. (Growth; 3–14 days; Application; Difficulty: 4)

HP-032. The answer is D. Feeding at night is normal and common. About 2/3 of infants 1–6 months old feed at night. It is always appropriate to breastfeed in response to the baby's cues 24 hours a day. (Growth; 4–6 months; Application; Difficulty: 3)

HP-033. The answer is C. Separation anxiety is very common around 8 months, the age of the child pictured. (Growth; 7–12 months; Application; Difficulty: 3)

HP-034. The answer is C. The tongue extrusion reflex fades (integrates) by 6 months. The child shown is 8 months old. Stepping at this age is not a reflex, but a deliberate behavior. (Growth; 7–12 months; Knowledge; Difficulty: 5)

HP-035. The answer is B. This child is 6 months old and has been experimenting with self-feeding of cooked yams. (Growth; 4–6 months; Application; Difficulty: 4)

HPN-036. The answer is B. There is no research evidence of increased risk to the baby's sleeping with a sober, nonsmoking breastfeeding mother on a safe surface. A, B, and D are well-documented benefits of breastfeeding at night. (Growth; 1–3 months; Application; Difficulty: 2)

HPN-037. The answer is C. Distractibility is common in the 4- to 6-month period. Most babies are not yet developmentally ready for solid foods at this time. The *Global Strategy for Infant & Young Child Feeding* recommends 6 months of exclusive breastfeeding. (Growth; 4–6 months; Application; Difficulty: 2)

HPN-038. The answer is C. The 2- to 4-week-old is not yet capable of reaching for objects. (Growth; 15–28 days; Application; Difficulty: 2)

HPN-039. The answer is B. Breastfeeding at night might not substantially change in the second 6 months of life. (Growth; 7–12 months; Application; Difficulty: 5)

HPN-040. The answer is C. Persistent biting is not common in nursing toddlers. Any attempts at biting should be immediately stopped by the mother. (Growth; > 12 months; Application; Difficulty: 3)

HPN-041. The answer is B. Sleeping through the night is least likely in this age child. "Gymnastic" nursing, pincer grasp and self-feeding, and separation anxiety are typical of the 7- to 12-month-old child. (Growth; 7–12 months; Application; Difficulty: 5)

HPN-042. The answer is D. Stools are usually more formed because of milk composition (higher casein:whey ratio) and addition of family foods. (Growth; 7–12 months; Application; Difficulty: 4)

HPN-043. The answer is B. One- to three-month-old, exclusively breastfed babies usually do not have long stretches without breastfeeding, even at night. About 1/3 of babies do not feed at night (10 PM to 4 AM). (Growth; 1–3 months; Application; Difficulty: 2)

Scoring:

Total number of questions in this section _____

Number of questions answered correctly _____

Percent correct (divide number correct by total number) _____

I. INTERPRETATION OF RESEARCH

In the 2000 exam blueprint, 4 to 8 questions are dedicated to interpretation of research.

SUBTOPICS INCLUDED IN THIS CATEGORY

1. Skills required for critical appraisal and interpretation of research literature

    a. Terminology
    b. Design, human rights
    c. Measurement tools

2. Terminology used in research

    a. Basic statistics
    b. Surveys and data collection
    c. Graphs and charts

3. Lactation consultant educational materials and consumer literature

CORE READING

Textbooks

Frank-Stromberg M, Olsen SJ. *Instruments for Clinical Health-Care Research.* 2nd ed. Sudbury, MA: Jones & Bartlett Publishers; 1997.
Lauwers J, Swisher A. *Counseling the Nursing Mother.* 4th ed. Sudbury, MA: Jones & Bartlett; 2003.
Lawrence RA, Lawrence RM. *Breastfeeding: A Guide for the Medical Profession.* 6th ed. St. Louis: Elsevier Mosby; 2005.
Polit D, Beck C. *Nursing Research: Principles and Methods.* Philadelphia: Lippencott; 2003.
Riordan J. *Breastfeeding and Human Lactation.* 3rd ed. Sudbury, MA: Jones & Bartlett Publishers; 2004.
Roberts K, Taylor B. *Nursing Research Processes: An Australian Perspective.* Melbourne: Nelson; 2002.

Internet Resources

The Cochrane Collection. Accessed Oct. 1, 2006. Available at www.cochrane.org.
Core Library for Evidence-Based Practice. Accessed Oct. 1, 2006. Available at www.shef.ac.uk/scharr/ir/core.html.
National Library of Medicine and National Institutes of Health. PubMed website. Accessed Oct. 1, 2006. Available at www.ncbi.nlm.nih.gov/PubMed.

Key Research Articles

Armstrong HC. International recommendations for consistent breastfeeding definitions. *J Hum Lact.* 1991;7:51–54.

Auerbach KG. Beyond the issue of accuracy: Evaluating patient education materials for breastfeeding mothers. *J Hum Lact.* 1988;4:108–110.

Evidence-based Medicine Working Group. Evidence-based medicine: A new approach to teaching the practice of medicine. *JAMA.* 1992;268(17):2420.

Fredrickson D. Breastfeeding study design problems—health policy, epidemiologic, and pediatric perspectives. In: Stuart-Macadam P, Dettwyler KA, eds. *Breastfeeding: Biocultural Perspectives.* New York: Aldine De Gruyter; 1995.

Greenhalgh T. How to read a paper: Assessing the methodological quality of published papers. *Br Med J.* 1997;315:305.

Greenhalgh T. How to read a paper: Getting your bearing (deciding what the paper is about). *Br Med J.* 1997;315:243.

Greenhalgh T. How to read a paper: The Medline database. *Br Med J.* 1997;315:180.

Greenhalgh T. How to read a paper: Papers that go beyond numbers (qualitative research). *Br Med J.* 1997;315:740.

Greenhalgh T. How to read a paper: Papers that summarize other papers (systematic reviews and meta-analyses). *Br Med J.* 1997;315:672.

Greenhalgh T. How to read a paper: Statistics for the non-statistician II: Significant relationships and their pitfalls. *Br Med J.* 1997;315:422.

Labbok M, Krasovek K. Toward consistency in breastfeeding definitions. *Stud Fam Plann.* 1990;21:226–230.

Riordan J. Readable, relevant, and reliable: The three Rs of breastfeeding pamphlets. *Breastfeed Abst.* 1985;5:5–6.

Smith L. A scoresheet for evaluating breastfeeding educational materials. *J Hum Lact.* 1995;11(4):307–311.

INTERPRETATION OF RESEARCH QUESTIONS

Notice on question numbering: I-000 means a basic question, with one correct answer and three wrong answers. IP-000, along with the camera icon, means there is a picture that needs to be viewed to answer the question. The pictures are located on the CD-ROM included with this book and are numbered to correspond with the questions. IN-000, along with the frowning face icon, means the question has a NEGATIVE stem; therefore, read the entire question very carefully to find the one WRONG answer among the choices. IPN-000, with both icons in the margin, means there is a picture associated with the question AND the question has a negative stem. See Appendix A for a fuller explanation of negative stem questions.

I-001. Which statement describes the most reliable research tool?

a. The tool has not broken in 5 years of continuous use.
b. Using the tool produces the same results, even when used by different people at different times.
c. The tool is quick to master and easy to use by multiple researchers.
d. The tool was developed by well-known researchers at a large, prestigious university.

I-002. When doing a review of the literature for a research study, which sources are most important to include?

a. review articles that analyze several studies
b. textbooks that explain basic concepts
c. peer-reviewed journal reports of research, written by the researcher
d. lectures given at large conferences by well-known speakers

I-003. A research report indicates that a sample of breastfed infants had no differences in illness rates than a comparable sample of artificially fed infants. While reading this report, the most important point to look for is:

a. the type of study used.
b. operational definitions.
c. the sample used.
d. the review of the literature.

I-004. A researcher is studying breastfeeding incidence in two neighboring community prenatal clinics. In one clinic, a new videotape is used to teach breastfeeding; the other continues to use an older videotape. At the follow-up, both clinics report similar increases in breastfeeding initiation. The most likely reason for this is:

a. all instructional videotapes are equivalent.
b. the Hawthorne effect.
c. changing the videotape had no effect.
d. the Nedelsky effect.

I-005. Which of the following citations is an example of a primary reference or source?

a. DeCoopman JM. *Pacifier Use in Breastfed Infants: Review and Recommendations* [master's thesis]. Ann Arbor: University of Michigan; 1996.

b. Als H, Lester BM, Tronick E, Brazelton TB. Manual for the assessment of preterm infants' behavior (AFPB). In: Fitzgerald JE, Lester BM, Jogman MW, eds. *Theory and Research in Behavioral Pediatrics.* Vol 1. New York: Plenum; 1982:64–133.

c. Fildes V. *Breasts, Bottles and Babies: A History of Infant Feeding.* Edinburgh: Edinburgh University Press; 1986.

d. Aarts C, Hornell A, Kylberg E, et al. Breastfeeding patterns in relation to thumb sucking and pacifier use. *Pediatrics.* 1999;104(4):e50.

I-006. Which of the following citations is a primary reference or source?

a. Anderson GC. Current knowledge about skin-to-skin (kangaroo) care for preterm infants: Review of the literature. *J Perinatol.* 1991;XI:216–226.

b. Als H, Lester BM, Tronick E, Brazelton TB. Manual for the assessment of preterm infants' behavior (AFPB). In: Fitzgerald JE, Lester BM, Jogman MW, eds. *Theory and Research in Behavioral Pediatrics.* Vol 1. New York: Plenum; 1982:64–133.

c. Ludington-Hoe SM, Golant SK. *Kangaroo Care: The Best You Can Do to Help Your Preterm Infant.* New York: Bantam Books; 1993.

d. Ludington-Hoe SM, Hadeed AJ, Anderson GC. Physiologic responses to skin-to-skin contact in hospitalized premature infants. *J Perinatol.* 1991; 11(1):19–24.

IN-007. Which statement is **FALSE** about experimental research designs?

a. Subjects receive the intervention, controls do not.
b. The dependent variable is manipulated to see what happens to the subjects.
c. The independent variable is manipulated to test the hypothesis.
d. Confounding variables will affect the results of the experiment.

I-008. A researcher plans to study the effect of giving breastfeeding mothers an herbal preparation to increase milk supply. The mothers are all from the same community, and their babies are in the same age range. Which of the following is the dependent variable in this study?

a. use of the herbal preparation
b. milk volume intake of the babies
c. amount of milk pumped
d. use of a placebo preparation

I-009. Which research study design is considered to be the most rigorous?

a. case-control
b. randomized, controlled trial
c. quasi-experimental
d. observational

I-010. Which term refers to the middle score in a range of scores?

a. mean
b. median
c. mode
d. meridian

I-011. Which statement describes a false negative (Type II) error in a breastfeeding research study?

a. The researcher decides there is a difference between groups when there is no real difference.
b. The researcher decides there is no difference between groups when there is a real difference.
c. The researcher fails to include a control group.
d. The researcher uses too small a sample size to detect differences between groups.

I-012. A research study concludes that an event happened purely by chance. Which probability value is most likely to show an effect by chance?

a. $p = 1.0$
b. $p = 0.10$
c. $p = 0.01$
d. $p = 0.001$

I-013. When revising or creating policies relating to breastfeeding, which of the following provides the strongest evidence for the policy?

a. meta-analyses
b. randomized, controlled trials
c. case-control studies
d. case reports

I-014. A research study found that when a baby has been given a pacifier for every sleep session but does not get one on a particular night, the baby may be more likely to die from SIDS (sudden infant death syndrome). Which conclusion can accurately be made from that report?

a. All babies should get pacifiers for every sleep session to prevent SIDS.
b. Pacifiers do not interfere with breastfeeding.
c. If a mother begins giving a pacifier, she may need to continue doing so.
d. Breastfed babies are protected from SIDS if they breastfeed all night long.

IP-015. Which conclusion can accurately be drawn from the data presented in this graph? (NH = non-Hispanic)

a. Hispanic babies are more likely to be breastfed for 6 months than black babies.
b. More white babies are breastfeeding at 12 months than black and Hispanic babies combined.
c. Twice as many black babies are weaned before 1 year than white or Hispanic babies.
d. Mothers of black babies are unable to produce enough milk for their babies.

IN-016. A research article reports that giving a baby 1 bottle of formula daily between the second and sixth weeks postpartum had no effect on breastfeeding outcomes at 6 weeks. All of the following aspects of the study are flaws that could bring the conclusions into question **EXCEPT:**

a. During the protocol period, the planned bottle group gave an average of 5 to 9 bottles per week compared with the total breastfeeding group's average of fewer than 2 bottles per week.
b. In both groups, babies received bottles (a mean of 2 bottles) in the first week postpartum.
c. No in-person, skilled follow-up care was provided to either group of mothers and babies.
d. The content of the bottles used (whether formula or mother's own milk) was not consistently documented.

IN-017. An effective, appropriate pamphlet promoting breastfeeding might contain all of the following features **EXCEPT:**

a. an accurate picture of a baby breastfeeding.
b. a comparison of breastfeeding with artificial feeding.
c. information about making enough milk.
d. local sources of breastfeeding help.

IN-018. You think you are seeing a certain phenomenon in your clients. In order to study this more thoroughly, you might do any of the following **EXCEPT**:

a. an observational study.
b. a qualitative survey.
c. case reports.
d. a clinical trial.

INTERPRETATION OF RESEARCH ANSWERS

The parenthetical material at the end of each answer includes the discipline and time period, indicates whether the question pertains to knowledge or application, and specifies the degree of difficulty.

I-001. The answer is B. Reliability of a test instrument means that the instrument produces consistent results regardless of user, time of use, use over a duration of time, and when applied to different subjects. (Research; General Principles; Knowledge; Difficulty: 2)

I-002. The answer is C. Original research (primary references) is the most important type of source to include in a literature review. Texts and review articles may help you locate primary references on a subject. Lectures also may direct you to primary references. (Research; General Principles; Application; Difficulty: 4)

I-003. The answer is B. Operational definitions, or how the authors define the term "breastfeeding," are critical. (Research; General Principles; Application; Difficulty: 3)

I-004. The answer is B. The Hawthorne effect means that observing a population for a specific behavior change often produces the desired change, independent of the intervention being studied. (Research; Prenatal; Application; Difficulty: 2)

I-005. The answer is D. A research article published in a peer-reviewed professional journal is a primary reference. A is a review, which is a secondary reference. B is a chapter in a book, which is a secondary or tertiary source. C is a book, interpreting other sources in its recommendations. (Research; General Principles; Application; Difficulty: 4)

I-006. The answer is D. A research article published in a peer-reviewed professional journal is a primary reference. A is a review article, which is a secondary reference. B is a chapter in a book, which is a secondary or tertiary source. C is a book for parents, interpreting other sources in its recommendations. (Research; Prematurity; Application; Difficulty: 4)

IN-007. The answer is B. The dependent variable is the result of the manipulation, not the part of the experiment that is changed. The other three statements about experimental research designs are true. (Research; General Principles; Knowledge; Difficulty: 2)

I-008. The answer is C. The amount of milk pumped is the dependent variable. Use of the herb or a placebo is the independent variable. Weight gain of the babies is a confounding variable, since milk volume intake may not reflect actual milk volume produced. (Research; General Principles; Knowledge; Difficulty: 3)

I-009. The answer is B. Randomized, controlled trials are considered the most rigorous evidence for a phenomenon. (Research; General Principles; Knowledge; Difficulty: 3)

I-010. The answer is B. The median score is the middle score, which may or may not also be the mean (average) or mode (most frequent) score. (Research; General Principles; Knowledge; Difficulty: 3)

I-011. The answer is B. False negative (Type II) errors occur when a real difference exists, but a flaw in the design or other aspect of the research does not identify the real difference. Inadequate sample size is one cause of Type II errors. Choice A is a Type I error, and a control group is necessary for any comparative analysis of groups. (Research; General Principles; Knowledge; Difficulty: 3)

I-012. The answer is A. The probability of a chance occurrence is usually established at 1.0. The smaller the probability value, the less likely the event happened by chance. (Research; General Principles; Knowledge; Difficulty: 3)

I-013. The answer is B. Systematic reviews and meta-analyses are the strongest forms of evidence for a policy or practice. Case reports are the weakest form of evidence. (Research; General Principles; Knowledge; Difficulty: 3)

I-014. The answer is C. Pollard and colleagues found that babies who are regularly given pacifiers may forget how to suck their own fingers. Sucking may help trigger respiration in some babies and be protective against SIDS. Babies suck on pacifiers, their own fingers, their mothers' fingers, and their mothers' breasts during breastfeeding. The findings of this article cannot be generalized to all babies or breastfeeding babies. (Research; General Principles; Application; Difficulty: 3)

IP-015. The answer is A. Hispanic babies are more likely to be breastfed at all and are more likely to be breastfed for 6 months than white or black babies are. (Research; 7–12 months; Application; Difficulty: 4)

IN-016. The answer is C. Both groups had the same care (or lack of care) before the study period began. The other choices are all significant flaws. (Research; 15–28 days; Application; Difficulty: 5)

IN-017. The answer is B. Comparing breastfeeding with artificial feeding suggests their equivalence, which is neither accurate nor helpful information. (Research; General Principles; Knowledge; Difficulty: 2)

IN-018. The answer is D. Clinical trials are rarely the first type of research done to investigate a phenomenon. Observational studies, qualitative surveys, and case reports establish the basis for possible later clinical trials. (Research; General Principles; Application; Difficulty: 2)

Scoring:

Total number of questions in this section   _____

Number of questions answered correctly   _____

Percent correct (divide number correct by total number)   _____

J. ETHICAL AND LEGAL ISSUES

In the 2000 exam blueprint, 4 to 8 questions are dedicated to ethical and legal issues.

SUBTOPICS INCLUDED IN THIS CATEGORY

1. IBLCE Code of Ethics

2. ILCA standards of practice

3. Scope of practice

4. Medical and legal responsibilities; informed consent

5. Report writing skills; charting and record keeping

6. Referrals and interdisciplinary relationships

7. Informed consent

8. Confidentiality

9. Battery

10. Conflict of interest

11. Ethics of equipment rental and sales

12. Maternal–infant neglect and infant abuse

CORE READING

Textbooks

Allain A, Chetley A. *Protecting Infant Health: A Healthworker's Guide to the International Code of Marketing of Breast-Milk Substitutes.* Penang, Malaysia: International Baby Food Action Network (IBFAN); 2003.

Bornmann P. A legal primer for lactation consultants. In: Walker M, ed. *ILCA Core Curriculum for Lactation Consultant Practice.* Sudbury, MA: Jones and Bartlett; 2001:465–516.

Clinical Competencies Checklist. Falls Church, VA: International Board of Lactation Consultant Examiners; 2003.

Code of Ethic for IBCLCs. Falls Church, VA: International Board of Lactation Consultant Examiners; 2004.

Competency Statements. Falls Church, VA: International Board of Lactation Consultant Examiners.

Palmer G. *The Politics of Breastfeeding*. 2nd ed. London: Pandora Press; 1993.

Protecting, Promoting and Supporting Breastfeeding: The Special Role of Maternity Services. A Joint WHO/UNICEF statement. Geneva, Switzerland: World Health Organization Nutrition Unit; 1989.

Scott J. The Code of Ethics for International Board Certified Lactation Consultants: ethical practice. In: Walker M, ed. *ILCA's Core Curriculum for Lactation Consultant Practice*. Sudbury, MA: Jones and Bartlett; 2001: 517–527.

Standards of Practice for Lactation Consultants. Raleigh, NC: International Lactation Consultant Association; 1999.

Key Research Articles

Arnold LDW. The ethics of donor human milk banking. *Breastfeeding Medicine*. 2006;1(1):3–13.

Bornmann P. Breastfeeding—a litigated issue. *J Hum Lact*. 1990;6(3):104.

Bornmann PG, Ross GL. Using the law of battery to protect and support breastfeeding. *J Hum Lact*. 2000;16(1):47–51.

Bornmann PG. Legal commentary: Cyberspace and the lactation consultant. *J Hum Lact*. 1997;13(3):191–192.

Rea MF, Marcolino FF, Colameo AJ, Trevellin LA. Protection of breastfeeding, marketing of human milk substitutes and ethics. *Adv Exp Med Biol*. 2004;554:329–332.

Smith LJ. Expert witness: What to emphasize. *J Hum Lact*. 1991;7(3):141.

Suhler A, Bornmann PG, Scott JW. The lactation consultant as expert witness. *J Hum Lact*. 1991;7(3):129–140.

ETHICAL AND LEGAL ISSUES QUESTIONS

Notice on question numbering: J-000 means a basic question, with one correct answer and three wrong answers. JP-000, along with the camera icon, means there is a picture that needs to be viewed to answer the question. The pictures are located on the CD-ROM included with this book and are numbered to correspond with the questions. JN-000, along with the frowning face icon, means the question has a NEGATIVE stem; therefore, read the entire question very carefully to find the one WRONG answer among the choices. JPN-000, with both icons in the margin, means there is a picture associated with the question AND the question has a negative stem. See Appendix A for a fuller explanation of negative stem questions.

J-001. In order to minimize your legal risk when practicing as a lactation consultant, it is most important for you to:

a. keep accurate financial records.
b. obtain detailed information from the primary care provider(s).
c. establish a respectful rapport with open communication.
d. accept the client's insurance payment plan.

J-002. Guidelines from the US Centers for Disease Control and Prevention state that healthcare workers should wear gloves when assisting breastfeeding mothers in which of the following situations?

a. when touching a mother's breast
b. when positioning a baby at breast
c. when helping a mother pump her milk
d. when processing donor human milk

J-003. Which of the following is considered fair use of published written material, according to international copyright law?

a. downloading or photocopying one copy of a published research article for your personal use
b. making copies of a research article for all participants in your for-profit breastfeeding course
c. using pictures downloaded from the Internet in your presentations or lectures
d. making lecture handouts that include reproductions of copyrighted images that you purchased

J-004. An 8-day-old infant has been at breast constantly since birth. His mother complains of nipple pain and states that her baby makes a clicking sound and loses his grasp of her nipple frequently during the feed. You have corrected her latch-on technique. Your next action should be:

a. provide her with a sterile nipple shield.
b. instruct her to use several different breastfeeding positions.
c. instruct her in suck training to correct the baby's sucking.
d. refer her to a health professional qualified to evaluate for tongue-tie.

JN-005. A mother's breast is very hard and painful. All of the following interventions are appropriate **EXCEPT**:

a. documenting her history leading up to this situation.
b. wearing gloves and assessing the degree of milk stasis in the breast tissue.
c. cleaning the incision and surrounding skin with an antiseptic solution.
d. gently teaching or assisting in expressing milk from the injured breast.

JP-006. When a breastfeeding baby has this condition, the first thing you would do is:

a. treat the baby and the mother's breast for a fungal infection.
b. check the child for other manifestations of allergic responses.
c. advise the mother to change the baby's diaper more frequently.
d. have the mother apply a cortisone ointment on the rash.

JP-007. The first thing that the lactation consultant should do for this mother's nipple condition is:

a. request that the primary provider culture the skin for infection.
b. wash off the white substance to examine the underlying skin.
c. position the baby deeper onto the breast to prevent friction on the nipple tip.
d. instruct the mother to massage expressed milk into the nipple tip.

 JPN-008. Documentation of this woman's breasts would include all of the following **EXCEPT**:

a. Breasts are asymmetric with a pinkish nipple/areola complex.
b. Right beast is very small; left breast is of moderate size and saggy.
c. Both breasts have scanty palpable glandular tissue.
d. Right breast has insufficient glandular tissue for lactation.

J-009. Which of the following practices is the most appropriate action to take in the hospital's labor and delivery (birthing) area?

a. Make sure the baby can take formula by bottle before attempting to breastfeed.
b. Read the hospital policies to the mother before she is admitted in labor.
c. Deep-suction the baby before feeding with oral fluids including breast milk or colostrum.
d. Give the baby only mother's own milk or colostrum unless medically indicated.

J-010. A disgruntled family files a malpractice suit after you provided lactation consultant services to them. The first thing you should do is:

a. call an attorney.
b. contact your professional insurance agent.
c. talk to the couple to find out why they are upset.
d. speak to the couple's physician.

J-011. Which of the following documents applies to lactation consultants?

a. *Global Strategy for Infant & Young Child Feeding*
b. IBLCE's *Standards of Practice*
c. ILCA's *Position Paper on Infant Feeding*
d. *International Code of Marketing of Breast-Milk Substitutes*

J-012. Which of the following actions is a violation of the *International Code of Marketing of Breast-Milk Substitutes*?

a. providing free samples of formula to all mothers who visit your clinic
b. teaching formula-feeding individually to mothers who have made the decision not to breast-feed
c. including bottles with the breast-pump kits you sell to mothers who are returning to work
d. recommending a teat-style feeding device for a baby with a sucking disorder

J-013. After giving your first lecture at a professional conference, you learn that the luncheon will be provided by an infant formula company. Your best response is to:

a. Eat the lunch quietly with other participants, because raising the issue would embarrass the conference sponsor.
b. Refuse to eat the luncheon and find another source for your food for that meal.
c. Announce from the speaker's stand that you are offended and refuse to give the rest of your lectures.
d. Thank the formula company publicly from the podium for their support of the conference.

J-014. Your client's baby is having problems breastfeeding and appears to have oral thrush. She requests that you NOT report your findings to the baby's pediatrician. Your best response is to:

a. Inform her that lactation consultants are required to communicate relevant information to the primary healthcare provider(s).
b. Agree to keep this information confidential.
c. Provide information on over-the-counter treatments for oral thrush.
d. Immediately discontinue providing breastfeeding care to this mother.

J-015. You are about to assess a breastfeeding mother–baby dyad. What should you do first?

a. Obtain written consent from the mother.
b. Weigh the baby on a sensitive scale.
c. Examine the mother's breasts.
d. Wash your hands for 2 minutes.

J-016. Which of the following educational opportunities violates the *International Code of Marketing of Breast-Milk Substitutes*?

a. conferences sponsored by breastfeeding-mother-support organizations or lactation consultant professional associations
b. college courses in lactation management
c. short courses and distance learning programs run by lactation education organizations
d. in-service programs presented by scientists employed by formula companies

J-017.   You recently read a published article by an International Board-Certified Lactation Consultant that sounds very much like something you wrote several years ago. Comparing the two documents confirms that you were correct. What is your next course of action?

a.   The article has already been published. There is nothing further you can do.
b.   Contact the writer directly to voice your concerns.
c.   Contact the publisher of the magazine to voice your concerns and request the material be properly cited in print.
d.   Begin legal proceedings against the writer for plagiarism.

J-018.   Which of the following situations is a violation of the ethical principle of role fidelity?

a.   An IBCLC in private practice tells her clients to take fenugreek to increase milk supply.
b.   A physician/IBCLC prescribes metoclopramide for low milk supply.
c.   An IBCLC instructs a mother on methods to increase a low milk supply and helps her to rent an electric breast pump.
d.   A nurse/IBCLC assists the mother of a preemie to increase her milk supply by increasing frequency of pumping and refers her to a physician for a prescription.

J-019.   A breastfeeding mother asks about taking an herbal remedy for migraine headaches. Your best response is:

a.   Herbs do not pass into milk, so whatever you take should be safe.
b.   Comfrey is a good choice.
c.   Please discuss this with your physician and a qualified herbalist.
d.   Migraines are best treated with prescription drugs.

J-020.   A pregnant mother is HIV-positive but otherwise healthy. Breastfeeding is expected in her culture and her family and is her personal strong desire. The first thing you should do is:

a.   tell her breastfeeding is contraindicated for HIV-positive mothers.
b.   tell her breastfeeding is safe for the first 6 weeks only.
c.   have her talk to her doctor and abide by that decision.
d.   share research and recommendations of WHO, CDC, and UNICEF.

J-021.   A lactation consultant operates a private breast-pump rental depot from her home and is employed by a hospital maternity unit. If a mother must leave the hospital without her baby, the lactation consultant tells the mother about her own rental depot but not others in the community. This behavior is:

a.   legal and ethical.
b.   illegal and unethical.
c.   a conflict of interest.
d.   a valuable service to patients.

J-022. You are planning to stock several kinds of breastfeeding equipment in your private practice. Which item most increases your professional liability?

a. cloth baby slings made by a commercial manufacturer
b. 30-ml syringes that have been altered for use as nipple-pulling devices
c. manual breast pumps distributed by a formula company
d. small plastic cups made for storing food

J-023. A speaker's lecture title is very similar to a lecture you've prepared and presented at a large conference recently. You have not given anyone else permission to use your particular lecture material. What is the first action you should take?

a. Report the speaker to the Ethics Committee of IBLCE.
b. Contact the speaker and find out if proper attribution is being made in the presentation.
c. Contact your attorney to investigate whether the speaker violated copyright laws.
d. Ignore the situation under the assumption that lactation consultants may independently create similar material.

J-024. You have a contract to lecture and you discover that the organizer of the event has created an electronic advertising flyer with a downloaded image from the Internet that links to a company that violates the *International Code of Marketing of Breast-Milk Substitutes*. What should be your first action?

a. Immediately cancel your contract.
b. Insist that the organizer remove the image and issue a disclaimer immediately.
c. Have your attorney contact the organizer regarding possible slander charges.
d. Ignore it—most people won't click on the image anyway.

JN-025. Which of the following situations **DOES NOT** require written documentation?

a. phone calls from clients
b. bedside contacts with mothers in a hospital
c. clinic or office visits when the primary care provider also sees the client
d. telephone inquiries about business hours or prices

JN-026. A mother is divorcing the father of her 7-month-old, breastfeeding child. The father wants her to wean immediately so the child will not miss his mother in the middle of the night when the child is with him. The lactation consultant has been asked by the mother to testify as an expert witness. Your lactation consultant's role would include all of the following actions **EXCEPT:**

a. charging your usual fees for this service.
b. preparing a written statement or deposition.
c. giving your professional opinion about the baby's needs.
d. encouraging the mother to comply with the father's wishes.

JN-027. Which of the following activities is **NOT** prohibited by the *International Code of Marketing of Breast-Milk Substitutes*?

a. giving gift packs containing samples and coupons for formula to new mothers at hospital discharge
b. providing detailed information on product composition to health workers
c. advertising toddler formula on local television stations
d. showing a picture of a happy baby on the label of infant formula containers

JN-028. Which of the following statements about the lactation consultant profession is **NOT TRUE?**

a. The lactation consultant profession began in 1985 with the first examination sponsored by IBLCE.
b. Lactation consultants must be licensed health professionals before entering the field.
c. The International Lactation Consultant Association is the professional association for lactation consultants.
d. The *Journal of Human Lactation* is a peer-reviewed journal dealing exclusively with breastfeeding topics.

JN-029. All of the following collaborations are appropriate for an IBCLC **EXCEPT**:

a. providing newsletters from the local mother-support group to mothers in your practice.
b. working closely with a registered dietitian in the case of a baby diagnosed with PKU (phenylketonuria).
c. obtaining a referral from a surgeon before providing breastfeeding help to the mother of a newborn with an unrepaired cleft palate.
d. discussing a feverish mother's inflamed breast with her physician to develop an appropriate care plan that preserves breastfeeding.

JN-030. Which of the following actions by an IBCLC is **NOT** within the lactation consultant's scope of practice?

a. examining a breastfeeding mother's breast
b. developing supplementing policies for the NICU
c. dispensing and instructing on the use of breast pumps
d. advising a mother that prescribed medication is safe to use during breastfeeding

☹ **JN-031.**   A mother tells you that the pediatrician has recommended that she give artificial baby milk after each breastfeeding to her slow-gaining, 9-week-old infant. What would **NOT** be an appropriate initial response?

a.   Offer alternative suggestions to frequent supplementation.
b.   Refer her to a different pediatrician.
c.   Refer her to a breastfeeding support group.
d.   Give information on how to provide supplemental feeding without compromising breastfeed-ing.

☹ **JN-032.**   A mother requests your help with her faltering milk supply. After ruling out breastfeed-ing management, which of the following would **NOT** be appropriate?

a.   Loan her a book about herbal preparations.
b.   Tell her to buy domperidone from an online pharmacy.
c.   Request that her physician conduct metabolic and endocrine tests.
d.   Suggest she discuss alternate therapies with her primary care provider.

☹ **JN-033.**   Which of the following actions by a healthcare worker is **NOT** a violation of the *International Code of Marketing of Breast-Milk Substitutes*?

a.   accepting a carton of a new, specialized formula for research at the institutional level
b.   distributing volu-feed bottles with formula logos to parents whose babies are in the neonatal intensive care unit
c.   using crib cards and measuring tapes with formula-company logos to cut hospital costs
d.   giving samples of two competing brands of formula to nonbreastfeeding mothers so they can test them

📷 ☹ **JPN-034.**   A mother reports painful nipples and asks about this white spot that she believes is a plugged nipple pore (bleb). You would do all of the following **EXCEPT**:

a.   carefully observe a full breastfeed, examine her breasts, and observe the baby's mouth.
b.   suggest she wash her nipples with water after every feed and massage the nipples' tip.
c.   use a sterile sharp instrument to open the plugged area of the nipple's tip.
d.   provide her with written material on plugged pores (nipple blebs) to discuss with her physi-cian.

ETHICAL AND LEGAL ISSUES ANSWERS

The parenthetical material at the end of each answer includes the discipline and time period, indicates whether the question pertains to knowledge or application, and specifies the degree of difficulty.

J-001. The answer is C. The most effective protection against legal actions is establishing a mutually respectful relationship and rapport. (Legal; General Principles; Knowledge; Difficulty: 4)

J-002. The answer is D. The US Centers for Disease Control does not require healthcare workers to wear gloves when assisting breastfeeding except in high-exposure situations such as donor milk banking. (Legal; General Principles; Knowledge; Difficulty: 5)

J-003. The answer is A. Making or downloading one copy of a copyrighted work for personal use is considered fair use. Making multiple copies without permission from the copyright holder violates copyright laws. Pictures and images posted on Internet sites are protected by international copyright laws. You may use legitimately purchased images in your presentations with proper attribution, but further distributing these images without specific permission, as in printed handouts, is not considered fair use. (Legal; General Principles; Application; Difficulty: 3)

J-004. The answer is D. This baby described is tongue-tied. Frenotomy (incision of the lingual frenulum) is an appropriate and effective treatment, especially when ordinary lactation techniques have not been helpful. The next action for the lactation consultant is to put the mother in contact with a professional who is qualified to evaluate and treat this anatomic condition of the infant. (Legal; 3–14 days; Application; Difficulty: 5)

JN-005. The answer is C. Wound cleaning is not a standard part of lactation consultant practice. The other actions are appropriate. (Legal; 7–12 months; Application; Difficulty: 3)

JP-006. The answer is B. This rash on the baby's thigh is one manifestation of allergic responses (atopic disease). A lactation consultant may not make a diagnosis nor prescribe, so A and D are inappropriate responses. (Legal; General Principles; Application; Difficulty: 5)

JP-007. The answer is A. This is a bacterial infection of the nipple; therefore, the lactation consultant should arrange for a medical provider to properly diagnose the infection. Washing with water and positioning the baby more deeply onto the breast are reasonable actions after medical diagnosis is in progress. Massaging expressed milk into the nipple is inappropriate because there is no benefit, and it could exacerbate the infection. (Legal; General Principles; Application; Difficulty: 4)

JPN-008. The answer is D. Determination of sufficient or insufficient glandular tissue for lactation cannot be determined by physical examination alone. This woman breastfed two children for over 2 years each. (Legal; General Principles; Application; Difficulty: 5)

J-009. The answer is D. Direct breastfeeding is the norm. All other feeding methods are considered interventions with known and unknown consequences. The Baby-Friendly Hospital Initiative clearly documents the acceptable reasons for supplementing a breastfed baby. (Legal; Labor/Birth; Knowledge; Difficulty: 3)

J-010. The answer is B. Professional malpractice insurance companies have access to qualified attorneys for their clients in ethical and legal matters. (Legal; General Principles; Knowledge; Difficulty: 3)

J-011. The answer is B. Standards of practice apply to lactation consultants. (Legal; General Principles; Knowledge; Difficulty: 4)

J-012. The answer is A. Providing free samples of infant formula to mothers is a violation of the International Code. (Legal; General Principles; Application; Difficulty: 4)

J-013. The answer is B. Lactation consultants are expected to avoid situations that would put them into an ethical conflict of interest. Refusal to eat the sponsored food is appropriate. Avoiding the issue simply supports the conflict of interest. Although refusing to participate in the rest of the meeting would strongly raise the issue to everyone at the meeting, that action may not be the best for that particular situation. Option D is inappropriate and violates the code of ethics for lactation consultants. (Legal; General Principles; Application; Difficulty: 3)

J-014. The answer is A. Communicating relevant information to primary care provider(s) is required of lactation consultants. (Legal; General Principles; Application; Difficulty: 3)

J-015. The answer is A. Consent must be obtained before touching the mother or baby or taking photographs. Unwanted touching could be considered battery. Written consent is preferred over verbal. The other actions are appropriate after obtaining consent from the mother. (Legal; General Principles; Knowledge; Difficulty: 2)

J-016.   The answer is D. Education provided by sources with a conflict of interest is inappropriate and is likely to be inaccurate and unhelpful. (Legal; General Principles; Knowledge; Difficulty: 2)

J-017.   The answer is C. Contacting the publisher is the next appropriate step to take. If the publisher does not respond, further legal action may be an option. Meanwhile, you may elect to lodge a formal complaint with the IBLCE for violation of intellectual property laws. (Legal; General Principles; Application; Difficulty: 5)

J-018.   The answer is A. Telling a client to take an herbal preparation for milk supply issues falls outside the legitimate scope of practice of IBCLCs. Role fidelity is one of the principles of biomedical ethics. Role fidelity means that individuals caring for patients/clients should practice within the scope of practice for which they are qualified. Operating outside one's scope of practice is a violation of an ethical principle that can lead to harm for the patient. (Legal; General Principles; Application; Difficulty: 2)

J-019.   The answer is C. Herbs can pass into milk and exert an effect on the baby. Giving pharmaceutical advice is not within the scope of practice of the lactation consultant. (Legal; General Principles; Application; Difficulty: 2)

J-020.   The answer is D. WHO, UNICEF, and other authorities support providing the mother with confidential and individualized information to help her make a fully informed decision regarding feeding her baby. The lactation consultant's role is to assist the primary care physician and mother by providing appropriate research and other literature on the topic. (Legal; Prenatal; Application; Difficulty: 5)

J-021.   The answer is C. Referring to one's self is a conflict of interest. (Legal; 3–14 days; Knowledge; Difficulty: 4)

J-022.   The answer is B. Products and equipment used or distributed by a lactation consultant must be covered by the product liability insurance of the manufacturer. Altered syringes would not be covered by product liability insurance and would put the LC at greatest liability. (Legal; General Principles; Application; Difficulty: 4)

J-023.   The answer is B. It may be a breach of the code of ethics if the speaker did not ask permission to use your material and does not properly attribute its source. IBCLCs are required to obtain permission from the original source of printed, visual, or other intellectual property. (Legal; General Principles; Application; Difficulty: 4)

J-024.   The answer is B. International board-certified lactation consultants are governed by the code of ethics. Cooperating in an event where intellectual property laws regarding images on the Internet were probably violated, and permitting a fraudulent link to a code-violating company, could put the IBCLC in violation of the code of ethics. (Legal; General Principles; Application; Difficulty: 3)

JN-025.   The answer is D. Inquiries about price, hours, or other business transactions do not require written documentation. All clinical contacts, including those by phone, should be documented. (Legal; General Principles; Knowledge; Difficulty: 2)

JN-026.   The answer is D. The lactation consultant may be asked to serve as an expert witness in divorce and custody situations involving a breastfed baby or lactating mother. The lactation consultant should always assist the mother in maintaining an intact and appropriate breastfeeding relationship with her child. (Legal; 7–12 months; Application; Difficulty: 2)

JN-027.   The answer is B. The International Code specifies that information on artificial feeding provided to health workers should be scientific and accurate. Detailed accurate information on product composition is appropriate marketing of products within the scope of the Code. (Legal; General Principles; Knowledge; Difficulty: 2)

JN-028.   The answer is B. The lactation consultant profession is open to individuals from a variety of backgrounds. As of this writing, holding a license in another health field is not a prerequisite for taking the IBLCE examination. (Legal; General Principles; Knowledge; Difficulty: 2)

JN-029.   The answer is C. The lactation consultant does not need a referral from a physician before assisting a baby with cleft palate to breastfeed. She should always work closely and collaboratively with the baby's physician(s) especially after any surgery for repair of the cleft. (Legal; General Principles; Knowledge; Difficulty: 2)

JN-030. The answer is D. Lactation consultants do not determine the safety of prescribed medications. It is within the IBCLC's scope of practice to provide references and written information to parents and providers of care. (Legal; General Principles; Knowledge; Difficulty: 2)

JN-031. The answer is B. The lactation consultant is expected to communicate relevant information to the primary care provider(s). Referring her to another physician as the first strategy in helping her is inappropriate, although if she asks for the names of other providers, the lactation consultant should follow appropriate referral guidelines and provide these names. (Legal; 1–3 months; Knowledge; Difficulty: 2)

JN-032. The answer is B. Lactation consultants may not prescribe nor directly refer the mother to sources of medications. The IBCLC may provide information to the mother, work with her physician to identify medical conditions, and/or discuss alternative therapies with her primary care provider. (Legal; 1–3 months; Application; Difficulty: 5)

JN-033. The answer is A. The *International Code of Marketing of Breast-Milk Substitutes*, Article 7.4, states that, "samples of infant formula or other products within the scope of this Code, or of equipment or utensil for their preparation or use, should not be provided to health workers except when necessary for the purpose of professional evaluation or research at the institutional level." (Legal; General Principles; Knowledge; Difficulty: 3)

JPN-034. The answer is C. It is not within the scope of practice of lactation consultants to perform procedures, diagnose illnesses, or prescribe medications, even over-the-counter preparations. All of the other actions are appropriate. (Legal; > 12 months; Application; Difficulty: 4)

Scoring:

Total number of questions in this section _____

Number of questions answered correctly _____

Percent correct (divide number correct by total number) _____

K. BREASTFEEDING EQUIPMENT AND TECHNOLOGY

In the 2000 exam blueprint, 10 to 16 questions are dedicated to breastfeeding equipment and technology.

SUBTOPICS INCLUDED IN THIS CATEGORY

1. Identification of breastfeeding devices and equipment

    a. Milk expression and removal devices
    b. Feeding devices
    c. Other devices, including social
    d. Appropriate use and technical expertise in using them properly

2. Donor human milk banking

    a. Handling and storage
    b. Protocols

CORE READING

Textbooks

Auerbach K, Riordan J. *Clinical Lactation: A Visual Guide.* Sudbury, MA: Jones & Bartlett Publishers; 2000.

Best Practice for Pumping, Storing and Handling of Mother's Own Milk in Hospital and at Home. Raleigh, NC: Human Milk Banking Association of North America; 2006.

Brodribb W, ed. *Breastfeeding Management.* Melbourne: Australian Breastfeeding Association; 2004.

Cadwell K, Turner-Maffei C. *Breastfeeding A–Z: Terminology and Telephone Triage.* Sudbury, MA: Jones & Bartlett Publishers; 2006.

Cadwell K, Turner-Maffei C. *Case Studies in Breastfeeding: Problem Solving Skills and Strategies.* Sudbury, MA: Jones & Bartlett Publishers; 2006.

Guidelines for the Establishment and Operation of a Donor Human Milk Bank. Raleigh, NC: Human Milk Banking Association of North America; 2006.

Lang S. *Breastfeeding Special Care Babies.* Edinburgh: Bailliere Tindall; 2002.

Lauwers J, Swisher A. *Counseling the Nursing Mother.* 4th ed. Sudbury, MA: Jones & Bartlett Publishers; 2003.

Lawrence RA, Lawrence RM. *Breastfeeding: A Guide for the Medical Profession.* 6th ed. St. Louis: Elsevier Mosby; 2005.

Morbacher N, Stock J. *The Breastfeeding Answer Book.* 3rd ed. Schaumburg, IL: La Leche League International; 2003.

The Royal College of Midwives, UK. *Successful Breastfeeding.* London: Churchill Livingstone; 2003.

Walker M. *Breastfeeding Management for the Clinician: Using the Evidence.* Sudbury, MA: Jones & Bartlett Publishers; 2006.

Wilson-Clay B, Hoover K. *The Breastfeeding Atlas.* 3rd ed. Austin, TX: Lactnews Press; 2005.

Key Research Articles

Alekseev NP, Ilyin VI, Yaroslavski VK, et al. Compression stimuli increase the efficacy of breast pump function. *Eur J Obstet Gynecol Reprod Biol.* 1998;77(2):131–139.

Chamberlain LB, McMahon M, Philipp BL, Merewood A. Breast pump access in the inner city: A hospital-based initiative to provide breast pumps for low-income women. *J Hum Lact.* 2006;22(1):94–98.

Chapman DJ, Young S, Ferris AM, Perez-Escamilla R. Impact of breast pumping on lactogenesis stage II after cesarean delivery: A randomized clinical trial. *Pediatrics.* 2001;107(6):E94.

Daley HK, Kennedy CM. Meta analysis: Effects of interventions on premature infants feeding. *J Perinat Neonatal Nurs.* 2000;14(3):62–77.

Dowling DA. Physiological responses of preterm infants to breast-feeding and bottle-feeding with the orthodontic nipple. *Nurs Res.* 1999;48(2):78–85.

Dowling DA, Madigan E, Siripul P. The effect of fluid density and volume on the accuracy of test weighing in a simulated oral feeding situation. *Adv Neonatal Care.* 2004;4(3):158–165.

Dowling DA, Meier PP, DiFiore JM, Blatz MA, Martin RJ. Cup-feeding for preterm infants: Mechanics and safety. *J Hum Lact.* 2002;18(1):13–20.

Groh-Wargo S, Toth A, Mahoney K, Simonian S, Wasser T, Rose S. The utility of a bilateral breast pumping system for mothers of premature infants. *Neonatal Netw.* 1995;14(8):31–36.

Jones E, Dimmock PW, Spencer SA. A randomised controlled trial to compare methods of milk expression after preterm delivery. *Arch Dis Child Fetal Neonatal Ed.* 2001;85(2):F91–F95.

Kent JC, Ramsay DT, Doherty D, Larsson M, Hartmann PE. Response of breasts to different stimulation patterns of an electric breast pump. *J Hum Lact.* 2003;19(2):179–186; quiz, 87–88, 218.

Kuehl J. Cup feeding the newborn: What you should know. *J Perinat Neonatal Nurs.* 1997;11(2):56–60.

Marinelli KA, Burke GS, Dodd VL. A comparison of the safety of cupfeedings and bottlefeedings in premature infants whose mothers intend to breastfeed. *J Perinatol.* 2001;21(6):350–355.

Meier P, Hurst N, Rodriguez N, et al. Comfort and effectiveness of the Symphony breast pump for mothers of preterm infants: Comparison of three suction patterns. *Adv Exp Med Biol.* 2004;554:321–323.

Mitoulas LR, Lai CT, Gurrin LC, Larsson M, Hartmann PE. Effect of vacuum profile on breast milk expression using an electric breast pump. *J Hum Lact.* 2002;18(4):353–360.

Mitoulas LR, Lai CT, Gurrin LC, Larsson M, Hartmann PE. Efficacy of breast milk expression using an electric breast pump. *J Hum Lact.* 2002;18(4):344–352.

Mitoulas LR, Ramsay DT, Kent JC, Larsson M, Hartmann PE. Identification of factors affecting breast pump efficacy. *Adv Exp Med Biol.* 2004;554:325–327.

Ramsay DT, Mitoulas LR, Kent JC, et al. Milk flow rates can be used to identify and investigate milk ejection in women expressing breast milk using an electric breast pump. *Breastfeed Med.* 2006;1(1):14–23.

Ramsay DT, Mitoulas LR, Kent JC, Larsson M, Hartmann PE. The use of ultrasound to characterize milk ejection in women using an electric breast pump. *J Hum Lact.* 2005;21(4):421–428.

Sisk PM, Lovelady CA, Dillard RG, Gruber KJ. Lactation counseling for mothers of very low birth weight infants: Effect on maternal anxiety and infant intake of human milk. *Pediatrics.* 2006;117(1):e67–e75.

BREASTFEEDING EQUIPMENT AND TECHNOLOGY QUESTIONS

Notice on question numbering: KA-000 means a basic question, with one correct answer and three wrong answers. KP-000, along with the camera icon, means there is a picture that needs to be viewed to answer the question. The pictures are located on the CD-ROM included with this book and are numbered to correspond with the questions. KN-000, along with the frowning face icon, means the question has a NEGATIVE stem; therefore, read the entire question very carefully to find the one WRONG answer among the choices. KPN-000, with both icons in the margin, means there is a picture associated with the question AND the question has a negative stem. See Appendix A for a fuller explanation of negative stem questions.

K-001.   In the global context, the foremost benefit of using an open cup for feeding a preterm baby who cannot yet breastfeed is that it:

a.   is inexpensive and readily available.
b.   has a low risk of fluid aspiration.
c.   fosters appropriate tongue motions.
d.   is easy to clean.

K-002.   The standard temperature and time for Holder pasteurization used in donor human milk banks are:

a.   87°C for 10 minutes
b.   70°C for 25 minutes
c.   62.5°C for 30 minutes
d.   60°C for 60 minutes

K-003.   A full-term baby 13 hours old has not yet been to breast. Your first choice to feed this baby is by:

a.   a curved-tip syringe.
b.   an open cup.
c.   a bottle with preemie nipple (teat).
d.   putting the baby to breast.

K-004.   Additional body contact, as when the mother uses a soft tie-on type carrier, is most likely to have which of the following effects?

a.   decreased total crying
b.   increased dependency
c.   delayed walking
d.   more night waking

K-005. A mother is collecting milk for her ill, premature baby. Which is the best container for her milk?

a. open plastic cups or bottles
b. soft plastic polyethylene (nurser) bags
c. large containers holding several feeds
d. glass containers with airtight lids

K-006. Which of the following is a result of pasteurizing donor human milk?

a. concentration of lipids
b. reduction in lactose
c. no change in secretory IgA
d. destruction of lactoferrin

K-007. An effective technique for hand expression of milk is to:

a. compress the breast behind the areola, then slide the fingers toward the nipple.
b. pinch the base of the nipple.
c. press deeply at the nipple-areolar juncture.
d. position fingers at the edge of the areola, press inward, and roll toward the nipple.

KN-008. During a routine examination in her second trimester of pregnancy, a woman is discovered to have nonprotractile nipples. All of the following increase the probability that she will successfully breastfeed **EXCEPT**:

a. wearing breast shells for increasing amounts of time per day throughout the remainder of her pregnancy.
b. appropriate positioning and latch-on techniques.
c. breastfeeding the baby during the first hour after birth.
d. nonpharmaceutical pain-relief strategies for labor and birth.

KN-009. Pacifier (dummy, soother) use is associated with all of the following **EXCEPT**:

a. improved dental development.
b. increase in ear infections.
c. increase in oral thrush.
d. shorter duration of breastfeeding.

KP-010. Breast shells would be most helpful for this mother to:

a. evert her nipples.
b. protect the damaged skin from clothing.
c. protect the nipple tip from the baby's palate.
d. reduce areolar edema.

KP-011. This mother just finished pumping her milk. The most likely explanation for the condition pictured is:

a. nipple thrush.
b. the pump flange was too small in diameter.
c. Reynaud's phenomenon.
d. the pump has everted her nipples.

KP-012. This mother has been using a piece of equipment to help resolve her breastfeeding problem. Which is the most likely product that she used?

a. nipple shields
b. breast shells
c. bottle teat placed over her nipple
d. breast pump

KP-013. The breastfeeding equipment shown in this photograph is most likely being used for:

a. provision of sufficient calories while increasing the milk supply.
b. training the baby at the breast to suck correctly and effectively.
c. ensuring adequate caloric intake because this baby is too small to obtain enough nourishment.
d. aiding this baby to attach correctly to the breast and continue sucking.

KPN-014. You would recommend this technique for all of the following **EXCEPT**:

a. premature baby.
b. separation of mother and baby for any reason.
c. mother taking a contraindicated medication.
d. a mother who has a history of sexual abuse.

KPN-015. This mother complains of sharp nipple pain. Your suggestions should include all of the following **EXCEPT**:

a. apply purified lanolin to the irritated area.
b. wear a silicone nipple shield during feeds.
c. wear breast shells between feeds.
d. bring the baby deeply onto the breast.

KN-016. An effective breast pump should have all of the following features **EXCEPT** that it:

a. transfers milk effectively.
b. is painless for the mother.
c. operates at 20–40 cycles per minute.
d. applies 100–250 mm Hg pressure.

KN-017. The use of teats (artificial nipples) should be avoided for all of the following reasons **EXCEPT**:

a. teats can alter the shape of the oral cavity.
b. the liquid can flow too rapidly.
c. the teat may stimulate the palate and trigger suck.
d. teats can change oral motor patterning.

KN-018. When selecting a device to assist breastfeeding, all of the following are principles to follow **EXCEPT**:

a. first, do no harm.
b. select the least expensive device.
c. use the least intervention for the shortest time.
d. obtain informed consent from the mother.

KN-019. Which is the **LEAST SIGNIFICANT** risk of using a nipple shield?

a. easy to misplace
b. changes in baby's oral-motor response
c. significant blockage of milk flow
d. shortened duration of breastfeeding

KP-020. This mother's baby is 4 days old. She is most likely using this equipment to:

a. remove excess milk.
b. stimulate the breast to make milk.
c. correct inverted nipples.
d. prevent mastitis.

KPN-021. The equipment shown in this picture could be appropriately used for all of the following **EXCEPT**:

a. inducing lactation when the baby is adopted.
b. supplementing an impaired baby at breast.
c. correcting a baby's dysfunctional sucking pattern.
d. aiding the mother to reestablish breastfeeding after an interruption.

KPN-022. Consequences of using this equipment include all of the following **EXCEPT**:

a. release of stress hormones in the baby.
b. neonatal hypothermia.
c. facilitation of maternal access to the infant.
d. increased crying.

KPN-023. Advantages of using this alternative feeding technique include all of the following **EXCEPT** that it:

a. is easy to clean the equipment.
b. can pace to the baby's ability.
c. prevents nipple confusion.
d. is inexpensive.

BREASTFEEDING EQUIPMENT AND TECHNOLOGY ANSWERS

The parenthetical material at the end of each answer includes the discipline and time period, indicates whether the question pertains to knowledge or application, and specifies the degree of difficulty.

K-001. The answer is D. Spoons and open cups are easier to clean than other feeding devices. (Equipment; Prematurity; Application; Difficulty: 4)

K-002. The answer is C. Holder pasteurization by donor human milk banks raises milk to 62.5°C for 30 minutes. (Equipment; General Principles; Knowledge; Difficulty: 5)

K-003. The answer is D. Direct breastfeeding should be tried first. Devices should only be considered when direct breastfeeding is impossible. (Equipment; 1–2 days; Application; Difficulty: 3)

K-004. The answer is A. Increased carrying when the baby is not fussy as well as when he is fussy reduces total crying per day. (Equipment; General Principles; Knowledge; Difficulty: 2)

K-005. The answer is D. Glass is a recommended storage container for mother's own milk. Hard plastic (polycarbonate or polypropylene) containers with lids are acceptable. (Equipment; General Principles; Knowledge; Difficulty: 2)

K-006. The answer is C. SIgA is stable to heat treatment and freezing. (Equipment; General Principles; Knowledge; Difficulty: 5)

K-007. The answer is D. The rolling action presses milk out of the milk duct sinuses toward the nipple. Little milk is stored in the ducts, but of the techniques listed, this is likely the most effective method for hand expressing. (Equipment; General Principles; Application; Difficulty: 3)

KN-008. The answer is A. Breast shells have not been found to be effective for correcting nonprotractile nipples. The other statements are all appropriate. (Equipment; Prenatal; Application; Difficulty: 2)

KN-009. The answer is A. Some allege that orthodontic shape pacifiers improve dentition, but research reveals more orthodontic problems in children who use pacifiers. (Equipment; 15–28 days; Knowledge; Difficulty: 2)

KP-010. The answer is B. Breast shells with wide backs will protect the injured skin from the rubbing of her bra or clothing. (Equipment; 3–14 days; Application; Difficulty: 3)

KP-011. The answer is B. The pump flange was too small in diameter for this mother's large, fibrous nipples. (Equipment; 1–2 days; Application; Difficulty: 4)

KP-012. The answer is B. The indentation visible on the areolar skin was caused by a breast shell placed over her nipple to allow air drying of the wound. (Equipment; 3–14 days; Application; Difficulty: 4)

KP-013. The answer is A. Nursing supplementers were designed to provide food at breast for an adopted baby so that the baby's sucking will help stimulate the mother's breast to make milk. There is no research evidence that feeding tube devices accomplish any of the other outcomes. (Equipment; 1–3 months; Application; Difficulty: 4)

KPN-014. The answer is D. A mother with a history of sexual abuse should first be encouraged to breastfeed. Only if direct breastfeeding is rejected should pumping be suggested. The other reasons for pumping are appropriate. (Equipment; 3–14 days; Application; Difficulty: 2)

KPN-015. The answer is B. A silicone nipple shield is the least helpful of the suggestions. The sore spot on her nipple tip is very tiny, and most often better positioning and latch will remedy the problem. (Equipment; 3–14 days; Application; Difficulty: 2)

KN-016. The answer is C. Pumps should have at least one setting operating at about the same number of cycles per minute as the baby would feed: 40–60 times per minute. (Equipment; General Principles; Knowledge; Difficulty: 3)

KN-017. The answer is C. Teats have significant drawbacks, yet in some circumstances can help stimulate a baby's suck response and aid in getting a baby to or back to breast. They should be used only rarely and only if other methods fail. (Equipment; Prematurity; Application; Difficulty: 2)

KN-018. The answer is B. The least expensive device may not be effective, nor is it necessarily the most appropriate device for the situation. (Equipment; General Principles; Application; Difficulty: 2)

KN-019. The answer is C. A thin silicone nipple shield has been found to permit adequate transfer of milk in most cases. Old, thick, or rigid designs blocked milk flow. A shield is fairly easy to keep clean and should be cleaned thoroughly after each use. However, the risk of contamination by pathogens is still present. The other risks listed are more significant. (Equipment; 3–14 days; Application; Difficulty: 5)

KP-020. The answer is A. On day 4, many mothers make more milk than their infants can consume. Use of a pump to remove excess milk can help prevent milk stasis and help the baby latch on and feed more effectively. (Equipment; 3–14 days; Application; Difficulty: 5)

KPN-021. The answer is C. Tube feeding devices do not correct a dysfunctional sucking pattern. The other answers could be appropriate uses. The device pictured is a Medela™ supplemental nursing system. (Equipment; 1–3 months; Application; Difficulty: 2)

KPN-022. The answer is C. Radiant warmers do not facilitate maternal access to the infant. Separation from the mother creates psychological and physical stress to the infant, including increased crying, more risk of hypothermia, and release of stress hormones. (Equipment; Labor/Birth; Application; Difficulty: 4)

KPN-023. The answer is C. Cup feeding may not necessarily prevent nipple confusion. The other answers are correct. (Equipment; 3–14 days; Application; Difficulty: 2)

Scoring:

Total number of questions in this section   _____

Number of questions answered correctly   _____

Percent correct (divide number correct by total number)   _____

L. TECHNIQUES

In the 2000 exam blueprint, 19 to 33 questions are dedicated to techniques.

SUBTOPICS INCLUDED IN THIS CATEGORY

1. Positioning, attachment/latch

2. Management skills

3. Assessing a breastfeed

    a. Observing; history
    b. Assessing infant suck, lactating breast, milk transfer
    c. Objective tools
    d. Care planning and following up

4. Kangaroo mother care (skin-to-skin care)

5. Normal feeding patterns

6. Milk expression

CORE READING

Textbooks

Auerbach K, Riordan J. *Clinical Lactation: A Visual Guide.* Sudbury, MA: Jones & Bartlett Publishers; 2000.

Brodribb W, ed. *Breastfeeding Management.* Melbourne: Australian Breastfeeding Association; 2004.

Cadwell K, Turner-Maffei C, O'Connor B, et al. *Maternal and Infant Assessment for Breastfeeding and Human Lactation: A Guide for the Practitioner.* 2nd ed. Sudbury, MA: Jones & Bartlett Publishers; 2006.

Cadwell K, Turner-Maffei C. *Breastfeeding A–Z: Terminology and Telephone Triage.* Sudbury, MA: Jones & Bartlett Publishers; 2006.

Cadwell K, Turner-Maffei C. *Case Studies in Breastfeeding: Problem Solving Skills and Strategies.* Sudbury, MA: Jones & Bartlett Publishers; 2006.

Clinical Competencies Checklist. Falls Church, VA: International Board of Lactation Consultant Examiners, 2003.

Kutner L, Barger J. *Clinical Experience in Lactation: A Blueprint for Internship.* Wheaton, IL: 1997.

Lauwers J, Swisher A. *Counseling the Nursing Mother.* 4th ed. Sudbury, MA: Jones & Bartlett Publishers; 2003.

Lawrence RA, Lawrence RM. *Breastfeeding: A Guide for the Medical Profession*. 6th ed. St. Louis: Elsevier Mosby; 2005.

Mohrbacher N, Kendall-Tackett KA. *Breastfeeding Made Simple: Seven Natural Laws for Nursing Mothers*. Oakland, CA: New Harbinger; 2005.

Morbacher N, Stock J. *The Breastfeeding Answer Book*. 3rd ed. Schaumburg, IL: La Leche League International; 2003.

Riordan J. *Breastfeeding and Human Lactation*. 3rd ed. Sudbury, MA: Jones & Bartlett Publishers; 2004.

Wilson-Clay B, Hoover K. *The Breastfeeding Atlas*. 3rd ed. Austin, TX: Lactnews Press; 2005.

Walker M. *Breastfeeding Management for the Clinician: Using the Evidence*. Sudbury, MA: Jones & Bartlett Publishers; 2006.

Wolf LS, Glass RP. *Feeding and Swallowing Disorders in Infancy: Assessment and Management*. San Antonio: Psych Corp; 1992.

Key Research Articles

Anderson GC, Moore E, Hepworth J, Bergman N. Early skin-to-skin contact for mothers and their healthy newborn infants. *Cochrane Database Syst Rev*. 2003(2):CD003519.

Bergman NJ, Linley LL, Fawcus SR. Randomized controlled trial of skin-to-skin contact from birth versus conventional incubator for physiological stabilization in 1200- to 2199-gram newborns. *Acta Paediatr*. 2004;93(6):779–785.

Conde-Agudelo A, Diaz-Rossello JL, Belizan JM. Kangaroo mother care to reduce morbidity and mortality in low birthweight infants (Cochrane review). *The Cochrane Library*. 2004(3).

Gray L, Miller LW, Philipp BL, Blass EM. Breastfeeding is analgesic in healthy newborns. *Pediatrics*. 2002;109(4):590–593.

Gray L, Watt L, Blass EM. Skin-to-skin contact is analgesic in healthy newborns. *Pediatrics*. 2000;105(1):e14.

Kent JC, Mitoulas LR, Cregan MD, Ramsay DT, Doherty DA, Hartmann PE. Volume and frequency of breast-feedings and fat content of breast milk throughout the day. *Pediatrics*. 2006;117(3):e387–e395.

Paul VK, Singh M, Deorari AK, Pacheco J, Taneja U. Manual and pump methods of expression of breast milk. *Indian J Pediatr*. 1996;63(1):87–92.

AUDIO-VISUAL

Frantz K. *First Attachment*. [DVD/videotape] Los Angeles: Geddes Productions; 2006.

Glover, Rebecca. *Follow Me Mum* [DVD/videotape]. Accessed Oct 1, 2006. Available at http://www.rebeccaglover.com.au

TECHNIQUES QUESTIONS

Notice on question numbering: L-000 means a basic question, with one correct answer and three wrong answers. LP-000, along with the camera icon, means there is a picture that needs to be viewed to answer the question. The pictures are located on the CD-ROM included with this book and are numbered to correspond with the questions. LN-000, along with the frowning face icon, means the question has a NEGATIVE stem; therefore, read the entire question very carefully to find the one WRONG answer among the choices. LPN-000, with both icons in the margin, means there is a picture associated with the question AND the question has a negative stem. See Appendix A for a fuller explanation of negative stem questions.

LN-001. A mother is planning for surgery to repair her 5-month-old child's cleft palate. Your suggestions would include all of the following **EXCEPT**:

a. wean your baby at least a week before the surgery.
b. prepare to stay with your baby around the clock.
c. practice expressing milk in case the baby cannot nurse directly.
d. expect your baby to nurse very frequently afterward for a while.

LN-002. Which is the **LEAST IMPORTANT** reason to use skin-to-skin (kangaroo mother care) for premature babies?

a. Mothers are more inclined to breastfeed and produce more milk.
b. Babies breastfeed from a younger gestational age and more frequently.
c. Babies can be discharged to home earlier and more fully breastfeeding.
d. The facility has a shortage of incubators (isolettes).

LP-003. This baby has been at breast about 20 minutes. What is your best recommendation to this mother?

a. Insert your finger to break the suction, then remove him.
b. Pull his buttocks in closer to you for a better latch.
c. Watch his sucking slow down as he prepares to self-detach.
d. Tickle his feet to wake him so he can finish the feed.

LP-004. This baby is having trouble feeding. Which suggestion is most likely to improve the situation?

a. Support your breast with your left hand.
b. Pull your baby's hips and legs in closer to your body.
c. Place a pillow under the baby's body.
d. Change to a horizontal position.

LP-005. This baby attaches to the breast, feeds steadily and comfortably for about 17 minutes, then releases the breast. Which of the following suggestions is most appropriate for mother?

a. Use your other hand to support your breast during feeds.
b. Bring your arm closer to your baby's neck.
c. No suggestions.
d. Pull your baby's legs closer to you.

 LP-006. The most important action to take in helping this mother breastfeed is:

a. have her wear a nipple shield during feedings.
b. have her hand-express milk before feeds to soften the large nipple area.
c. help the baby latch on to the breast deeply.
d. have her apply an antifungal preparation to the nipples after every feed.

 LP-007. Which actions are most likely to support the baby breastfeeding?

a. Lift the mother's breast into the baby's mouth.
b. Ask the mother to sit up and bring her baby to breast.
c. Support the baby while he crawls to the mother's breast.
d. Have the mother compress her breast and tickle the baby's lips.

 LP-008. The most appropriate advice you can give this mother on feeding patterns is:

a. your milk supply is very high, so use only one breast per feed.
b. start on the fuller breast for about 10 minutes, then switch to the other.
c. let the baby nurse on the first breast until he releases the breast on his own.
d. switch sides several times during a feed to make sure both sides get stimulated.

 LP-009. This mother complains of sudden-onset sore nipples. The first suggestion you would make or question you would ask is:

a. whether her baby has teeth.
b. tell the mother to roll the baby inward toward her, so the baby's entire front side is facing hers.
c. tell the mother to pull the baby's legs in closer to her.
d. whether she has taken an antibiotic recently.

LP-010. This condition has persisted for 2½ months. What is the most helpful action you could take for this mother?

a. Thoroughly examine the baby's nursing technique at breast.
b. Refer her to a dermatologist for further evaluation.
c. Provide her with moist wound-healing preparations.
d. Recommend she pump or express and feed the baby with a device.

LP-011. Which visual element of this baby's latch is most likely to indicate a problem?

a. deep puckering at the naso-labial crease
b. eyes closed
c. chin driven into the breast
d. nose barely touching the breast

LPN-012. Which is the **LEAST** appropriate treatment for this condition?

a. antifungal therapy
b. continued breastfeeding
c. breast binder for the mother
d. antibiotic therapy

L-013. A 38-week neonate with a birth weight of 3573 grams (7 lbs, 12 oz) is referred to you with a discharge weight of 3171 grams (6 lbs, 12 oz) at 72 hours postdelivery. The first thing you should do is:

a. weigh the infant to see if the hospital's scale was correct.
b. tell the mother that the weight loss is within normal range.
c. take a thorough history of the dyad's breastfeeding practices.
d. suggest she discuss any interventions with her baby's doctor.

L-014. A mother calls you complaining of breast pain. Her breasts are hot, hard, knotty, and painful to the touch. She is 3 days postpartum. The first suggestion you should give her is:

a. don't worry; your breasts will feel better in 24 hours.
b. use a nipple shield during feedings.
c. express or pump at least every 2–3 hours if your baby can't nurse well.
d. restrict your fluid intake.

L-015. Which of the following feeding patterns would be most likely in a 2-month-old, exclusively breastfed baby?

a. clustering feeds in the late morning
b. no feeding for 6–8 hours at night
c. feeds about every 3–4 hours during the day and one or two at night
d. 8–12 or more feeds spaced throughout the 24-hour day

L-016. Which component of human milk is destroyed by freezing?

a. lactoferrin
b. macrophages
c. lysozyme
d. secretory IgA

L-017. Twelve-hour-old Rose was born after 15 hours of hard labor and pushing, with forceps and vacuum extractor, deep-suctioned for meconium above the cords, and molded cranium and puncture mark from an internal monitor probe. Her mother is anxious to bond and breastfeed within the first hour after delivery. Rose is very sleepy. Your first intervention will be to:

a. bring Rose horizontally to her mother's breast level.
b. rub Rose's face with a cold washcloth.
c. pull Rose's chin down for a latch-on.
d. place Rose skin to skin with her mother and turn down the lights.

L-018. A baby begins sucking on his fists about 45 minutes after the last feed ended. His mother should:

a. give the baby a pacifier.
b. nurse the baby again.
c. change the baby's diaper.
d. wait until he cries, then feed him.

LN-019. An 18-hour-old baby has not yet successfully breastfed. He cues to feed but cannot stay on the breast. In order to help him suck better, which would be the **LEAST** effective strategy?

a. Bottle-feed him to help organize his suck.
b. Cup-feed him to increase calorie intake.
c. Use a nipple shield to increase sensation to his palate.
d. Use a supplementer at breast so his suck increases milk volume.

🙁 **LN-020.** A mother contacts you for help weaning her baby because she's going back to work in 4 weeks and has no place to express and store her milk. Your responses should include all of the following **EXCEPT**:

a. discussion of milk expression techniques and/or equipment.
b. information on storing milk at room temperature.
c. encouragement to wean completely.
d. support for partial breastfeeding during her off-work hours.

🙁 **LN-021.** You are working with a baby who has a unilateral cleft of the hard palate. The **LEAST** desirable intervention to suggest is:

a. to instruct the mother on proper attachment, showing her how to fill up the cleft with her breast.
b. to have her supplement with a bottle of artificial baby milk if the baby has difficulty maintaining proper suction at breast.
c. to instruct the mother on proper breast pumping frequency and technique to support her milk supply.
d. to have her feed the baby in upright positions to avoid nasopharyngeal reflux.

📷 **LP-022.** The most likely explanation for what this mother is doing is:

a. a pinch test for retraction.
b. a nipple rolling technique.
c. measuring the size of her areola.
d. hand-expressing her milk.

📷 **LP-023.** The mother in this picture is preparing to breastfeed her baby. Your first suggestion or comment would be:

a. great technique to firm your nipples!
b. move your hand back behind the areola to support your breast.
c. place the nipple tip in the baby's mouth.
d. pinching your nipple can injure the tissue.

📷 **LP-024.** This mother is 36 weeks pregnant. Your best recommendation would be:

a. rub your nipples with a towel twice a day.
b. be sure to breastfeed in the first hour postbirth.
c. pull and roll the nipple to stretch it.
d. you won't be able to breastfeed.

📷 **LP-025.** What is this mother doing?

a. expressing colostrum
b. doing a pinch test
c. everting her retracting nipple
d. nipple rolling to firm the tip

📷 **LP-026.** What technique is being shown in this picture?

a. checking for cleft palate
b. suck training
c. performing a digital oral assessment
d. checking for short frenulum

📷 **LP-027.** How is the baby pictured responding to this technique?

a. Baby is stressed.
b. Baby is shut down.
c. Baby is relaxed.
d. Baby is agitated.

📷 **LP-028.** This mother and baby are having difficulty breastfeeding. Your first suggestion to the mother should be to:

a. have her sit more upright.
b. lower her hand on the baby's back so the baby's head can extend slightly.
c. have her support her breast with her right hand.
d. swaddle the baby so the baby's hands don't interfere.

📷 **LP-029.** What is the first thing you would do to assist this mother?

a. Correct positioning and latch-on technique.
b. Apply an antibacterial ointment.
c. Apply an antifungal preparation.
d. Provide her with a silicone nipple shield.

📷 **LP-030.** This mother's baby is 4 months old. The most important thing you would do to help relieve this mother's discomfort is:

a. teach her how to keep her baby from squirming during feeds.
b. assist her baby to take more of the breast during latch-on.
c. provide a silicone nipple shield to reduce abrasion on the nipple skin.
d. help her get treatment for a probable nipple thrush infection.

LP-031. To relieve the condition pictured, your best recommendation is:

a. hand-express for a few minutes before each feed.
b. soak your nipples in warm water, then gently massage the tip.
c. wear breast shells between feeds.
d. apply an antifungal preparation after each feed.

LP-032. Which action or statement would be most helpful to this mother?

a. Try to get all of your areola into the baby's mouth.
b. Remove your bra so the baby can get a deep latch.
c. Support your breast from underneath, between your thumb and first finger.
d. Center your nipple in the baby's mouth, and lean forward to help him latch.

LP-033. What would be the most appropriate use for this technique?

a. helping a baby less than 24 hours old and not yet nursing
b. helping a 6-month-old refusing solid foods
c. assisting a baby with poor suck and a mother with damaged nipples
d. supplementing a 4-day-old baby who is 7% below birth weight

LP-034. This mother's baby is 20 hours old and has not yet effectively latched on and breastfed. What would be your first strategy to help them?

a. Place a silicone nipple shield over her nipples during feeds.
b. Have the mother pump her breasts to firm and evert the nipple tissue.
c. Remove her clothing and place the baby skin to skin on her chest.
d. Suggest she begin suck training to coordinate the baby's suck.

LP-035. This woman is in her third trimester of pregnancy. What is the most important action you could take to help her prepare to breastfeed?

a. Teach her good positioning and latch-on technique, using a doll as a model.
b. Provide her with breast shells to wear several hours a day.
c. Teach her Hoffman's techniques to prepare her nipples.
d. Instruct her to rub her nipples with a towel several times a day.

LP-036. This mother says she has been hand-expressing her milk as shown in the picture. Which is the most likely result of her using the technique pictured?

a. Milk is easily expressed.
b. Little or no milk flows.
c. The areola is bruised.
d. The nipple and areola become more elastic.

LP-037. This mother complains of pinpoint pain at the 1:00 position on her nipple. Your first suggestion to her would be:

a. use a sterile instrument to lift the flap of skin over that pore.
b. soak the nipple tip in warm water, then try to pop out the plug.
c. coat the nipple with an antifungal preparation.
d. nurse on that side as often as the baby is willing.

LP-038. This mother is preparing to feed. The next action she should take is to:

a. rub the nipple to make it firmer and more projectile.
b. move the bottom hand closer to the areola to better support the breast.
c. stop pulling back with the top hand.
d. bring the baby onto the breast.

LP-039. This baby is 2 weeks old and still under his birth weight. The mother's nipples are cracked, scabbed, and painful. Feeds are 30–45 minutes long every 2 hours around the clock. The mother is exhausted. The first recommendation you would give to his mother is:

a. have the baby's pediatrician or dentist evaluate his frenulum.
b. he's obviously upset—give him a pacifier to calm him before trying to breastfeed.
c. are you willing to try feeding him some expressed milk in a cup?
d. go to bed with him and try nursing lying down in a darkened room.

LP-040. This baby's mother is concerned about a clicking, smacking sound that occurs during nursing. Her nipples are mildly tender. Your first intervention would be to:

a. refer her for evaluation of the baby's tongue musculature.
b. assure good alignment and deep latch at breast.
c. perform a digital exam to assess tongue movement.
d. reassure her that some nipple tenderness is normal in early lactation.

LP-041. What is the first suggestion you would make to help this mother breastfeed more comfortably?

a. Place a nipple shield over your nipple until the baby's suck improves.
b. Wear a supportive bra 24 hours a day.
c. Support your breast with your hand during feeds.
d. Put some lanolin on your nipple before feeds.

LP-042. The adult's hand is most likely doing which of these procedures?

a. suck training or reorganization
b. digital oral exam or assessment
c. finger feeding
d. pacifying a crying/upset baby

LP-043. This baby had trouble latching and staying on breast and was not gaining weight. The mother's nipples were very painful at every feed. Attempting a deeper latch and better positioning did not improve the situation. The practitioner shown is most likely performing which of the following procedures?

a. frenectomy
b. frenotomy
c. tonsillectomy
d. myringotomy

LP-044. This picture was taken immediately after a baby ended a feeding. Which option most likely describes the preceding feed?

a. comfortable, with good milk transfer
b. comfortable, but with poor milk transfer
c. painful, but with good milk transfer
d. painful, with poor milk transfer

LP-045. What, if anything, would you suggest to this mother regarding her baby's position and latch?

a. Everything looks good.
b. Try uncurling his lower lip with your finger.
c. Tickle his feet so he wakes up during feeds.
d. Press down on your breast so his nostrils are clear.

LP-046. Which of the following suggestions is most likely to be helpful for the condition pictured?

a. Air-dry after feedings.
b. Expose the breast to a sunlamp placed about 1 ft (0.3 m) away.
c. Use moist wound-healing techniques or preparations.
d. Cover with a breast shell between feeds.

LP-047. A mother and baby are most likely to prefer the underarm (vertical) position for which of the following reasons?

a. The infant has greater head stability.
b. There is a stronger let-down reflex.
c. There is less chance of plugged milk ducts.
d. It reduces infant colic.

LP-048. This mother complains of severe pain beginning at latch-on and continuing during the entire feed. What is the first thing you would do?

a. Suggest that the mother attempt deeper attachment at breast.
b. Make sure the mother breaks the baby's suction at the end of feeds.
c. Weigh the baby before and after the next two consecutive feeds.
d. Have the mother try nursing lying down instead of sitting up.

LP-049. What is this mother doing with the hand that is not holding the device?

a. Tapping the breast to aid milk let-down.
b. Massaging milk toward the nipple to increase collected volume.
c. Pressing her breast more deeply into the flange.
d. Stroking the skin surface to increase milk synthesis.

LP-050. This mother is 4 days postpartum. Your first suggestion to assist her in breastfeeding should be:

a. support your breast and bring the baby to you.
b. use warm compresses to soften the areola.
c. use cool compresses to reduce edema.
d. express some milk to soften the breast.

LP-051. What is the first thing you would do to support this 5-hour-old baby and her mother?

a. Make sure she and her baby are undisturbed and comfortable in bed together.
b. Raise the side rails of the bed so the baby doesn't fall out.
c. Monitor the mother every 15 minutes to prevent her rolling onto her baby.
d. Remove the baby at the end of the feed so the mother can better rest.

LP-052. What is your best recommendation for the condition pictured?

a. Rub cocoa butter into the sore area.
b. Rinse with hydrogen peroxide several times a day.
c. Use a dressing designed for moist wound healing on the wound.
d. Apply vitamin E oil to the nipple tip.

LPN-053. You have just observed this mother feeding her baby. She describes nipple pain all throughout the feed. At the next feed, you would suggest all of the following **EXCEPT**:

a. bring the baby onto the breast more deeply.
b. wait until the baby's mouth is very wide open before latching.
c. everything looks good—do what you've been doing all along.
d. make sure the baby's lip is turned outward (flanged).

LPN-054. This baby has difficulty latching on to the breast and cannot sustain a sucking pattern for more than a few minutes. Which of the following suggestions would be **LEAST LIKELY** to help this baby breastfeed?

a. Position the baby in a vertical position with his head higher than his shoulders.
b. Reduce light and sound in the room.
c. Feed expressed mother's milk with an orthodontic shaped teat (nipple).
d. Handle the baby gently and slowly as if he has a headache.

LPN-055. Which visual aspect of this baby's latch is **LEAST LIKELY** to be a problem?

a. angle of the lips/mouth is about 90 degrees
b. puckering along the naso-labial crease
c. chin barely touches the breast
d. areola is nearly completely in the baby's mouth

LPN-056. This mother's baby is 4 months old. The **LEAST** appropriate suggestion you would offer this mother is:

a. see your doctor or a dermatologist for a diagnosis of these rashes.
b. have your baby's mouth cultured for possible infectious organisms.
c. keep a diary of all the foods you and your baby are eating.
d. start using a breast pump and feed the collected milk to the baby by another means.

LPN-057. This breastfeeding baby might demonstrate any of the following feeding patterns **EXCEPT**:

a. self-feeding with pincer grasp.
b. sipping liquids from an open cup.
c. self-weaning from the breast.
d. breastfeeding 8–16 times a day.

LPN-058. This technique is recommended for all of the following conditions **EXCEPT**:

a. Down syndrome.
b. premature baby.
c. mother with nipple thrush.
d. medicating the infant.

LPN-059. This 6-day-old baby has been nursing about every 4 hours during the day and once at night and has not returned to birth weight. The mother has asked for help breastfeeding. At the time this picture was taken, the baby had been sleeping since his last feed ended 3 hours ago. Your recommendations to the mother should include all of the following **EXCEPT**:

a. try giving him some expressed breast milk with a spoon right now.
b. please undress him so we can check his weight.
c. take him to his physician's office or an emergency room immediately.
d. let's see what he does at breast, even while he's sleepy.

L-060. Risks of using nipple shields may include all of the following **EXCEPT**:

a. reduction of milk flow.
b. changes in baby's oral-motor response.
c. reduced prolactin levels.
d. shortened duration of breastfeeding.

TECHNIQUES ANSWERS

The parenthetical material at the end of each answer includes the discipline and time period, indicates whether the question pertains to knowledge or application, and specifies the degree of difficulty.

LN-001. The answer is A. Hospitalization is usually a traumatic experience for the child, and the emotional comfort from breastfeeding is especially important at that time. (Techniques; 4–6 months; Application; Difficulty: 2)

LN-002. The answer is D. Although a shortage of equipment led to the development of kangaroo mother care, research now supports the other reasons as far more important. (Techniques; Prematurity; Application; Difficulty: 4)

LP-003. The answer is C. This baby is nearing the end of the feed on this breast and should be allowed to self-detach at his own pace. He is correctly positioned. (Techniques; 15–28 days; Application; Difficulty: 4)

LP-004. The answer is B. The baby's head is too extended relative to his trunk, so pulling the legs closer to the mother will better align the hips and shoulders. Supporting the breast will not correct the infant's position. The horizontal position and use of a pillow are not likely to help. (Techniques; 15–28 days; Application; Difficulty: 2)

LP-005. The answer is C. This baby is adequately attached and positioned for feeding, and the pattern is normal in length and comfortable for both mother and baby. While A, B, and D would be appropriate if the feeding pattern were uncomfortable or ineffective, suggesting too many technique changes could undermine the mother's confidence in breastfeeding. (Techniques; 15–28 days; Application; Difficulty: 2)

LP-006. The answer is C. Assuring proper positioning and latch is always the first action. This mother's bifurcated nipple was fully functional and the baby fed from this breast easily and effectively. (Techniques; 1–2 days; Application; Difficulty: 4)

LP-007. The answer is C. This baby is capable of crawling to the breast unassisted. Self-attachment suggests that the baby has completed the required behavioral sequencing and will suck normally and effectively. There is no indication that any of the other actions are necessary or even appropriate. (Techniques; Labor/Birth; Application; Difficulty: 3)

LP-008. The answer is C. Allowing the baby to set the pace of feeds is most appropriate. This mother has very large breasts, and the baby may even want to feed more than one time from one breast before switching sides. (Techniques; 3–14 days; Application; Difficulty: 4)

LP-009. The answer is B. The most likely explanation for sudden-onset soreness is poor positioning, causing pulling or tugging on the nipple skin. The first intervention would be correcting positioning and latch. The other choices are possibilities after poor positioning has been ruled out. (Techniques; 4–6 months; Application; Difficulty: 5)

LP-010. The answer is A. Always evaluate the baby's breastfeeding technique first. This mother's baby was tongue-tied, and friction from his tongue was causing the persistent nipple wound. (Techniques; 3–14 days; Application; Difficulty: 4)

LP-011. The answer is A. Deep puckering suggests poor tongue position or motion. In this case, the baby was tongue-tied. Feeding with the eyes closed is a lesser indicator of a problem. The chin and nose are well-positioned. (Techniques; 3–14 days; Application; Difficulty: 3)

LPN-012. The answer is C. Breast binders have not been found to be safe or effective for inflammatory conditions of the lactating breast. (Techniques; 3–14 days; Application; Difficulty: 5)

L-013. The answer is C. Assessing the dyad's current feeding patterns is the first step. After that, the other strategies may be appropriate. (Techniques; 3–14 days; Knowledge; Difficulty: 4)

L-014. The answer is C. The mother is experiencing milk stasis and inflammation, a common event on day 3. Removal of milk and control of edema are top priorities. (Techniques; 3–14 days; Application; Difficulty: 3)

L-015. The answer is D. The 1- to 3-month-old's feeds are usually spaced throughout the day and night. Clustering is more likely in the late afternoon or early evening. B and C are unusual patterns for a thriving, exclusively breastfed 2-month-old. (Techniques; 1–3 months; Knowledge; Difficulty: 4)

L-016. The answer is B. Living cells including macrophages are killed by freezing. The other components are not significantly affected by freezing. (Techniques; General Principles; Knowledge; Difficulty: 2)

L-017. The answer is D. Skin-to-skin contact with reduced sensory stimulation is the first intervention, and it is usually successful. Once that is done, A could help. B is harsh and usually unnecessary. Pulling down a baby's chin may cause jaw clenching. (Techniques; Labor/Birth; Application; Difficulty: 4)

L-018. The answer is B. Sucking on fists is a feeding cue, which should be responded to by offering the breast. (Techniques; 3–14 days; Application; Difficulty: 2)

LN-019. The answer is D. Using a supplementer at breast to increase milk volume is only effective when the baby's suck is effective. (Techniques; 1–2 days; Application; Difficulty: 5)

LN-020. The answer is C. The lactation consultant supports the breastfeeding relationship, including helping the mother to explore all her options in any given situation. (Techniques; 15–28 days; Application; Difficulty: 2)

LN-021. The answer is B. Artificial feeding carries substantial risks that are only compounded by the infant's vulnerability to upper respiratory infection. (Techniques; 3–14 days; Application; Difficulty: 2)

LP-022. The answer is D. This mother is hand-expressing her milk. The retracted nipple is not causing a problem. (Techniques; 3–14 days; Knowledge; Difficulty: 4)

LP-023. The answer is A. This mother is gently and correctly rolling her retracted nipples to firm them prior to feeding. (Techniques; 1–2 days; Application; Difficulty: 4)

LP-024. The answer is B. Early breastfeeding is the most important action when a mother has flat nipples or, for that matter, for all mothers. Prenatal nipple preparation has not been shown to significantly improve flat nipples. (Techniques; Prenatal; Application; Difficulty: 3)

LP-025. The answer is C. She is attempting to pull the nipple tip outward. (Techniques; Prenatal; Application; Difficulty: 2)

LP-026. The answer is C. The mother is doing a digital oral assessment to feel her own baby's palate. This also explains why she is not wearing gloves. (Techniques; 3–14 days; Knowledge; Difficulty: 4)

LP-027. The answer is C. This 7-day-old baby is relaxed and feeding well from the cup, which is being used correctly. (Techniques; 3–14 days; Application; Difficulty: 2)

LP-028. The answer is B. The hand on the baby's back should be slightly lower, allowing the baby to extend her head for easier coordination of suck-swallow-breathe. Supporting the breast might help if the first suggestion is ineffective. (Techniques; 1–2 days; Application; Difficulty: 3)

LP-029. The answer is A. Correcting positioning is nearly always the first and most important intervention. This mother's nipple is sore and abraded from positional soreness, which was completely relieved when her technique was corrected. (Techniques; 1–3 months; Application; Difficulty: 4)

LP-030. The answer is D. The crack at the base of the nipple plus the shiny, reddish skin are common signs of nipple thrush. The other suggestions may provide some relief until the nipple thrush is dealt with. (Techniques; 4–6 months; Application; Difficulty: 5)

LP-031. The answer is B. The most effective treatment for a plugged nipple pore, also known as a "bleb" or "white spot," is softening the plugged area in warm water, then massaging or expressing the duct opening. Hand-expressing before feeds is a technique for softening the entire breast; wearing shells does not treat a plugged pore, and there is no other indication of nipple thrush in this mother's situation. (Techniques; 4–6 months; Application; Difficulty: 4)

LP-032. The answer is C. Supporting this soft breast from underneath is the MOST helpful suggestion. This mother's areolae are very large and may not be fully covered by the baby's mouth. Removing the bra is not necessary. Leaning forward is usually uncomfortable at best. (Techniques; 1–2 days; Application; Difficulty: 3)

LP-033. The answer is C. Finger-feeding is considered one appropriate technique for improving a baby's suboptimum suck, providing food, allowing nipples to heal, and behavior modification. (Techniques; 3–14 days; Application; Difficulty: 4)

LP-034. The answer is C. Skin-to-skin contact is the first and least invasive intervention of the strategies suggested, and it is often the most effective. (Techniques; 1–2 days; Application; Difficulty: 4)

LP-035. The answer is A. Teaching her how to position her baby for breastfeeding is the most important action. Her nipples are not retracted, so B and C are incorrect. Rubbing the skin with rough fabric is inappropriate and can damage areolar structures. (Techniques; Prenatal; Application; Difficulty: 4)

LP-036. The answer is B. The hand is pinching the base of the nipple, cutting off milk flow. This could also bruise the areola. There is no published evidence that nipple rolling will improve nipple elasticity. (Techniques; > 12 months; Application; Difficulty: 4)

LP-037. The answer is D. Frequent nursing on the affected side is the first, least complicated approach to opening a plugged nipple pore. C is not appropriate, since the plug is a mechanical problem. B is the next-best strategy, with A being the riskiest recommendation. (Techniques; > 12 months; Application; Difficulty: 4)

LP-038. The answer is D. The hand positions shown are adequate. The next appropriate action is bringing the baby to breast. (Techniques; 1–2 days; Application; Difficulty: 5)

LP-039. The answer is C. This baby's most immediate need is for calories. His skin is slightly yellow, suggesting some amount of jaundice. That fact, combined with 2 weeks of poor feeding at breast, indicates inadequate milk transfer. The baby needs calories immediately while other approaches to remedy this situation are explored. (Techniques; 3–14 days; Application; Difficulty: 5)

LP-040. The answer is B. Assuring good alignment and deep latch is the first action to take. After that, C would be the next step to take. Nipple tenderness is not normal during any stage of lactation, and referral for evaluation of the tongue musculature would rarely be needed. (Techniques; 3–14 days; Application; Difficulty: 4)

LP-041. The answer is C. The first suggestion to prevent nipple damage is to support the large, pendulous breasts and help the baby attach deeply onto the breast. A nipple shield is not appropriate for this mother. (Techniques; 3–14 days; Application; Difficulty: 2)

LP-042. The answer is B. An oral exam is considered a basic lactation assessment. Suck training is considered an advanced therapy and is rarely needed. During finger feeding, a thin tube is held against the adult's finger. The baby in the picture is being held and appears to be asleep; therefore, D is unlikely. (Techniques; 1–2 days; Application; Difficulty: 5)

LP-043. The answer is B. The practitioner is performing a frenotomy, an incision of the baby's lingual frenulum, which was short and tight. Frenectomy is removal of tissue, not a simple incision. Tonsillectomy (removal of the tonsils) would have no relationship to the breastfeeding problem, and myringotomy is ear surgery. (Techniques; 3–14 days; Application; Difficulty: 3)

LP-044. The answer is A. The nipple is a normal shape and the breast is not full postfeed. Both of these suggest maternal comfort with effective milk transfer. If milk transfer were poor, there should be breast fullness postfeed. If the mother experiences pain, there is usually nipple distortion visible postfeed. (Techniques; 3–14 days; Application; Difficulty: 3)

LP-045. The answer is B. The baby's lower lip is curled in and needs to be turned (flanged) outward. Tickling the baby's feet is ineffective, and there is no need to press down on the breast to clear his nostrils. (Techniques; 3–14 days; Application; Difficulty: 4)

LP-046. The answer is C. Moist wound healing is most effective. Choice D is the second–best response. A and D are unhelpful strategies because they dry the skin surface and retard healing. (Techniques; 1-2 days; Application; Difficulty: 4)

LP-047. The answer is A. The vertical position is helpful when the baby has a head injury or needs help maintaining good alignment. Let-down reflex is not affected by a baby's position; the "colic hold" is holding the baby prone on the mother's forearm. Plugged milk ducts are rarely found in the upper quadrant. (Techniques; 15–28 days; Application; Difficulty: 2)

LP-048. The answer is A. Attempting a deeper latch is the first and usually most effective intervention. If that does not eliminate the pain and result in better feeding, further investigation is needed. (Techniques; 3–14 days; Application; Difficulty: 4)

LP-049. The answer is B. Massaging the breast toward the nipple during pumping or feeding may help move milk from the alveoli toward the nipple. (Techniques; 1–2 days; Knowledge; Difficulty: 4)

LP-050. The answer is A. Large breasts often need to be supported while the baby feeds. This mother's breast is large, but there is no evidence of milk stasis, edema, or excessive fullness. (Techniques; 15–28 days; Application; Difficulty: 3)

LP-051. The answer is A. Mothers and babies thrive when 24-hour rooming-in with safe bedding-in is practiced. This mother is on a firm surface, is awake and is alert, and is holding her baby at breast in a protective position. The other actions are unnecessary or inappropriate. (Techniques; 1–2 days; Application; Difficulty: 4)

LP-052. The answer is C. Dressings designed for moist wound healing are appropriate treatments for nipple wounds. The source of the damage needs to be identified and corrected. The other suggestions are inappropriate. (Techniques; 15–28 days; Application; Difficulty: 2)

LPN-053. The answer is C. The peaked shape of the nipple does not look good—it suggests a shallow latch and/or poor sucking technique, both of which need attention and correction. A, B, and D are all reasonable and appropriate suggestions. (Techniques; 15–28 days; Application; Difficulty: 2)

LPN-054. The answer is C. Birth injuries such as this wound from a vacuum extractor may cause head pain in the baby. Direct breastfeeding should be tried first; if unsuccessful, other methods could be explored. (Techniques; 1–2 days; Application; Difficulty: 2)

LPN-055. The answer is D. The amount of areola in the mouth is the least important indicator of a problem latch. In this picture, the pursed lips, puckering at the naso-labial crease, and chin failing to touch the breast are all strong indications of a poor latch and positioning. The baby in this picture was tongue-tied. (Techniques; 3–14 days; Application; Difficulty: 4)

LPN-056. The answer is D. There is no indication for interrupting breastfeeding in this situation. The rash could be bacterial, yeast, eczema, or some other organic condition. A, B, and C are all appropriate suggestions. (Techniques; 4–6 months; Application; Difficulty: 3)

LPN-057. The answer is C. This 9-month-old baby may self-feed with a pincer grasp, sip liquids from an open cup, and/or breastfeed 8–16 times a day or as often as a newborn. It is highly unlikely that she would self-wean at this age. (Techniques; 7–12 months; Application; Difficulty: 3)

LPN-058. The answer is C. The mother can breastfeed directly if she has nipple thrush. All of the other answers are appropriate uses for cup feeding. (Techniques; 3–14 days; Application; Difficulty: 2)

LPN-059. The answer is C. Emergency action is not warranted for this baby as there are no obvious indications of a life-threatening condition. The baby is slightly yellow (jaundiced) and sleepy, so the other choices are appropriate. (Techniques; 3–14 days; Application; Difficulty: 2)

L-060. The answer is C. Prolactin levels are unaffected by thin, silicone nipple shields. (Techniques; 3–14 days; Knowledge; Difficulty: 5)

Scoring:

Total number of questions in this section _____

Number of questions answered correctly _____

Percent correct (divide number correct by total number) _____

M. PUBLIC HEALTH

In the 2000 exam blueprint, 4 to 8 questions are dedicated to public health and advocacy.

SUBTOPICS INCLUDED IN THIS CATEGORY

1. Breastfeeding promotion and community education

2. Vulnerable populations (groups with low breastfeeding rates)

3. Creating and implementing clinical protocols

4. International tools and documents

5. WHO Code (International Code of Marketing of Breast-Milk Substitutes)

6. Baby-Friendly Hospital Initiative (BFHI) implementation

7. Skills (advocacy)

8. Interaction with policy makers; changing public policy

9. Prevalence, surveys, and data collection for research purposes

CORE READING

Textbooks

Allain A, Chetley A. *Protecting Infant Health: A Healthworker's Guide to the International Code of Marketing of Breast-Milk Substitutes.* Penang, Malaysia: IBFAN; 2003.

Armstrong HC, Sokol E: *The International Code of Marketing of Breast-Milk Substitutes: What It Means for Mothers and Babies World-Wide.* Raleigh, NC: International Lactation Consultant Association; 2001.

Baby Milk: Destruction of a World Resource. London: Catholic Institute for International Relations; 1993.

Evidence for the Ten Steps to Successful Breastfeeding. Geneva, Switzerland: World Health Organization, Division of Child Health and Development; 1998.

The International Code of Marketing of Breast-Milk Substitutes: A Common Review and Evaluation Framework. Geneva, Switzerland: World Health Organization; 1996.

Out of the Mouths of Babes: How Canada's Infant Foods Industry Defies WHO Rules and Puts Infant Health at Risk. Toronto: INFACT Canada; 2002.

Selling Out Mothers and Babies: Marketing of Breast-Milk Substitutes in the USA. Weston, MA: NABA REAL; 2001.

Shealy KR, Li R, Benton-Davis S, Grummer-Strawn LM. *The CDC Guide to Breastfeeding Interventions.* Atlanta, GA: Centers for Disease Control and Prevention; 2005.

Sokol E, Allain A. *Complying with the Code: A Manufacturers' and Distributors' Guide to the Code.* Penang, Malaysia: IBFAN; 1998.

Key Research Articles

Ball TM, Wright AL. Health care costs of formula-feeding in the first year of life. *Pediatrics.* 1999;103(4):870–876.

Berman S, Rannie M, Moore L, Elias E, Dryer LJ, Jones Jr. MD. Utilization and costs for children who have special health care needs and are enrolled in a hospital-based comprehensive primary care clinic. *Pediatrics.* 2005;115(6):e637–e642.

DiGirolamo A, Thompson N, Martorell R, Fein S, Grummer-Strawn L. Intention or experience? Predictors of continued breastfeeding. *Health Educ Behav.* 2005;32(2):208–226.

DiGirolamo AM, Grummer-Strawn LM, Fein SB. Do perceived attitudes of physicians and hospital staff affect breastfeeding decisions? *Birth.* 2003;30(2):94–100.

DiGirolamo AM, Grummer-Strawn LM, Fein S. Maternity care practices: Implications for breastfeeding. *Birth.* 2001;28(2):94–100.

Edmond KM, Zandoh C, Quigley MA, et al. Delayed breastfeeding initiation increases risk of neonatal mortality. *Pediatrics.* 2006;117(3):e380–e386.

Labbok MH, Clark D, Goldman AS. Breastfeeding: maintaining an irreplaceable immunological resource. *Nat Rev Immunol.* 2004;4(7):565–572.

Leung GM, Lam TH, Ho LM, Lau YL. Health consequences of breast-feeding: Doctors' visits and hospitalizations during the first 18 months of life in Hong Kong Chinese infants. *Epidemiology.* 2005;16(3):328–335.

Smith JP, Thompson JF, Ellwood DA. Hospital system costs of artificial infant feeding: Estimates for the Australian Capital Territory. *Aust N Z J Public Health.* 2002;26(6):543–551.

Taveras EM, Li R, Grummer-Strawn L, et al. Mothers' and clinicians' perspectives on breastfeeding counseling during routine preventive visits. *Pediatrics.* 2004;113(5):e405–e411.

Taveras EM, Li R, Grummer-Strawn L, et al. Opinions and practices of clinicians associated with continuation of exclusive breastfeeding. *Pediatrics.* 2004;113(4):e283–e290.

Wright AL, Bauer M, Naylor A, Sutcliffe E, Clark L. Increasing breastfeeding rates to reduce infant illness at the community level. *Pediatrics.* 1998;101(5):837–844.

Internet Resources

Baby-Friendly Hospital Initiative. UNICEF Web site. Available at www.unicef.org/programme/breastfeeding/baby.htm

Innocenti Declaration of 2005. Available at http://innocenti15.net

PUBLIC HEALTH QUESTIONS

Notice on question numbering: M-000 means a basic question, with one correct answer and three wrong answers. MP-000, along with the camera icon, means there is a picture that needs to be viewed to answer the question. The pictures are located on the CD-ROM included with this book and are numbered to correspond with the questions. MN-000, along with the frowning face icon, means the question has a NEGATIVE stem; therefore, read the entire question very carefully to find the one WRONG answer among the choices. MPN-000, with both icons in the margin, means there is a picture associated with the question AND the question has a negative stem. See Appendix A for a fuller explanation of negative stem questions.

M-001. A well-balanced diet with sufficient calories accompanied by early and regular prenatal care significantly reduces the incidence of:

a. infants with diabetes.
b. low birth weight.
c. maternal gestational diabetes.
d. lactation failure.

M-002. Which of the following is permissible under the terms of the World Health Organization's International Code of Marketing of Breast-Milk Substitutes?

a. gift packs containing samples and coupons for formula given to new mothers at hospital discharge
b. detailed information on artificial feeding product composition provided to health workers
c. advertisements for toddler formula on local television stations
d. a picture of a happy baby on the label of infant formula containers

M-003. If a mother cannot provide her milk to her baby, the World Health Organization recommends that the next-best food for her baby is:

a. soy-based formula.
b. cow's-milk-based formula.
c. pasteurized donor human milk.
d. milk of another mother.

MN-004. Safe motherhood initiatives include breastfeeding because it protects women's health in all of the following ways **EXCEPT**:

a. reduced postpartum bleeding.
b. reduced risk of reproductive cancers.
c. reduced postpartum fertility.
d. reduced libido during breastfeeding.

MN-005. The World Health Organization's International Code of Marketing of Breast-Milk Substitutes applies to all of the following products **EXCEPT**:

a. breast pumps.
b. infant formula.
c. feeding bottles and teats.
d. weaning foods.

MN-006. The existing policy on the maternity unit at your hospital is to supplement all breast-feeding babies with 1 oz (30 cc) glucose water by bottle after every breastfeed. Which strategy is **LEAST** likely to be effective in changing this policy?

a. Include pediatricians, nursing staff, and neonatalogists on the policy planning committee.
b. Distribute copies of research articles from peer-reviewed journals on the subject.
c. Plan a series of in-service meetings for all affected staff to carefully educate them on the risks and benefits of supplementing breastfeeding babies.
d. Develop the new policy with a small core group, then tell the staff that they must follow the new policy.

MN-007. The WHO/UNICEF Ten Steps to Successful Breastfeeding (Baby-Friendly Hospital Initiative) prohibits the use of all of the following devices **EXCEPT**:

a. artificial teats (nipples).
b. pacifiers (dummies, soothers).
c. breast pumps.
d. feeding bottles.

MN-008. Implementation of the Baby-Friendly Hospital Initiative has been demonstrated to have all **EXCEPT** which one of the following outcomes?

a. decreased rates of infant abandonment during the hospital stay
b. decreased risk of upper respiratory tract infection in the first year of life
c. increased rates of breastfeeding initiation, duration, and exclusivity
d. decreased risk of gastrointestinal infection in the first year of life

MP-009. How soon after birth should this activity take place for a birth facility to comply with BFHI guidelines?

a. after the baby has been transitioned in the newborn nursery
b. after the baby has been examined by a physician or midwife
c. within the first hour after birth, before other procedures are done
d. after the baby has been bathed, weighed, and measured

M-010. What is the recommended duration of exclusive breastfeeding described in the WHO/UNICEF Global Strategy for Infant and Young Child Feeding?

a. 4 months
b. 6 months
c. 12 months
d. until the child self-weans

M-011. A mother has begun breastfeeding successfully and is leaving the hospital with her 3-day-old son. Your best action is to:

a. call her in a week to see how things are going.
b. refer her to a local mother support group such as La Leche League.
c. enroll her in a food supplement program in case she needs infant formula.
d. make sure she has a written pamphlet on breastfeeding.

M-012. The WHO/UNICEF Ten Steps to Successful Breastfeeding include which one of the following steps?

a. Train all maternity staff with 3 hours of breastfeeding education.
b. Give only breast milk to premature infants under 37 weeks' gestation.
c. Use at-breast supplementers for supplementing breastfed infants.
d. Encourage breastfeeding on demand when teaching.

MN-013. All of the following activities would be appropriate for celebrating World Breastfeeding Week **EXCEPT**:

a. setting up a display showing environmental hazards associated with formula manufacturing.
b. instituting a hospital policy that all mothers must breastfeed their babies at least once before the hospital staff will assist them with formula feeding.
c. publishing a directory of local lactation support services in the community.
d. printing "Breastfeeding Welcome Here" stickers/signs for local businesses and employers.

MN-014. Which of the following is **NOT** an example of breastfeeding promotion?

a. assisting in developing legislation to protect breastfeeding in public
b. opening a private lactation consultant practice
c. presenting a lecture on breastfeeding to a civic organization
d. wearing breastfeeding buttons, jewelry, or T-shirts in social situations

MN-015. The Innocenti Declaration of 1990 contains all of the following operational targets **EXCEPT**:

a. appointment of a national breastfeeding coordinator and committee.
b. adherance to the Ten Steps to Successful Breastfeeding by every maternity facility.
c. implementation of the International Code of Marketing of Breast-Milk Substitutes.
d. passage of legislation protecting a mother's right to breastfeed in public.

MN-016. Health policies that are affected by breastfeeding rates include all of the following **EXCEPT**:

a. food security.
b. environmental protection.
c. reduction in family violence.
d. economic development.

MN-017. Which of the following provisions was **NOT** part of the International Labor Organization's Maternity Protection Convention of 2000?

a. 14 weeks of maternity leave
b. one or more nursing breaks
c. on-site (workplace) child care
d. job protection after maternity leave

MN-018. Breastfeeding is a core strategy of child survival programs because it provides all of the following health advantages **EXCEPT**:

a. baby's first immunization.
b. best nutrition for first 12 months.
c. lower rates of infant mortality.
d. long-term reduction in diabetes risk.

MN-019. International agencies that have official position papers or programs supporting breast-feeding include all of the following **EXCEPT**:

a. World Bank Family Planning branch
b. World Health Organization
c. United Nations Children's Fund
d. International Monetary Fund

PUBLIC HEALTH ANSWERS

The parenthetical material at the end of each answer includes the discipline and time period, indicates whether the question pertains to knowledge or application, and specifies the degree of difficulty.

M-001. The answer is B. A good maternal diet during pregnancy significantly reduces the incidence of low-birth-weight infants. Diet may have a relationship to the development of gestational diabetes. Maternal diet does not directly affect A or D. (Public Health; Prenatal; Knowledge; Difficulty: 3)

M-002. The answer is B. The code specifies that information on artificial feeding provided to health workers should be scientific and accurate. Detailed, accurate information on product composition provided to health workers is appropriate marketing of products within the scope of the code. (Public Health; General Principles; Knowledge; Difficulty: 2)

M-003. The answer is D. The options for this question are listed in reverse order of WHO recommendations for prioritizing other foods. (Public Health; General Principles; Knowledge; Difficulty: 4)

MN-004. The answer is D. Libido is not addressed in safe motherhood initiatives. Libido is not necessarily lower during breastfeeding. (Public Health; General Principles; Knowledge; Difficulty: 2)

MN-005. The answer is A. Breast pumps are not currently covered by the International Code. However, feeding bottles (baby bottles) not used as collection containers attached to breast pumps are included in the scope of the Code. (Public Health; General Principles; Knowledge; Difficulty: 2)

MN-006. The answer is D. Involving all pertinent staff, planning sufficient education, and providing substantial evidence of the safety and effectiveness of the new policy are all successful strategies for changing policies. Forcing new policies on staff is likely to result in open and covert resistance. (Public Health; 1–2 days; Application; Difficulty: 2)

MN-007. The answer is C. The Baby-Friendly Hospital Initiative, Step 9, is "Give no artificial teats or pacifiers (also called dummies or soothers) to breastfeeding infants." This step also includes prohibition of feeding bottles. Bottles that are attached to breast pumps are not addressed. (Public Health; 1–2 days; Knowledge; Difficulty: 2)

MN-008. The answer is B. Of the conditions listed, evidence is weakest for lower risk of respiratory infections following implementation of BFHI policies. (Public Health; General Principles; Knowledge; Difficulty: 3)

MP-009. The answer is C. The newborn should be placed at breast immediately postbirth and assisted (if needed) to begin breastfeeding within the first hour. The expanded BFHI guidelines recommend that all non–life-saving procedures be delayed until after the first effective breastfeed. (Public Health; Labor/Birth; Application; Difficulty: 2)

M-010. The answer is B. Exclusive breastfeeding for 6 months is recommended by WHO, UNICEF, and virtually all health professional associations around the world. (Public Health; 4–6 months; Knowledge; Difficulty: 5)

M-011. The answer is B. Step 10 of the Baby-Friendly Hospital Initiative addresses the importance of referring new mothers to peer support groups. The other actions are less likely to result in her continuing to breastfeed successfully. (Public Health; 3–14 days; Application; Difficulty: 5)

M-012. The answer is D. Breastfeeding on demand, or "on cue," is Step 8, also described as "Encourage unrestricted breastfeeding." Step 2 addresses staff training of at least 18 hours; feeding only breast milk (Step 6) applies only to healthy term babies. Step 9 calls for avoidance of teats or pacifiers for breastfed babies. Step 9 does not specify which other devices may be used. (Public Health; General Principles; Knowledge; Difficulty: 5)

MN-013. The answer is B. World Breastfeeding Week themes focus on benefits of breastfeeding and positive changes to facilitate breastfeeding. Forcing mothers to breastfeed is inappropriate. World Breastfeeding Week celebrates the signing of the Innocenti Declaration on the Protection, Promotion and Support of Breastfeeding on August 1, 1990. (Public Health; General Principles; Knowledge; Difficulty: 2)

MN-014. The answer is B. Clinical services are considered breastfeeding support, not promotion. The other activities are considered advocacy or promotion. (Public Health; General Principles; Knowledge; Difficulty: 2)

MN-015. The answer is D. The fourth provision of the 1990 Innocenti Declaration protects the breastfeeding rights of working women, not their right to breastfeed in public. (Public Health; General Principles; Knowledge; Difficulty: 2)

MN-016. The answer is C. Family violence has not yet been linked to breastfeeding at the policy level. One study suggests that violence in the home is a barrier to women breastfeeding. (Public Health; General Principles; Knowledge; Difficulty: 2)

MN-017. The answer is C. The ILO convention of 2000 did not specifically address on-site child care. On-site child care is beneficial to all parents, especially breastfeeding mothers. (Public Health; General Principles; Knowledge; Difficulty: 2)

MN-018. The answer is B. Child survival programs advocate exclusive breastfeeding as the best nutrition for the first 6 months, and breastfeeding as an excellent staple food for 2 years or more. (Public Health; General Principles; Knowledge; Difficulty: 3)

MN-019. The answer is D. The International Monetary Fund is the only agency listed that to date does not have a statement or program supporting breastfeeding. (Public Health; General Principles; Knowledge; Difficulty: 3)

Scoring:

Total number of questions in this section   _____

Number of questions answered correctly   _____

Percent correct (divide number correct by total number)   _____

PART 2 Practice Exams

EXAM A QUESTIONS

1. During normal breastfeeding, where does the mother's nipple tip lie in the infant's mouth?

    a. at the junction of the hard palate and the alveolar ridge
    b. at the junction of the hard and soft palates
    c. at the junction of the soft palate and the uvula
    d. at the junction of the uvula and the epiglottis

2. When commencing oral feeds for the preterm infant, which is the most important infant factor to consider?

    a. cardiorespiratory stability
    b. toleration of enteral feedings
    c. ability to suck well on a bottle
    d. developmental age

3. A mother is concerned that tandem nursing may be harmful to her new baby or older breastfeeding child. Your first recommendation would be:

    a. wean the older child.
    b. tandem breastfeeding is not harmful to either child.
    c. reduce the time the older child is at breast.
    d. feed the new baby first, before breastfeeding the older child.

4. Why is it vital for the baby to breastfeed immediately postbirth, before any other substance is ingested?

    a. The gut is relatively high in pH.
    b. The newborn gut is sterile and permeable.
    c. Any residual amniotic fluid remaining must be neutralized.
    d. The baby needs caloric support as soon as the cord is cut.

5. You are on a team preparing clinical policies for a maternity unit. Which action is most important in preventing postpartum breast engorgement?

    a. prenatal expression of colostrum
    b. immediate breastfeeding in the first hour or so postbirth
    c. begin milk expression if the baby has not breastfed by 12 hours
    d. restriction of the mother's fluid intake in the first 48 hours postpartum

6. Which drug property results in more transfer of the drug into mother's milk?

   a. milk-plasma ratio < 1.0
   b. molecular weight > 300
   c. high protein binding
   d. lipid solubility

7. According to studies of breastfed babies in an industrialized society, which of the following feeding patterns most closely approximates that of an exclusively breastfed 3-month-old baby?

   a. 4–6 feeds per day, total 60 minutes or more
   b. 6–8 feeds per day, total 100 minutes or more
   c. 8–10 feeds per day, total 120 minutes or more
   d. 10–12 feeds per day, total 140 minutes or more

8. A baby born very prematurely (weight 1500 g or less) is ready to breastfeed when he:

   a. has successfully taken breast milk by bottle.
   b. has first fed by spoon or cup.
   c. is showing sucking movements.
   d. is able to mouth a pacifier.

9. A research study is designed to determine whether or not breastfeeding decreases the incidence of asthma in 5-year-olds. Pregnant women are asked whether or not they plan to breastfeed. Five years later their children are examined for signs and symptoms of asthma. This type of research design is called:

   a. intent to treat.
   b. double blind.
   c. crossover.
   d. meta-analysis.

10. Your job at a hospital includes determining what items patients are given upon discharge. A formula company representative is pressuring you to include their breastfeeding bag, which contains samples of powdered formula, coupons for more samples, and pictures that idealize that company's product. What is your best course of action?

   a. Accept the bags as generous gifts because some mothers may need the supplement.
   b. Accept the bags, but remove the samples and coupons before distributing them.
   c. Refuse the bags because giving samples violates BFHI Step 6 and the International Code of Marketing of Breast-Milk Substitutes.
   d. Accept the bags and a competing company's bags so mothers will have a choice.

11. Which feeding device is most appropriate if a preterm baby cannot yet breastfeed but can tolerate oral feedings?

    a. syringe
    b. cup
    c. tube against a finger (finger feeding)
    d. teat

12. A mother birthed by cesarean surgery after a 36-hour labor with pitocin and intravenous fluid support. At the 6-day visit, the baby is still losing weight. The baby is urinating adequately and stooling adequately. The pediatrician asks that the baby be supplemented. The lactation consultant's first action is:

    a. ask about medications and IV fluids during labor.
    b. observe the mother breastfeeding her baby.
    c. supplement the baby with expressed breast milk.
    d. wait one more day because of adequate infant output.

13. According to the WHO/UNICEF "Ten Steps to Successful Breastfeeding," a mother should:

    a. remain in the hospital with her baby for 48 hours after delivery.
    b. express colostrum or milk within 6 hours after birth.
    c. place her baby skin-to-skin immediately afterbirth.
    d. keep her premature baby skin to skin as many hours as possible.

14. Which policy document was adopted on August 1, 1990, in Florence, Italy, and contains specific national action steps to promote, protect, and support breastfeeding?

    a. Innocenti Declaration
    b. International Code of Marketing of Breast-Milk Substitutes
    c. Convention on the Rights of the Child
    d. Baby-Friendly Hospital Initiative

15. Which cranial nerve is responsible for the gag response and, if triggered, may inhibit the infant's deep latch?

    a. hypoglossal
    b. vagus
    c. trigeminal
    d. glossopharyngeal

16. Which breastfeeding behavior is most likely practiced by women using the Lactational Amenorrhea Method (LAM) of family planning?

    a. The baby sleeps 6 or more hours alone at night.
    b. The mother feeds the baby every 2–3 hours during the day.
    c. The baby breastfeeds on cue 8 or more times in 24 hours.
    d. The mother gives water between feeds in hot weather.

17. Which component of milk varies most with maternal diet?

    a. lactose
    b. immunoglobulins
    c. vitamins
    d. protein

18. Which of the following components of bovine milk is most likely to cause an allergic reaction in babies?

    a. lactose
    b. beta-lactoglobulin
    c. alpha-lactalbumin
    d. lactoferrin

19. Which of these sets of symptoms is most likely to culture positive for mammary candidosis?

    a. burning nipple pain
    b. shiny nipple skin and stabbing breast pain
    c. flaky nipple skin with nonstabbing breast pain
    d. shiny and flaky nipple skin with breast pain

20. A 3-month-old, exclusively breastfed baby is suddenly hospitalized for treatment of a cardiac abnormality. The mother is told she must stop breastfeeding because the baby's intake and output need to be carefully measured. Of the following options, which is most supportive of her desire to continue breastfeeding?

    a. Mother expresses her milk and gives it by an alternative feeding device.
    b. Weigh the baby before and after feeds.
    c. Weigh the mother before and after feeds.
    d. Carefully count the baby's swallows, and record the duration of breastfeeding.

21. You are asked to teach formula feeding and breastfeeding to expectant parents. Which approach is most supportive of breastfeeding?

    a. Refuse to teach formula feeding and refer students to other resources.
    b. Teach breastfeeding during the class, and offer a separate 1:1 session on formula feeding upon request.
    c. Teach both during the group sessions, and offer additional information on breastfeeding separately.
    d. Schedule separate classes for breastfeeding and formula feeding.

22. Which of the following actions best describes the Babinski reflex?

    a. grasping an object when the palm is stimulated
    b. turning the mouth toward the source of stimulation
    c. bearing partial weight of the body while standing on a flat surface
    d. flaring the toes when the sole of the foot is stimulated

23. A 5-month-old, breastfed baby's mother feels that her baby should learn how to sleep for at least eight hours straight at night. Your best response to her is:

    a. at this age, she needs frequent contact for reassurance and comfort.
    b. she is old enough to self-soothe now.
    c. she has already learned how to manipulate you; you had better train her to sleep.
    d. now that she is not a newborn, you do not need to respond quickly when she cries.

24. Banked donor human milk has been used clinically to treat many diseases and conditions. Which of the following is the most common and traditional use of banked donor milk?

    a. treatment of adult gastrointestinal problems such as ulcers or colitis
    b. treatment for infantile botulism
    c. nutrition and immunological therapy for premature infants
    d. therapy for inborn errors of metabolism

25. Which is the primary or main immunoglobulin found in human milk?

    a. IgA
    b. IgE
    c. IgG
    d. IgM

26. A mother complains that her baby is clamping down on her nipple with his lips. Which muscle is responsible for closing the lips around the nipple?

    a. masseter
    b. temporal
    c. obicularis oris
    d. internal pterygoid

27. Which part of the infant skull most often presents during birth?

    a. occipital bone
    b. parietal bone
    c. frontal bone
    d. sphenoid bone

28. Which is most likely to put a premature infant at risk of evaporative water loss?

    a. lower brown fat reserves
    b. immature thyroid control of metabolic rate
    c. relatively large skin surface area
    d. poor insulin response leading to hyperglycemia

29. During the first 24 hours, about how much fluid volume does the average normal newborn consume per breastfeeding session?

    a. 90 ml (3 oz)
    b. 60 ml (2 oz)
    c. 3 ml (1 oz)
    d. 7 ml (0.2 oz)

30. What is the approximate risk reduction for leukemia conferred by breastfeeding?

    a. 9%
    b. 19%
    c. 29%
    d. more than 30%

31. A breastfeeding mother calls to report waking up with a high fever, chills, and flulike aches. Her left breast is red and painful. Which is the most likely condition causing these symptoms?

    a. blocked milk duct
    b. inflammatory mastitis
    c. infectious mastitis
    d. breast abscess

32. When considering whether a breastfeeding mother should take a certain medication, which is the first question to consider?

    a. Is the drug regarded as safe in the neonatal period?
    b. How much drug would the infant receive per day via the milk?
    c. Is systemic maternal therapy needed?
    d. Is it really necessary for the mother to take this drug now?

33. Which drug would most likely inhibit lactation?

    a. bromocriptine
    b. metoclopramide
    c. domperidone
    d. cimetidine

34. A baby is having difficulty sucking after a long, difficult labor. Which drug administered during labor is most likely to cause breastfeeding problems in the baby?

    a. nalbuphine (Nubain)
    b. fentanyl (Sublimaze)
    c. butorphanol (Stadol)
    d. lidocaine or mepivicaine

35. The most important consequence of adding fortifiers to human milk given to premature babies is:

    a. better long-term bone mineralization.
    b. increased risk of allergic reaction from bovine protein in fortifiers.
    c. increased iron transport.
    d. decreased gut transit time.

36. A mother expressing milk for premature twins notices that her milk is slightly green-colored on the second day postpartum. What should she do with the milk?

    a. Ask the laboratory to run bacteriological tests.
    b. Examine her diet for the presence of foods high in chlorophyll.
    c. Discard the milk until the greenish color is no longer present.
    d. Feed it to her babies as usual.

37. A mother is concerned about an odd smell in a container of milk that she pumped 2 days ago and that has been stored in her refrigerator in a closed container. The milk smelled normal when she collected it. The most likely cause of this odd smell is:

   a.   the protein has been changed by amylase.
   b.   the minerals have been changed by bile salt-stimulated lipase.
   c.   the fats have been changed by lipase.
   d.   the lactose has been changed by lysozyme.

38. A mother asks you when her baby will likely wean from breastfeeding. Your best response is:

   a.   she should wean at 12 months to prevent dental decay.
   b.   continue to at least 24 months and as long as you and your baby desire.
   c.   your baby will begin weaning at 6 months and complete weaning by 1 year.
   d.   she'll probably want to continue exclusive breastfeeding until 12 months, then begin weaning.

39. A dark-skinned, 3-month-old exclusively breastfed baby lives in a location with limited sunlight many months of the year. Which suggestion is most appropriate?

   a.   Give the child multivitamin supplements containing at least 200 I.U. of vitamin D daily.
   b.   Expose the baby's face and hands to direct sunlight at least 30 minutes per week.
   c.   Supplement your diet with 2000–4000 I.U. of vitamin D per day.
   d.   Feed the child two servings of dark green or orange vegetables daily.

40. At what point in the suck-swallow-breathe cycle does most of the milk flow into the baby?

   a.   when the jaw rises and collects the milk from the nipple and areola
   b.   as the baby draws the nipple into his mouth using negative pressure
   c.   as the posterior tongue and jaw drops vertically, opening the oral space
   d.   during the wave-like motion of the tongue stripping the milk sinuses

41. Lack of sensation in the nipple and areola is most likely caused by damage to the:

   a.   fourth intercostal nerve.
   b.   supraclavicular nerve.
   c.   thoracic intercostal nerve.
   d.   spinal accessory nerve.

42. What event triggers Lactogenesis II (onset of copious milk secretion)?

   a.   stimulation from baby at breast
   b.   drop in progesterone from placenta separation
   c.   rise in oxytocin from uterine contractions
   d.   change in blood pH when the umbilical cord is cut

43. Which of the following components found in breast milk may be particularly important as an energy source for the rapidly developing brain of the infant?

    a. lactose
    b. taurine
    c. choline
    d. iron

44. A baby gained 19 oz in the past 5 days but is fussy and gassy much of the day. His mother feeds him on both breasts at each feed. Your best suggestion to her is:

    a. cut down your own fluid intake, because you have too much milk.
    b. let him finish nursing on the first breast before you offer the other one.
    c. stop drinking cow's milk for the next 2 weeks.
    d. try giving him some lactose-free supplement 3 times a day.

45. Where is most of the glandular tissue of the breast located?

    a. deep in the breast, close to the chest wall
    b. clustered on the distal ends of the milk ducts
    c. interspersed throughout the breast fairly evenly
    d. within a 30-mm radius of the nipple base

46. The most common cause of inadequate milk supply is:

    a. impaired let-down reflex.
    b. restricted maternal fluid intake.
    c. inadequate or infrequent milk removal.
    d. inadequate maternal diet.

47. A breastfeeding mother is also pregnant. She asks the lactation consultant if she needs special dietary considerations to eat for three while she's pregnant. Which suggestion or question is irrelevant?

    a. Double your protein intake.
    b. Eat enough calories of a basic mixed diet.
    c. Gain weight within the same parameters as if you were pregnant and not breastfeeding.
    d. Do you ordinarily have special dietary needs, such as avoiding meat (suggesting a possible need for vitamin B_{12} supplements)?

48. Which statement is most accurate about human milk after 1 year of lactation?

a. Total fat is 14% lower than at 6 months of lactation.
b. Total energy is 34% lower than at 6 months.
c. Lactose is 8% higher in proportion to minerals.
d. Creamatocrit (fat) levels are up to 28% higher.

49. Which statement is most accurate regarding breastfeeding longer than 2 years?

a. It provides no immune protection to the child.
b. It provides health benefits to mother and child.
c. It prolongs the child's dependency on her mother.
d. It increases the incidence of tooth decay.

50. Which maternal medication is most likely to require temporary discarding of the mother's milk?

a. tetracycline
b. iodine 131
c. diazepam
d. prednisone

51. A woman had breast reduction surgery when she was a teenager. Now that she has a new baby, she may need to use:

a. a breast pump to relieve engorgement.
b. a nipple shield to enhance nipple stimulation.
c. a feeding tube system because of lactation insufficiency.
d. breast shells to enhance nipple eversion.

52. Using the WHO 2006 growth standards, which statement best describes the growth of exclusively breastfed babies in the first 6 months?

a. Breastfed babies gain more weight.
b. Breastfed babies are shorter in length.
c. There is no difference in weight gain.
d. By height, breastfed babies are leaner.

53. Banking of donated human milk has been practiced in the United States since the early 1900s. Which factor is most important in dispensing banked donor milk?

a. being financially able to afford its purchase
b. acquiring a prescription from the physician
c. being under the age of 3
d. availability of abundant supply of donor milk

54. What is the most likely number of milk ducts terminating on the nipple?

    a. fewer than 6

    b. 9 or 10

    c. 15 to 20

    d. more than 20

55. About an hour after collection, bacterial counts in freshly expressed human milk are lower than immediately after collection. The most likely explanation for this is:

    a. the cooler temperature in the container is unsuitable for growth of bacteria.

    b. macrophages in milk are actively phagocytic.

    c. gangliosides in milk disrupt the cell walls of bacteria.

    d. bifidus factor starves the bacteria of nutrients.

56. A pregnant woman reports seeing a sticky greenish discharge come from her nipple during a bath. The most likely cause of this discharge is:

    a. an intraductal papilloma.

    b. a breast abscess.

    c. an infected Montgomery tubercle.

    d. mammary duct ectasia.

57. You are writing a pamphlet on breastfeeding for new mothers. The best advice on whether to use one or both breasts is:

    a. use only one breast per feed.

    b. be sure to use both breasts per feed.

    c. let the baby finish one breast before offering the second breast.

    d. switch breasts several times per feed.

58. Which maternal factor is most responsible for the amount of milk consumed by a baby at a feed?

    a. size of the breast

    b. number of milk ejections

    c. number of milk ducts

    d. amount of fat in the breast

59. A mother is 3 days postbirth and is worried that her milk is not flowing out, even though her breasts feel very full. She pumps 5 cc from one breast and 10 cc from the other. Your first action should be:

    a. provide her with oxytocin nasal spray.
    b. perform alternate breast massage.
    c. apply cold packs to her breasts.
    d. apply hot compresses to her breasts.

60. During pregnancy, which characteristic of the breasts is most relevant to lactation capacity?

    a. breast growth (size change) during pregnancy
    b. one breast is markedly different in size from the other
    c. colostrum can be expressed from the breasts
    d. tubular shape of the breasts

61. A mother is concerned because her areola is over 4 in (10 cm) in diameter, and drops of milk appear on the areola when her milk lets down. How will this affect her ability to breastfeed?

    a. The areola is too large to fit completely inside the baby's mouth.
    b. The milk duct openings on the areola will make it difficult for her baby to latch.
    c. Very large areolae are associated with milk oversupply.
    d. Her breasts are normal, and she should easily be able to breastfeed.

62. Which is the most effective strategy for increasing milk supply?

    a. Take fenugreek tea or capsules.
    b. Drink more fluids.
    c. Eat more food.
    d. Express milk after feeds.

63. A healthy, thriving, 10-day-old baby is diagnosed with a bilirubin level of 120 mg/dl (17mmol/L). The first suggestion for his care should be:

    a. replace most of the breastfeeds with artificial baby milk.
    b. institute phototherapy except during feedings.
    c. continue his 10–12 effective breastfeedings every day.
    d. he should have several sessions undressed in a sunny window.

64. A mother complains that her baby is not fitting the feeding schedule recommended by a book she has read. Your best response to her is:

a. it's acceptable to limit your baby's feeds to 10 minutes per side.
b. you can give a pacifier to help your baby space out his feeds.
c. breastfeeding on cue, or when your baby signals hunger, is always best.
d. giving water between feeds will get him onto a better pattern.

65. How long does it take the infant gut to recover its normal flora after one bottle of artificial baby milk?

a. 2 feedings
b. 2 days
c. 2 weeks
d. 2 months

66. Which fetal structure may remain open or be reopened by excessive infant crying?

a. ductus venosus
b. ductus arteriosus
c. foramen ovale
d. portal sinus

67. Which infant disease/condition is incompatible with breastfeeding?

a. hypothyroidism
b. Down syndrome
c. phenylketonuria
d. galactosemia

68. A breastfeeding mother sustained a broken leg in an automobile injury. Which of the following actions is most supportive of breastfeeding after acute care is finished?

a. Provide her with a hospital-grade electric breast pump.
b. Encourage family to bring her baby to her for feeding.
c. Collaborate in selecting pain-relief medications compatible with breastfeeding.
d. Help the family select an infant formula to use during her hospitalization.

69. A mother 12 days postbirth complains of a firm, tender area in her right breast that has persisted for 3 days, despite application of cool cabbage compresses, ice packs, and frequent milk expression using a hospital-grade electric breast pump. Your next action should be:

    a. suggest she continue this strategy for another 48 hours.
    b. switch to warm compresses before pumping.
    c. ask for a more thorough medical evaluation by a breast specialist.
    d. apply a breast binder and ask her to restrict fluids.

70. A mother is concerned that her 1-week old baby is passing one black, tarry stool per day. The baby nurses about every 3 hours for 15–20 minutes. Your first recommendation is:

    a. relax, the baby is still passing meconium stools.
    b. your baby needs to be examined by a physician today.
    c. stop drinking milk because your baby is reacting to the protein.
    d. begin supplementing, because the baby is not getting sufficient fluids.

71. A mother expresses fear that her milk supply is faltering. She is nursing on cue at least 12 times per 24 hours and is feeling tired and chilly. Which is the most likely cause of these signs?

    a. low serum prolactin levels
    b. low thyroid level
    c. anemia
    d. chronic fatigue syndrome

72. A mother has treatment-controlled hyperthyroidism. The best recommendation is:

    a. the baby should not be breastfed.
    b. the baby may be breastfed, but he should be monitored for hyperthyroidism.
    c. the baby may breastfeed normally.
    d. the baby will need thyroid medication.

73. A mother is exclusively breastfeeding her 5-month-old, and her menses have not yet returned. What is her chance of pregnancy?

    a. 7–8%
    b. 5–6%
    c. 3–4%
    d. 1–2%

74. An article published in a women's magazine says that women who breastfeed feel better bonded to their infants compared to women who don't breastfeed. The article concludes that breastfeeding is desirable because of the effect of breastfeeding on the mother's attitude. Because women choose whether or not to breastfeed, the conclusion may be considered flawed because of:

   a. sociocultural influences.
   b. confounding variables.
   c. lack of a placebo group.
   d. sample size.

75. Gastroesophageal reflux may be caused by a defect in the infant's:

   a. esophagus.
   b. trachea.
   c. small intestine.
   d. large intestine.

76. A lactating mother noticed two raised bumps on her areola that drip milk when her baby is nursing on the other breast. These bumps are most likely:

   a. Montgomery glands.
   b. milk duct pores.
   c. warts.
   d. insect bites.

77. An 18-hour-old infant breastfed successfully in the first hour. Since then, he has not fed. The baby is healthy and full term and is not showing any signs of hypoglycemia. To help this baby begin breastfeeding, your first action should be to have the mother:

   a. start using a nursing supplementer at breast.
   b. use a nipple shield.
   c. keep her baby skin to skin for the next 3 hours.
   d. give 2 oz of formula, then try breastfeeding again.

78. A 10-hour-old healthy, full-term baby has a blood sugar level of 36 mg/dL (2 mmol/L). The best treatment is to:

   a. ask the mother to breastfeed her baby.
   b. do nothing.
   c. give the baby a bottle of glucose water.
   d. give the baby 30 ml (1 oz) of artificial baby milk.

79. A 3-week-old, exclusively breastfed baby nurses every 1.5 to 2 hours in the late afternoon and evenings. She is gaining over 1 oz per day with 5–6 profuse, yellow stools and 8+ wet diapers per day. The most likely explanation for this frequent nursing pattern is:

    a. normal behavior for this age.
    b. low milk supply.
    c. the baby is becoming too dependent.
    d. the baby is ready for solid foods.

80. A breastfeeding mother of a 3-week-old baby needs oral surgery for an abscessed tooth. Her dentist is concerned that the anti-inflammatory drug he plans to prescribe may appear in her milk and cause problems for her baby. Which of the following statements is true?

    a. Anti-inflammatory drugs cause severe bleeding in breastfed babies.
    b. Most drugs appear in high concentrations in milk.
    c. Breastfeeding will retard healing of her surgical incision.
    d. Anti-inflammatory drugs are generally compatible with breastfeeding.

81. A mother asks when she can start giving her baby bovine-based formula so she can go out to a movie. Based on your knowledge of gut closure, your best answer is:

    a. after the baby is 6 months old.
    b. after she breastfeeds the baby.
    c. any time, as long as a bottle is not used as the device.
    d. after 1 year of age.

82. When does the mammary secretory glandular tissue develop?

    a. during puberty
    b. gradually with each menstrual period
    c. in the first trimester of pregnancy
    d. during pregnancy and the early weeks postbirth

83. The tail of Spence is mammary glandular tissue that:

    a. is only present with supernumerary nipples.
    b. does not produce milk.
    c. extends into the axilla.
    d. is not connected to the breast's duct system.

84. Which reference indicates a study design that presents the strongest evidence for kangaroo mother care?

    a. Influence of feeding patterns and other factors on early somatic growth of healthy, preterm infants in home-based kangaroo mother care: A cohort study. *J Pediatr Gastroenterol Nutr.* 2005;41(4):430–437.

    b. Implementation of kangaroo mother care: A randomized trial of two outreach strategies. *Acta Paediatr.* 2005;94(7):924–927.

    c. Getting to know you: Mothers' experiences of kangaroo care. *MCN Am J Matern Child Nurs.* 2005;30(5):338.

    d. Early skin-to-skin contact for mothers and their healthy newborn infants. *Cochrane Database Syst Rev.* 2003;(2):CD003519.

85. When selecting a drug to be given to a breastfeeding woman, which of the following drug properties is most important to consider?

    a. absorption from the GI tract

    b. protein binding

    c. milk/plasma ratio

    d. pediatric half-life

86. A breastfeeding mother must receive a radioactive isotope for diagnostic testing. How long should she wait before breastfeeding her baby again?

    a. 5 days

    b. 48 hours

    c. 5 half-lives

    d. She must completely wean.

87. Which statement best describes the role of the father and the exclusively breastfed baby?

    a. Breastfeeding increases the father's jealousy of the mother–baby relationship.

    b. Fathers of breastfed babies miss out on the opportunity to bond during feeding.

    c. Breastfeeding is not a barrier to father–child bonding.

    d. The baby may attempt to feed from the father's breasts.

88. Which of these research designs has the highest internal validity?

    a. quasi-experimental group studies

    b. case-control studies

    c. cross-sectional surveys

    d. pretest followed by posttest

89. A mother asks how to maximize the amount of milk connected with an automatic-cycling electric breast pump. Your best suggestion is:

    a. pump for 10 minutes on the first breast, then 10–15 minutes on the other breast.
    b. use the maximum tolerable vacuum pressure.
    c. set the speed to cycle as fast as possible.
    d. use a narrow-diameter flange for maximum nipple stimulation.

90. You work in a large clinic with a lactation consultant who advises mothers to toughen up their nipples by rubbing them with a rough washcloth during pregnancy. The first action you should take is:

    a. lodge a complaint with the IBLCE Discipline Committee.
    b. bring in research evidence of the harmful nature of this practice, and discuss it with the lactation consultant.
    c. form a committee to develop written protocols on all aspects of lactation practice for your clinic.
    d. try to intercept all of the clients seen by this lactation consultant and correct the misinformation.

91. The management of mother–baby dyads addressed in the WHO/UNICEF Baby-Friendly Hospital Initiative (Ten Steps to Successful Breastfeeding) applies to:

    a. all babies, no matter how fed.
    b. all artificially fed babies.
    c. only breastfed babies.
    d. breastfed babies who room-in.

92. A mother is concerned that her baby has suddenly lost interest in breastfeeding. Your best action is:

    a. do nothing. Breastfeeding mothers are usually overprotective.
    b. reassure her that the baby's appetite may change abruptly.
    c. carefully investigate the situation.
    d. instruct her how to give her milk in a bottle.

93. Which aspect of maternal–infant bonding with mothers of multiple infants is most likely to occur first?

    a. The mother bonds with the unit.
    b. The mother bonds with the firstborn.
    c. The mother bonds with the lastborn.
    d. The mother has delayed bonding with all of her babies.

94. A lactation consultant working on a postpartum unit notices that a physician routinely prescribes Depoprovera for all of his patients to prevent pregnancy before the 6-week postpartum return visit. The IBCLC knows that this drug may inhibit establishment of adequate and abundant milk supply. Ethically, the lactation consultant should:

    a. follow the doctor's orders and assume he has told each patient about the potential hazards of the medication.
    b. discuss potential side effect on the milk supply with each mother prior to her receiving the injection.
    c. ask breastfeeding mothers if they know the potential problems with milk supply that may be related to this medication.
    d. report the physician to the ethics committee of the hospital for not using a medication according to the package insert.

95. A mother tells you that a lactation consultant in your city took a course in a manipulative therapy and used her new skills on the mother's baby, without informing the mother or the baby's primary care provider. What should you do next?

    a. Report the lactation consultant to the medical licensing board in your jurisdiction.
    b. Contact the lactation consultant and discuss what the mother reported to you.
    c. Express doubt to the mother that your colleague would ever do such a thing.
    d. Write a letter to the mother's doctor, explaining the nature of the training taken by your colleague.

96. The most important determinant of drug penetration into milk is the mother's:

    a. plasma level.
    b. body weight.
    c. blood type.
    d. milk storage capacity.

97. Which drug taken by a breastfeeding mother is most likely to have an effect on her baby?

    a. insulin
    b. digoxin
    c. caffeine
    d. warfarin

98. A breastfeeding mother with insulin-dependent diabetes mellitus (IDDM) is at increased risk for which of the following conditions?

    a. insufficient milk supply
    b. mastitis
    c. oversupply
    d. plugged milk ducts

99. "Exclusive breastfeeding" means that the baby:

    a. breastfeeds directly and without restriction day and night.

    b. receives expressed or pumped breast milk plus supplemental vitamins.

    c. receives less than 2 oz (60 ml) of other fluids per day.

    d. receives no formula or solid foods but is given a pacifier daily.

100. Which drug decreases rapidly in the breast milk after the mother stops taking the drug?

    a. marijuana

    b. cocaine

    c. amphetamines

    d. alcohol

101. A breastfeeding mother who is 40 years old is also pregnant. She is worried about her bones being depleted of calcium due to the overlap. What is the most accurate response?

    a. Make sure you are getting the amount of calcium recommended for adult women.

    b. The more calcium in your diet, the lower your risk of osteoporosis later in life.

    c. Even with increased dietary calcium, overlapping breastfeeding and pregnancy is likely to result in a long-term loss of bone mineral density.

    d. Focus on plant sources of calcium, like oranges and kale, and reduce your intake of dairy products.

102. Which is the most appropriate suggestion for a pregnant woman concerned about eating well enough for her own body growth and her developing baby?

    a. Take prenatal vitamins every day.

    b. Eat fruits, vegetables, and protein-rich food 5 times a day.

    c. Plan your meals and snacks so you eat every few hours.

    d. Plan to gain 25–35 pounds (11.4–15.9 kg) by the end of your pregnancy.

103. A mother of a 10-week-old adopted baby consults you inquiring about induced lactation. The first thing you would tell her is:

    a. adoptive breastfeeding is possible.

    b. the baby is the deciding factor.

    c. you will need to know how to provide supplementary feeds.

    d. you won't have a full milk supply.

104. What effect does at least 7 months of breastfeeding have on urinary tract infections?

    a. higher risk of infections unless water is given, because less urine is produced by the breastfed child

    b. lower risk of infection up to 2 years because of sIgA antibodies and lactoferrin in milk

    c. no difference in the risk of infection after supplements and family foods are started

    d. no difference in boys, but breastfed girls have increased risk after 6 months of breastfeeding

105. A mother is struggling to maintain milk supply for her premature baby. After trying increased frequency and thoroughness of milk removal, which preparation would be most likely to increase milk supply?

    a. metronidazole

    b. beer

    c. domperidone

    d. theophylline

The next section of questions is constructed with a NEGATIVE STEM format. Be prepared to do a "mental shift" to think in negative terms, and read the stem and responses especially carefully before answering. There will be one **WRONG** answer among several correct answers.

106. A pregnant mother has heard that letting epidural anesthesia wear off prior to delivery will avoid anesthesia-related breastfeeding problems. You should tell her all of the following **EXCEPT**:

    a. drugs can take much longer to clear the baby's system, so there is still possible breastfeeding risk with this approach.

    b. the combination of drugs used in epidural anesthesia makes it difficult to determine which medications cause breastfeeding problems.

    c. epidural anesthesia has minimal or no effect on the baby regardless of how long before delivery it is administered.

    d. epidural anesthesia increases the likelihood of other birth interventions that can affect breastfeeding.

107. The lymphatic system associated with the lactating breast serves all of the following functions **EXCEPT**:

    a. it drains extracellular fluid from breast tissue.

    b. it filters bacteria that have entered ducts.

    c. it provides local responses to infection.

    d. it supplies lymphocytes present in milk.

108. A mother has been having migraine headaches and asks about various remedies and their effect on her nursing 3-week-old. The remedy **LEAST LIKELY** to affect her baby is:

    a. acetaminophen.
    b. an herbal preparation.
    c. a homeopathic remedy.
    d. a caffeinated beverage.

109. A mother is having trouble keeping her 40-hour-old son awake. The **WORST** thing you would suggest is:

    a. try putting a cool cloth on his face.
    b. flick his feet with your finger.
    c. gently massage his back, arms, and legs.
    d. place him on your chest skin to skin.

110. All of the following components are found in the whey portion of milk **EXCEPT**:

    a. secretory IgA.
    b. lactoferrin.
    c. docosahexaenoic acid.
    d. bifidus factor.

111. Which is the **LEAST LIKELY** cause of low milk volume at 3 weeks postpartum in a mother with a normal newborn?

    a. breast surgery
    b. retained placental fragments
    c. breastfeeding mismanagement
    d. environmental estrogenic compounds

112. Which statement about complementary feeding is **INCORRECT**?

    a. Parents should feed their babies a variety of foods including meat, poultry, fish, and eggs daily.
    b. Vegetarian diets can meet a child's nutrient needs after 12 months.
    c. Vitamin A-rich foods should be eaten daily.
    d. Whole fruits are more nutritious for children than fruit juices.

113. A mother has recently been diagnosed with gestational diabetes. Following the birth of her infant, which of the following is **LEAST LIKELY**?

   a. The infant is more at risk of hypoglycemia and hyperbilirubinemia.
   b. Onset of copious milk secretion may be delayed about 24 hours.
   c. Breastfeeding may help protect the infant against Type II diabetes.
   d. Lactation will increase the mother's chance of developing adult-onset diabetes.

114. For an 18-month-old child, breastfeeding is **LEAST** significant as a source of:

   a. calories.
   b. immunities.
   c. comfort.
   d. bonding.

115. Which of the following does **NOT** occur routinely in the processing of banked donor human milk in the United States?

   a. pasteurization of milk prior to dispensing
   b. bacteriological screening of milk
   c. screening of milk for environmental contaminants
   d. serum screening of all donors

116. A mother of a 4-month-old is worried that her baby is constipated. Earlier, he stooled several times a day. Starting a few days ago, he stools 2–3 times in the morning only, but passes some gas during the day. The mother is currently restricting her food intake to a few carbohydrate foods because of a religious celebration. What is the **LEAST LIKELY** cause of the baby's stool pattern?

   a. The mother's carbohydrate diet is constipating.
   b. Her milk has a higher casein:whey ratio than earlier in lactation.
   c. The baby absorbs over 90% of the milk components, leaving little residue to be eliminated as stool.
   d. Breastfed babies of this age often pass stool less often, but the consistency remains normal.

117. Which body system is **LEAST** affected by breastfeeding?

   a. oro-facial musculature
   b. gastrointestinal functioning
   c. urogenital system
   d. speech and language

118. Which is the **LEAST** important function of colostrum?

    a. It coats the immature gut and prevents adherence of pathogens.
    b. It provides high-calorie food for energy.
    c. It blocks the transmission of allergens.
    d. Beta-endorphins reduce infant pain.

119. Mothers of twins are **LEAST** likely to experience which of the following circumstances?

    a. premature birth
    b. cesarean birth
    c. intrauterine growth retardation
    d. insufficient milk supply

120. Twenty-four-hour rooming-in from birth has been shown to have all the following effects **EXCEPT**:

    a. increased maternal–infant bonding (attachment).
    b. increased duration of breastfeeding.
    c. decreased abandonment or neglect of infant.
    d. decreased interaction between grandparents and baby.

121. Accessory nipple or breast tissue is **LEAST LIKELY** to be found in which of the following locations?

    a. axilla
    b. inguinal region
    c. near the umbilicus
    d. outer thigh

122. A preterm infant of 1361 g (3.0 lb) has stable cardiac and respiratory systems. All of the following are appropriate **EXCEPT**:

    a. beginning breastfeeding without equipment or devices.
    b. breastfeeding with nasogastric tube in place.
    c. cup feeding and allowing the baby to suck at an empty breast for comfort.
    d. bottle feeding with human milk before breastfeeding.

123. Mary has just delivered her baby at 32 weeks' gestation. Which of the following statements is **LEAST LIKELY** to empower her?

 a. Don't worry dear. Your baby is in good hands; we'll take good care of her.
 b. There are a lot of noisy machines and it may seem scary, but don't let that come between you and your baby.
 c. Your baby seems so much calmer when you're nearby. Would you like to touch and hold her?
 d. Your milk is so important for your baby. It's great that you're expressing milk for her!

124. "External gestation" includes all of the following behaviors **EXCEPT**:

 a. the baby sleeps through the night in his own room.
 b. the mother carries the baby in a sling or tie-on carrier many hours a day.
 c. frequent breastfeeding around the clock.
 d. the mother takes her baby to work with her.

125. Which condition is **LEAST LIKELY** to be associated with bottle feeding?

 a. need for orthodontia
 b. weak masseter muscles
 c. speech and articulation disorders
 d. broadly arched palate

The following questions require the candidate to view a photograph or diagram to answer the question. The pictures (images) for these questions are on the CD in this book. Be sure to check the reference number of the image against the number of the question you are attempting to answer.

126. This mother is concerned about breastfeeding her second baby. Her first baby had jaundice and did not thrive until supplements were given. From the picture shown, your first line of inquiry would be concerning:

 a. breast changes during pregnancy.
 b. length of gestation.
 c. age at her first menstrual period.
 d. history of breastfeeding failure in female relatives.

127. This mother has not completed Stage III of her labor. Her baby is healthy. The next action you should take is :

 a. get her to a hospital.
 b. help the mother put the baby to breast.
 c. give her oxygen for her exhaustion.
 d. have her assume a supine position.

128. Which of the following statements best describes the exclusively breastfed baby of this age?

    a. The baby will need complementary (solid) food soon.

    b. The baby consumes about 2/3 of available milk over the course of a day.

    c. The baby needs vitamin D supplements.

    d. The baby is at highest risk of SIDS.

129. This exclusively breastfed baby's mother became ill with rubella, and her doctor suggested she stop breastfeeding. She asks you to discuss the situation with her physician. Your best response to the physician is:

    a. the baby will likely get the disease, because the virus is transmitted in breast milk.

    b. the baby is likely to get a mild case or no infection at all because of disease-specific antibodies being released into her mother's milk.

    c. the mother should wean immediately to prevent the baby from becoming infected through skin-to-skin contact.

    d. the medications used to treat German measles are considered by the AAP to be compatible with breastfeeding.

130. The first thing you would suggest to the mother whose nipple looks like this is:

    a. have your doctor culture the nipple skin for thrush.

    b. wash your nipple with plain, cool water after feeding.

    c. use a nipple shield for the next day or two.

    d. keep the nipple warm, especially after feeds.

131. The drugs used in this procedure are most likely to have which effect on the newborn?

    a. fewer spontaneous kneading movements on the mother's chest

    b. depressed respiration in the first 5 minutes postbirth

    c. no effect on the infant

    d. transient bradycardia

132. What is the first thing you should say to this mother?

    a. Bring the baby on the right more deeply onto your breast.

    b. Shall I help restrain one baby's hands so he doesn't interfere with the other baby?

    c. How do you like breastfeeding both twins at once?

    d. Be sure to make eye contact with both babies during each feed.

133. At which age does this interaction between an adult and baby begin?

    a. 1 day

    b. 1 week

    c. 2 weeks

    d. 1 month

134. The chart shows the mean axillary and skin temperatures between 15 and 90 minutes after birth in healthy, full-term babies. The closed circles represent the babies cared for skin to skin with their mother. The open circles stand for babies who spent the time in the warming bed. What conclusion can be drawn from this chart?

    a. At 90 minutes, the babies who were cared for skin to skin were cooler than the babies in the warming bed.

    b. At 90 minutes, all the babies were cooler as measured at all three locations—axillar, interscapular, and thigh outside.

    c. At 90 minutes, all the babies were warmer as measured at all three locations—axillar, interscapular, and thigh outside.

    d. At 90 minutes, the interscapular temperature of the skin-to-skin babies is the same as the outside thigh temperature of the warming-bed babies.

135. This condition has not improved with the application of antifungal ointment, antibacterial ointment, or several nonmedicated nipple creams. What is your next course of action?

    a. Suggest the mother wear a silicone nipple shield during feeds.

    b. Examine the baby's mouth for signs of infection.

    c. Recommend breast shells between feeds to keep the sore area from crusting over.

    d. Refer the mother for a medical evaluation of the white areas on her nipple.

136. What is the most likely reason this device is being used?

    a. The baby has a weak suck and cannot stay latched at breast.

    b. The mother adopted this baby 3 weeks ago and is building up her milk supply.

    c. The baby has a cardiac defect and tires easily when breastfeeding.

    d. The mother is giving a prescribed medication during each feed.

137. The most appropriate action for the lactation consultant to take with this mother–baby pair is:

    a. instruct the mother to stop compressing the breast, as she is causing milk to flow too forcefully.

    b. help the mother use a more upright position to reduce nasal regurgitation.

    c. teach the mother to use a special slow-flow teat to prevent aspiration.

    d. show the mother how to use a bulb syringe to aspirate the baby's nose after feeds.

138. This exclusively breastfed child is falling below the pre-2006 NCHS growth curve that he has been following for 4 months. Your first action would be to recommend:

   a. giving him solid food.
   b. supplementing with infant formula.
   c. pumping the breasts after feeds to increase milk supply.
   d. continued exclusive breastfeeding for at least 2 more months.

139. What is the most likely condition pictured?

   a. abscess in the lower inner quadrant of the left breast
   b. bilateral primary engorgement
   c. large breasts with accessory breast tissue in both axilla
   d. bilateral mastitis extending to the axilla

140. The most likely reason for this infant's low weight gain is:

   a. a hyperextended neck, which prevents comfortable swallowing.
   b. hypertonia, as demonstrated by the baby's position.
   c. breast hypoplasia and insufficient glandular tissue.
   d. damage to the milk ducts and sensory tissue under the scarred area of the breast.

141. This mother is worried about her full-term baby's skin color. Your best recommendation is:

   a. have the baby's bilirubin checked by the pediatrician.
   b. adjust her positioning and encourage breastfeeding every 1–3 hours.
   c. begin supplementing feeds with expressed breast milk.
   d. give the baby water between breastfeeds.

142. This child's mother wonders why her child recently became ill with a respiratory illness. Your best response is:

   a. the immune factors in human milk decrease after 6 months.
   b. as his mobility increases, he is exposed to more pathogens.
   c. teething lowers his resistance to infection.
   d. placentally acquired immunity is wearing off.

143. This mother complains of sore nipples and this rapidly growing condition on her nipple. What would be your best course of action?

   a. Give the mother information on *Candida* infections of the nipple.
   b. Refer her to a qualified medical care provider immediately.
   c. Suggest she wash her nipples with water after each feed.
   d. Inquire about the red line on the lateral side of the breast.

144. What is the most likely explanation for the color of this milk, which was collected on day 5 post-birth?

    a.   The mother is taking prenatal vitamins containing beta carotene.

    b.   The milk contains pus from the mother's breast infection.

    c.   Transitional milk normally contains significant amounts of colostrum.

    d.   The mother had carrots and sweet potatoes for dinner last night.

145. This mother is becoming annoyed with her child's behavior during nursings, including the action shown in the photo. Your first response to her should be:

    a.   well, then it's time to think about weaning him.

    b.   many children try to nurse while they play with toys.

    c.   driving his toy truck across your chest during nursing really bothers you.

    d.   grab his hand and don't let him play with your body during feeds.

146. This baby now refuses to take a bottle from her daycare provider. Your best recommendation to her mother is that the provider should:

    a.   give milk in a cup.

    b.   wait until the child is really hungry.

    c.   try an orthodontic-shaped teat (nipple).

    d.   give the bottle in a dark room.

147. Using the 2006 WHO growth standards, this child gained weight faster than expected in the first 3 months, and now is lean for his length. All of his developmental milestones are normal. Your best recommendation to his mother is:

    a.   continue what you are doing. His growth pattern is normal for breastfed babies.

    b.   begin feeding him more solid foods to increase his weight.

    c.   take away his chewing toys and pacifiers as they are distracting him from eating.

    d.   supplement with a cow's-milk-based infant formula because he needs more calcium for growth.

148. If a lactation consultant sees this condition in a breastfeeding mother, which is the most important course of action to take?

    a.   Instruct the mother to use a lotion or oil to lubricate her skin.

    b.   Apply cold green cabbage leaves.

    c.   Contact her primary care provider to rule out cancer.

    d.   Ask about any history of polycystic ovarian syndrome.

149. The most important reason to use this feeding position and device is to:

   a. simulate a breastfeeding position.
   b. prevent the tongue from falling back into the airway.
   c. prevent milk from being lost into the cleft.
   d. increase the baby's muscle tone.

150. The first action you would do to assist this baby is:

   a. Have the mother attempt direct breastfeeding, correcting positioning as needed.
   b. Send the baby to an oral surgeon for a frenotomy.
   c. Cup feed 2 oz of expressed mother's milk.
   d. Have the mother place the baby skin to skin for 30 minutes.

151. This woman is planning to become pregnant. She is concerned about her nipple size and worried that her baby will have difficulty breastfeeding. Your best response to her is:

   a. yes, your small nipples may be a problem.
   b. normal nipples vary in size, and your nipples appear normal.
   c. be sure to pull and roll your nipples daily throughout pregnancy.
   d. wear breast shells during your pregnancy to increase eversion.

152. This mother asks for advice on family planning. She wishes to continue breastfeeding yet does not want to become pregnant again. Your best response to her is:

   a. begin taking a progestin-only oral contraceptive.
   b. use a condom every time you have intercourse.
   c. an intrauterine device is your best option.
   d. breastfeed exclusively around the clock without supplements or pacifiers.

153. This exclusively breastfed baby's behavior as shown is most likely to be caused by:

   a. overfeeding at breast.
   b. too-vigorous burping after feeds.
   c. allergy to something in the mother's diet.
   d. gastroesophageal reflux.

154. This mother's baby is teething, has recently started solid foods, and is taking an antibiotic for strep throat. The most likely cause of this condition is:

   a. an allergic reaction to a food the baby consumed.
   b. an allergic reaction to the medication being taken by her infant.
   c. psoriasis exacerbated by the infant's saliva.
   d. a baterial infection of the nipple skin.

155. This activity is appropriate or necessary during which of the following maternal conditions?

    a. chicken pox

    b. infectious mastitis

    c. breast abscess near the nipple

    d. toxoplasmosis

156. Mother support groups are very effective for which of the following reasons?

    a. Groups meet in members' homes.

    b. The group leader is highly trained.

    c. Cost for support groups is usually low.

    d. Mothers hear other mothers' ideas.

157. This mother tells you that her child loves the device pictured and sleeps best this way. The most likely reason for this is:

    a. the child has become too dependent because of prolonged breastfeeding.

    b. overuse of the baby carrier has delayed the child's ability to sleep alone.

    c. the mother is using her child to meet her own needs for companionship.

    d. this is normal behavior for this age child.

158. Which conclusion can be drawn from this chart?

    a. Baby A will always be smaller than baby D.

    b. Baby B gained weight faster than the others.

    c. Baby C is failing to thrive.

    d. Baby D gained the most weight in 1 month.

159. What is the most appropriate documentation of the appearance of this woman's breast?

    a. red circular area on the areola near the nipple margin

    b. red lesion 1/2-in (1-cm) diameter on the areola at the 7:00 position

    c. bacterial infection on the areolar skin in the lower, outer quadrant

    d. painful nipples with reddened area below the nipple base

160. To properly use this device, the mother should:

    a. cycle the pressure rapidly in the beginning, then slower as milk flows.

    b. hold the pressure steady for up to 5 minutes.

    c. cycle the pressure about 80–100 times per minute.

    d. use the pump vacuum to stretch the nipple forward into the flange.

161. At the age shown, what is the most appropriate recommendation for this child's nutrition?

    a. exclusive breastfeeding 24 hours a day
    b. breastfeeding with added carbohydrates
    c. breastfeeding with complementary family foods
    d. breastfeeding supplemented with infant formula

162. The most likely gestational age of this baby is:

    a. 36 weeks.
    b. 38 weeks.
    c. 40 weeks.
    d. 42 weeks.

163. When would this mother's baby get milk with the highest fat content?

    a. the last 5 minutes of each feed on either breast
    b. after nursing several times on one breast
    c. in the middle of the night
    d. when the mother is eating a high-fat diet

164. According to the Ten Steps to Successful Breastfeeding, this baby should be:

    a. taken to the admission nursery after 1 hour.
    b. moved to the central nursery only if the mother had a cesarean birth.
    c. given eye prophylaxis after 2 hours of age.
    d. kept with the mother 24 hours a day.

165. This baby breastfeeds at least 10 times a day, including 2–3 feeds at night. Her grandmother has advised her mother that she should be feeding her rice cereal and strained fruits. Your best response to the mother is:

    a. this pattern of breastfeeding is normal for a baby of this age.
    b. if she has been nursing this frequently for several days, then you apparently cannot make enough milk for her.
    c. she does not need solids, but she should be sleeping through the night.
    d. if she is 4 months old, it is good to start her on supplemental foods.

166. What is the most likely age of this baby?

    a. 36 weeks' gestational age
    b. 38 weeks' gestational age
    c. 2 days postbirth
    d. 4 days postbirth

167. This condition began when the child started taking solid foods. What would be your first management strategy?

    a. Discontinue all solid foods until the rash clears up.
    b. Mother should stop consuming dairy products.
    c. Take a thorough history of the mother's and baby's food intake.
    d. Refer the dyad to a dermatologist.

168. This mother's baby keeps bobbing on and off the breast and can't quite latch on. The first action the mother should take is:

    a. place a nipple shield over her nipple.
    b. let her baby suck on her finger to calm him.
    c. express some milk to soften the breast.
    d. burp him first before trying again.

169. The condition pictured appeared suddenly several days ago, when the baby began spending several hours daily in a child-care facility. The most likely cause of the condition pictured is:

    a. the baby's mother recently began taking an antibiotic.
    b. the baby recently ingested two bottles of artificial baby milk.
    c. the baby shared teething toys with other children.
    d. the baby began using a pacifier at the daycare center.

170. This baby's mother calls you, worried because for the past 2 days her baby has been nursing much more frequently than previously. The most likely reason for the change in nursing pattern is:

    a. teething.
    b. an illness.
    c. a growth spurt.
    d. a need for supplemental foods.

171. This exclusively breastfed baby's weight has dropped a bit on the NCHS standardized growth charts that were in use prior to 2000. Her development in other areas is completely normal to advanced, and she is content and happy most of the time. The most likely reason for this apparent growth faltering is:

    a. The mother's milk is too low in fat.
    b. The baby is physiologically ready for solid foods.
    c. Breastfeeding requires extra energy intake at this age.
    d. Breastfed babies tend to be leaner than artificially fed babies at this age.

172. This mother complains of nipple pain while pumping. The most likely cause is:

    a. she has a fungal infection on her nipples.
    b. the pump flange is not centered over her nipple.
    c. the pressure on the pump is too high.
    d. her lower hand is pulling the breast away from the pump.

173. What is the first action you would recommend to increase this mother's comfort during breast-feeding?

    a. Bring the baby more deeply onto the breast.
    b. Use an antifungal cream on your nipples.
    c. Apply lanolin after nursings.
    d. Use a different brand of absorbent bra pad.

174. What is the most likley condition shown in this picture?

    a. unpigmented areola
    b. poison ivy
    c. normal breast
    d. fungal infection

175. According to the Baby-Friendly Hospital Initiative, when will this event most likely occur?

    a. less than 5 minutes after birth
    b. within the first hour after birth
    c. within 6 hours after birth
    d. within 12 hours after birth

176. This 4-week-old, exclusively breastfed baby was 6 lbs, 3 oz at birth. The most likely reason for her appearance at this age is:

    a. her mother's milk is too high in fat.
    b. she is taking steroid drugs for a medical condition.
    c. her mother feeds her on cue, 24 hours a day, without a pacifier.
    d. her mother's milk is too high in lactose.

177. What is the average volume of milk consumed per 24 hours by a breastfed baby of this age?

    a. 550–600 ml (18–20 oz)
    b. 650–700 ml (21.5–23 oz)
    c. 750–800 ml (25–26.5 oz)
    d. 850–900 ml (28–30 oz)

178. Which of the following findings is most likely to be related to this mother's breastfeeding problem?

    a. Her husband has an oral yeast infection.
    b. The baby recently had strep throat.
    c. Her baby is 7 months old and teething.
    d. The mother has many allergies, including atopic dermatitis.

179. This baby's mother complains of sore nipples. Of the following, which is the first question you should ask?

    a. How did you prepare your nipples during pregnancy?
    b. May I watch you breastfeed right now?
    c. Are you feeling a stinging, burning sensation?
    d. How long do you intend to breastfeed?

180. The asymmetry of this woman's breasts is most likely due to:

    a. normal development.
    b. low milk supply in the smaller breast.
    c. insufficient glandular tissue in the smaller breast.
    d. hypermastia in the larger breast.

181. This woman says the condition pictured on her inner thigh becomes tender about once a month. It is most likely:

    a. a skin tag responding to varying estrogen levels.
    b. a wart that is sensitive to her clothing.
    c. a mole that should be examined by a dermatologist.
    d. an accessory nipple with sensitivity paralleling menstrual cycles.

182. This breastfed baby's mother comments that he should learn how to sleep for at least 8 hours straight at night. Your best response to her is:

    a. most babies of this age still need to breastfeed around the clock.
    b. he is too young now, but he should be sleeping through the night soon.
    c. if you don't go to him for a few nights, he will learn to sleep longer.
    d. he does not need to breastfeed at night if he weighs at least 12 pounds (5.4 kg).

183. How would you document this baby's oral configuration?

    a. The baby has a normal tongue position.
    b. The tongue is not moving normally.
    c. The tongue stays behind the inferior alveolar ridge.
    d. The baby has a poor tongue position.

184. To comfortably breastfeed, this mother may want to use:

   a. a breast pump to remove excessive milk before feeding.
   b. ice packs to reduce swelling.
   c. a nipple shield to help her baby latch on.
   d. a well-fitting bra to support her large breasts.

185. What would you do next to help this baby breastfeed?

   a. Put him to the mother's breast while he is alert.
   b. Put him under a radiant warmer for 2 hours to stabilize his temperature.
   c. Put him upright on his mother's bare chest, covered with a loose blanket.
   d. Swaddle him tightly with a small blanket to contain extraneous movements.

The next section of questions is constructed with a NEGATIVE STEM format. Be prepared to do a mental shift to think in negative terms, and read the stem and responses especially carefully before answering. There will be one **WRONG** answer among several correct answers. Continue using the pictures (images) on the CD in this book.

186. This mother brings her baby to a well-child clinic for a routine visit and nurses in the position shown. Your first response should be any of the following **EXCEPT**:

   a. how is breastfeeding going for you both?
   b. turn your baby's body to face your body.
   c. has your baby shown any interest in family foods?
   d. what family planning method are you using or planning to use?

187. The mother of this baby is practicing the Lactation Amenorrhea Method of family planning. Which behavior would **NOT** diminish the effectiveness of the method?

   a. intercourse more than twice a week
   b. relief bottle every other day
   c. baby sleeping through the night
   d. return of menstruation

188. The kind of care being given to this laboring woman results in all of the following **EXCEPT**:

   a. reduced involvement by her husband (partner).
   b. longer duration of breastfeeding.
   c. lower risk of cesarean birth.
   d. less infant asphyxia.

189. Which is the **LEAST** appropriate reason to offer this child family (complementary) foods in addition to breast milk?

    a. She is about 6½ months old.
    b. She is reaching for table foods.
    c. The nutritional quality of mother's milk is diminishing.
    d. She enjoys the social aspects of family mealtimes.

190. The nursing baby in this picture has not yet shown any interest in eating any family foods. Your **LEAST** appropriate response is:

    a. his growth is faltering, so you'll need to try harder to get him to eat family food.
    b. exclusive breastfeeding for longer than 6 months is a normal and desirable behavior.
    c. with your family history of allergies, it's not surprising that he's avoiding other foods.
    d. your other child is probably distracting him at mealtimes.

191. Which statement is **LEAST LIKELY** to be true concerning this mother's breast and nipple?

    a. The nipple is flat.
    b. The nipple/areolar complex has poor elasticity.
    c. The nipple tip is very soft and pliable.
    d. The nipple inverts between feeds.

192. The support being received by this mother helps foster all of the following **EXCEPT**:

    a. improved maternal–infant bonding.
    b. breastfeeding duration.
    c. fewer postpartum complications.
    d. increased maternal dependency.

193. Which situation is **LEAST LIKELY** to cause the condition shown?

    a. baby has a short, tight frenulum
    b. shallow latch
    c. flat, inelastic nipple tissue
    d. biting during nursing

194. Which of the following is the **LEAST LIKELY** condition pictured?

    a. galactocele
    b. areolar edema
    c. abscess
    d. milk stasis

195. Which of the following is this mother–twins triad **LEAST** likely to experience?

    a. mutual enjoyment of breastfeeding
    b. sibling rivalry for the breast
    c. babies' interaction with each other during feeds
    d. uninterrupted sleep for 8 hours at night

196. This device should have all of the following features **EXCEPT**:

    a. cycling power of 40–60 times per minute.
    b. creation of vacuum pressure in the range of 100–300 mm Hg.
    c. a flange diameter that easily accommodates the mother's nipple.
    d. sterilization required after every use.

197. This practice has all of the following results on the infant's physiology **EXCEPT**:

    a. higher infant metabolism.
    b. reduction of infant pain.
    c. stabilized infant temperature.
    d. increased infant oxygen saturation.

198. This technique might be used for all of the following **EXCEPT**:

    a. massaging a plugged nipple pore.
    b. firming the nipple tip before feeding.
    c. expressing milk.
    d. increasing tissue elasticity.

199. In a Baby-Friendly Hospital™, all of the following are standard care practices **EXCEPT**:

    a. mothers and babies room-in 24 hours per day.
    b. infant formula is never administered to breastfed babies.
    c. all maternity staff are competent in teaching hand expression of breast milk.
    d. mothers are never instructed to time feedings.

200. This feeding technique and equipment are a possible solution for all of the following situations **EXCEPT**:

    a. increased sensory input to palate.
    b. skin-to-mouth contact.
    c. prevents nipple confusion/flow preference.
    d. immediately after cleft palate repair.

EXAM A ANSWERS

The parenthetical material at the end of each answer includes the discipline and time period, indicates whether the question pertains to knowledge or application, and specifies the degree of difficulty.

1. The answer is B. At rest, the nipple tip is under the juncture of the hard and soft palate. (A. Anatomy; General Principles; Knowledge; Difficulty: 5)

2. The answer is A. Cardiorespiratory stability is most important when beginning oral feeds. Skin-to-skin contact and human milk both contribute to cardiorespiratory stability, especially in preterm infants. (B. Physiology; Prematurity; Knowledge; Difficulty: 4)

3. The answer is B. There is no evidence that continuing to breastfeed both children is harmful to either child or the mother. (B. Physiology; General Principles; Application; Difficulty: 3)

4. The answer is B. The newborn gut is sterile and should be protected by colostrum before anything else is ingested or inhaled. Colostrum paints the gut, sealing it from potential pathogens. (D. Immunology; Labor/Birth; Application; Difficulty: 4)

5. The answer is B. Immediate effective breastfeeding in the first hour or so, followed by 24-hour rooming-in, is the most important strategy. Prenatal expression of colostrum has not been researched. If the baby cannot breastfeed, milk expression should begin soon after birth. Restricting the mother's fluids is inappropriate and dangerous. (E. Pathology; 1–2 days; Application; Difficulty: 4)

6. The answer is D. Lipid solubility facilitates transfer of drugs into the mother's milk. The other factors inhibit drug transfer to milk. (F. Pharmacology; General Principles; Knowledge; Difficulty: 5)

7. The answer is D. Experience and research show that 8–12 feeds totaling 140–160 minutes or more are most typical in industrialized cultures. Less than 100 minutes at breast per day may indicate a problem. (H. Growth; Labor/Birth; Application; Difficulty: 4)

8. The answer is C. Research has established that a premature baby can go to breast earlier than he can feed from devices. (H. Growth; Prematurity; Application; Difficulty: 2)

9. The answer is A. The intent to treat design allocates research participants to groups according to a planned intervention. Whether or not the mothers actually breastfeed is not considered in the group assignment. (I. Research; General Principles; Knowledge; Difficulty: 4)

10. The answer is C. Discharge bags containing formula samples or coupons violate BFHI Step 6 and the international code. They are a marketing tool that has been clearly found to undermine breastfeeding. Furthermore, powdered formula is not sterile, which could put babies at risk and therefore your hospital at legal risk. (J. Legal; Labor/Birth; Application; Difficulty: 3)

11. The answer is B. Cup feeding has been researched better than any other alternative feeding device for preterm babies. Caution should be used to avoid pouring milk down the baby's throat, and spillage may occur. The baby should be watched closely for signs of stress in all cases. (K. Equipment; Prematurity; Application; Difficulty: 4)

12. The answer is B. It is always best to evaluate breastfeeding problems in person, because you can weigh the baby, observe the breastfeeding, and do more. (L. Techniques; 1–2 days; Application; Difficulty: 4)

13. The answer is C. Place babies in skin-to-skin contact with their mothers immediately following birth for at least an hour and encourage mothers to recognize when their babies are ready to breastfeed, offering help if needed. Research indicates that most babies will begin breastfeeding within the first hour if left undisturbed on the mother's chest/abdomen following birth. The BFHI includes no requirements for length of stay, when expressing milk should begin if the baby cannot breastfeed, or for care of premature babies other than expressing milk for them (Step 5). (M. Public Health; Labor/Birth; Knowledge; Difficulty: 5)

14. The answer is A. The Innocenti Declaration was adopted in 1990 and signed by representatives of many nations. It was modified and reconfirmed in November 2005. The other documents also support breastfeeding. The action steps of the Innocenti are more specific. (M. Public Health; General Principles; Knowledge; Difficulty: 4)

15. The answer is D. The glossopharyngeal nerve (C IX) controls the gag response in the soft palate and posterior tongue. (A. Anatomy; General Principles; Application; Difficulty: 5)

16. The answer is C. Women who choose LAM practice closer to optimal breastfeeding behaviors. Feeding on cue day and night is the most optimal of the above behaviors. Sleeping alone and giving water are likely to weaken the effect of LAM on fertility. Feeding on a schedule (every 2–3 hours) is less appropriate and suboptimal. (B. Physiology; 1–3 months; Application; Difficulty: 3)

17. The answer is C. Water-soluble vitamins vary with maternal intake. Fat-soluble vitamins vary slightly with maternal intake and when exposed to sunlight. Deficiencies are rare except for B_{12} in mothers who consume no animal products and vitamin D in women who lack sunlight exposure. Supplementing the mother in both cases increases these components in her milk. (C. Biochemistry; General Principles; Application; Difficulty: 3)

18. The answer is B. Beta-lactoglobulin isn't even found in human milk and is the most likely of the given options to cause allergic reactions in babies. Alpha-lactalbumin is not found in bovine milk. Lactose and lactoferrin are found in both milks. (D. Immunology; General Principles; Application; Difficulty: 4)

19. The answer is D. Three or more key symptoms are found in 70% of diagnosed *Candida* infection of the nipples. According to Morrill's research, key symptoms strongly correlated to *Candida* infections are burning pain, stabbing pain, nonstabbing pain, shiny skin, and flaky skin. Other symptoms can also occur. (E. Pathology; Labor/Birth; Knowledge; Difficulty: 5)

20. The answer is B. Checking pre- and postfeed weight on a sensitive scale is the most accurate and least disruptive of the options listed. Expressing is disruptive. Weighing the mother and counting swallows are less accurate. (L. Techniques; 1–3 months; Application; Difficulty: 4)

21. The answer is B. Breastfeeding can and should be taught in a group setting and with 1:1 instruction. Formula feeding should only be taught individually to those mothers who will not breastfeed for various reasons. (G. Psychology; Prenatal; Application; Difficulty: 2)

22. The answer is D. The Babinski reflex, flaring of the toes, is triggered when the sole of the foot is stimulated. (H. Growth; 1–2 days; Knowledge; Difficulty: 4)

23. The answer is A. A baby's trust develops by consistently and promptly responding to her needs. Close frequent contact at night helps develop trust. Forcing a baby to cry it out destroys the baby's growing sense of trust. Once broken, trust is difficult to repair. Over time, her needs diminish and the baby can tolerate delays in her mother's response. (H. Growth; 4–6 months; Application; Difficulty: 2)

24. The answer is C. Nutrition and immunological therapy for premature infants are the most common historical use of banked donor milk. The other uses of donor milk may occur, depending on availability of donors. (K. Equipment; Prematurity; Knowledge; Difficulty: 5)

25. The answer is A. Secretory IgA is found in large quantities in human milk, protecting the entire GI tract. The other immunoglobulins are also present in human milk, in lower proportions. (D. Immunology; 1–2 days; Knowledge; Difficulty: 5)

26. The answer is C. The obicularis oris is a circular sphincter-like muscle that circles the mouth and closes the lips around an object in the mouth. Masseter muscles close the jaw, temporal muscles also close the jaw and are visible during sucking, and the internal and external pterygoids move the jaw sideways, as in grating the teeth. (A. Anatomy; General Principles; Application; Difficulty: 5)

27. The answer is A. The occiput, or occipital bone, most often presents during a normal vaginal birth. At birth, the occipital bone is in four segments that adjust during the birth process. The second most common bone presenting is the frontal bone, which leads in a brow presentation. The frontal bone is in two segments at birth. Babies have more trouble breastfeeding after a difficult birth. (A. Anatomy; Labor/Birth; Knowledge; Difficulty: 4)

28. The answer is C. Preterm and very-low-birth-weight babies may have higher evaporative water loss because of their relatively large skin surface area. Keeping a baby skin to skin with the mother and feeding with human milk reduce excess water loss. (A. Anatomy; Prematurity; Application; Difficulty: 4)

29. The answer is D. On the first day, newborns take an average of 7-10 ml per feed, which matches the physiological capacity of the newborn stomach at birth. On the first day, total intake ranges from 7 to 122.5 ml (0.2–4.1 oz) and averages 37.1 ml (1.2 oz). Larger feed volumes overwhelm the newborn. (B. Physiology; Labor/Birth; Knowledge; Difficulty: 3)

30. The answer is B. Breastfeeding reduces risk of childhood acute lymphocytic leukemia by 19% and acute myleogenous leukemia by 15%. (D. Immunology; General Principles; Knowledge; Difficulty: 5)

31. The answer is C. The symptoms are most likely infectious mastitis. She needs medical evaluation and treatment with an antibiotic, bed rest, and continued breastfeeding and/or increasing milk drainage from the affected breast. She would greatly benefit from help with her baby. (E. Pathology; General Principles; Application; Difficulty: 5)

32. The answer is D. The first question should be, "Is it really necessary to take this drug at all, or at this time?" If the answer is clearly yes, then the other questions are appropriate in selecting a compatible medication for the mother's condition. (F. Pharmacology; General Principles; Application; Difficulty: 5)

33. The answer is A. Bromocriptine (Parlodel, Bromolactin, Kripton, Bromohexal) has been used to suppress lactation. (F. Pharmacology; General Principles; Knowledge; Difficulty: 2)

34. The answer is B. Fentanyl, especially in higher doses, is related to breastfeeding problems and early weaning. (F. Pharmacology; Labor/Birth; Application; Difficulty: 5)

35. The answer is B. Allergic reactions to fortifiers based on bovine milk are a significant problem for preterm babies. (D. Immunology; Prematurity; Knowledge; Difficulty: 2)

36. The answer is D. Human milk varies in color with mother's diet, medications, and other factors. Colored milk has never been shown to be detrimental or harmful to babies. No testing needs to be done, and no dietary changes are needed. (C. Biochemistry; Prematurity; Application; Difficulty: 3)

37. The answer is C. Lipase present in human milk digests and breaks down the fatty acids and may change the taste and smell of stored milk. The stored milk is still safe and healthy for the baby. (E. Pathology; General Principles; Application; Difficulty: 3)

38. The answer is B. There is no age beyond which breastfeeding is inappropriate. Complementary foods should begin some time in the second 6 months of life. (H. Growth; 1–2 days; Knowledge; Difficulty: 4)

39. The answer is C. If the mother's skin pigment and limited sun exposure cause a deficiency in her own vitamin D levels, then her milk may have low levels. Supplementing the mother with 2000 or more I.U. of vitamin D protects her own health and increases levels of D in her milk, thus protecting her and her baby. Exposing the baby and mother to sunlight will help a little. The other two choices undermine the benefit of exclusive breastfeeding. (C. Biochemistry; 1–3 months; Application; Difficulty: 5)

40. The answer is C. Ultrasound studies confirm that a large bolus of milk flows when the posterior tongue and jaw drop, creating a negative pressure inside the baby's mouth. (A. Anatomy; General Principles; Knowledge; Difficulty: 5)

41. The answer is A. The fourth intercostal nerve innervates the nipple and areola. Damage to this nerve can result in loss of sensation at the nipple and resultant lack of nerve feedback for lactation. (A. Anatomy; Prenatal; Application; Difficulty: 4)

42. The answer is B. Lactogenesis II is triggered by the withdrawal of progesterone when the placenta separates from the uterus. (B. Physiology; 1–2 days; Knowledge; Difficulty: 4)

43. The answer is A. Lactose is an especially important carbohydrate needed for brain development, and it is found in abundance in human milk. The other components are also found in milk and have importance to the infant. (C. Biochemistry; General Principles; Knowledge; Difficulty: 5)

44. The answer is B. The baby should be allowed to feed in his own preferred pattern, which may be one breast per feed or even several feeds on one breast before switching to the other. Getting too little fat-rich hind milk is one possible factor in rapid weight gain with fussy, gassy behavior. (E. Pathology; 15–28 days; Application; Difficulty: 4)

45. The answer is D. A large proportion (~ 70%) of the glandular tissue is located within a 30-mm radius of the nipple, according to recent ultrasound studies. (A. Anatomy; Prenatal; Knowledge; Difficulty: 5)

46. The answer is C. Persistent milk stasis is the chief cause of suppressed lactation (inadequate milk supply). Frequent, thorough removal of milk is necessary to sustain lactation. The other factors listed are old myths and not central to maintaining milk synthesis. (B. Physiology; 3–14 days; Knowledge; Difficulty: 5)

47. The answer is A. Pregnant women do not need extra protein if they are lactating. The other three responses are appropriate for helping her to assess her needs. (C. Biochemistry; Prenatal; Application; Difficulty: 5)

48. The answer is D. Fat levels, measured by creamatocrit, are up to 28% higher than levels in the milk of a woman who lactated 2–6 months. Total energy contributed by fat might be significant to the infant who continues to breastfeed more than 1 year. (C. Biochemistry; > 12 months; Knowledge; Difficulty: 2)

49. The answer is B. Breastfeeding for more than 2 years has no documented risks for mother or baby, and it has many benefits for both. (H. Growth; 7–12 months; Knowledge; Difficulty: 3)

50. The answer is B. Iodine 131 is a radioactive isotope requiring temporary cessation of breastfeeding. The mother should express her milk to maintain supply until the isotope is out of her system. (F. Pharmacology; General Principles; Knowledge; Difficulty: 5)

51. The answer is C. Her breast reduction surgery may have severed the nerves and ducts needed for adequate lactation. Close follow-up is essential. (K. Equipment; 1–2 days; Application; Difficulty: 3)

52. The answer is D. Breastfed babies initially gain more weight and by 6 months have begun to be leaner by height. By 12 months, there is a significant difference—the breastfed babies are even more lean by height than artificially fed babies. (H. Growth; 1–3 months; Knowledge; Difficulty: 3)

53. The answer is B. Donor milk is dispensed by prescription only. Regardless of the amount of milk available, its dispensation is prioritized (ranked) according to severity of need by the recipient. (K. Equipment; General Principles; Knowledge; Difficulty: 3)

54. The answer is B. Current ultrasound research on healthy, normal lactating breasts reveals an average of 9 ducts (range 4–18) terminating on the nipple. (A. Anatomy; General Principles; Knowledge; Difficulty: 4)

55. The answer is B. Macrophages and possibly neutrophils and T-lymphocytes actively kill microbes by phagocytosis. (K. Equipment; Prematurity; Knowledge; Difficulty: 4)

56. The answer is D. Mammary duct ectasia is the most likely cause of nipple discharge in pregnancy. The other conditions do not cause greenish discharge. (E. Pathology; 1–2 days; Knowledge; Difficulty: 4)

57. The answer is C. Allowing the baby to finish the first breast first allows the baby's appetite to best determine the balance of nutrients he obtains during a feed. Enforcing other patterns may result in less-than-optimal intake of nutrients and calories. (B. Physiology; 1–2 days; Application; Difficulty: 5)

58. The answer is B. The number of milk ejections strongly correlates to the amount of milk consumed by the infant at a feed. Multiple milk ejections are common. (A. Anatomy; 15–28 days; Knowledge; Difficulty: 2)

59. The answer is C. Cold packs will reduce edema, the most likely cause of impeded milk flow in early postpartum. There is no research supporting the use of hot compresses to improve milk flow. (L. Techniques; 3–14 days; Application; Difficulty: 3)

60. The answer is A. Breast growth (size change) indicates the growth of glandular secretory tissue. Growth patterns may vary widely and still be within normal ranges. Different size breasts are common; expression of colostrum during pregnancy is not expected; and breast shape is rarely relevant to lactation capacity. (A. Anatomy; Prenatal; Knowledge; Difficulty: 3)

61. The answer is D. This mother's breasts are entirely normal. Dripping milk from duct openings is unlikely to have any effect on the baby's latch. Areolar size is unrelated to milk supply and ability to breastfeed. (A. Anatomy; 3–14 days; Application; Difficulty: 3)

62. The answer is D. The most important regulatory mechanism for milk synthesis is frequent and thorough milk removal. (B. Physiology; 15–28 days; Application; Difficulty: 4)

63. The answer is C. Prolonged elevated bilirubin in a healthy, thriving baby at the level listed is not considered pathological. The best suggestion is continued appropriate breastfeeding practices. (B. Physiology; 3–14 days; Application; Difficulty: 3)

64. The answer is C. Babies feed for varying lengths and at varying intervals according to their hunger, emotional needs, growth and developmental stages, and other physiological factors. Placing restrictions on length or frequency or offering substitutes disrupts the breastfeeding relationship and interferes with fulfillment of infant needs. (B. Physiology; 1–3 months; Application; Difficulty: 2)

65. The answer is C. The infant gut takes up to 2 weeks to recover from damage caused by a reaction to a single bottle of artificial baby milk. (E. Pathology; 1–2 days; Knowledge; Difficulty: 4)

66. The answer is C. The foramen ovale may remain open or be reopened by excessive infant crying, which produces a Valsalva effect and increases thoracic pressure. (E. Pathology; Prenatal; Application; Difficulty: 5)

67. The answer is D. Babies with galactosemia cannot metabolize lactose, which is in high amounts in human milk. If the inability to metabolize lactose is complete, the baby cannot have any breast milk at all. (E. Pathology; 1–2 days; Knowledge; Difficulty: 4)

68. The answer is B. Keeping the dyad together is the most supportive action. (E. Pathology; 15–28 days; Application; Difficulty: 4)

69. The answer is C. When standard, appropriate treatments for breast engorgement do not quickly resolve the problem, a thorough medical evaluation is warranted to confirm or rule out serious pathology. (E. Pathology; 3–14 days; Application; Difficulty: 3)

70. The answer is B. Passing black, tarry stools after day 4 is abnormal. The baby needs a thorough medical evaluation to rule out gastrointestinal bleeding. By day 7, the baby should be passing 3–5 or more profuse, loose, yellow stools every day. (E. Pathology; 3–14 days; Application; Difficulty: 4)

71. The answer is B. Low thyroid levels can cause suppressed milk synthesis, fatigue, and chilliness. The mother should have a full medical evaluation. (E. Pathology; 1–3 months; Knowledge; Difficulty: 5)

72. The answer is C. The baby may breastfeed normally. Maternal thyroid disease that is properly treated is compatible with breastfeeding. (E. Pathology; 1–2 days; Knowledge; Difficulty: 3)

73. The answer is D. When baby is exclusively breastfeeding day and night without long periods away from the breast, the baby is under 6 months old, and her menses have not returned, there is only a 1–2% chance of pregnancy. (B. Physiology; 3–14 days; Knowledge; Difficulty: 3)

74. The answer is B. Confounding variables are factors that could influence the outcome of research that were not described or eliminated by the research design. (I. Research; General Principles; Knowledge; Difficulty: 3)

75. The answer is A. Reflux may be caused by an esophageal defect at the upper sphincter, where the esophagus meets the stomach. (A. Anatomy; Prenatal; Application; Difficulty: 2)

76. The answer is B. Milk ducts sometimes terminate on the areola, causing milk to be released during the milk-ejection reflex. This is a normal breast configuration. (A. Anatomy; 3–14 days; Knowledge; Difficulty: 3)

77. The answer is C. Skin-to-skin contact helps babies initiate breastfeeding. (L. Techniques; 1–2 days; Application; Difficulty: 3)

78. The answer is A. Colostrum is the treatment of choice for asymptomatic hypoglycemia. A small amount of colostrum stabilizes blood sugar. Some methods of testing blood sugar are not accurate. Direct breastfeeding is always the first and best course of action. A newborn normally breastfeeds every 1–3 hours in the first 24 hours, and nothing in this question indicates when, if ever, the baby had previously been fed. (E. Pathology; 1–2 days; Application; Difficulty: 4)

79. The answer is A. This is a normal pattern. (H. Growth; 15–28 days; Knowledge; Difficulty: 2)

80. The answer is D. Anti-inflammatory drugs are generally compatible with breastfeeding. The other statements are false. (F. Pharmacology; 15–28 days; Knowledge; Difficulty: 3)

81. The answer is A. Gut closure occurs around 6 months in the full-term baby. The risk of allergic sensitization from bovine protein is higher before gut closure. (D. Immunology; 15–28 days; Application; Difficulty: 4)

82. The answer is D. Lactocyctes (mammary secretory cells, also called glandular tissue) develop on the basement membrane of the duct structure starting during pregnancy. Growth continues for several weeks postbirth. (A. Anatomy; Prenatal; Knowledge; Difficulty: 5)

83. The answer is C. The tail of Spence is normal mammary glandular tissue extending into the axilla. (A. Anatomy; General Principles; Knowledge; Difficulty: 3)

84. The answer is D. A systematic review is the strongest level of research evidence. The next strongest of the listed research methods is B, a randomized trial. A cohort study is the weakest of those three. The MCN article is qualitative research, while the others are quantitative methods. (B. Physiology; General Principles; Application; Difficulty: 4)

85. The answer is A. In order for a maternal medication to affect the baby, it must pass into milk and be ingested by the baby. Drugs that are not absorbed from the GI tract are very low-risk because the baby's GI tract would not absorb the drug even if the drug is in the milk. (F. Pharmacology; General Principles; Knowledge; Difficulty: 5)

86. The answer is C. After 5 half-lives have passed, approximately 98% of the drug or isotope has been eliminated. Each drug or isotope has a specific half-life. (F. Pharmacology; General Principles; Knowledge; Difficulty: 3)

87. The answer is C. Fathers easily bond with their exclusively breastfed babies. (G. Psychology; General Principles; Application; Difficulty: 3)

88. The answer is A. Quasi-experimental studies are more likely to show that the explanation really did cause the outcome; therefore, these designs have the highest internal validity. (I. Research; General Principles; Knowledge; Difficulty: 3)

89. The answer is B. The higher the vacuum pressure, the more milk collected during the let-down (milk-ejection) reflex. Timing the sessions is less effective than monitoring milk ejections. Fast speed may trigger a milk ejection but then should be slowed during high flow periods. Narrow-diameter flanges may pinch the nipple and may be detrimental. (K. Equipment; General Principles; Application; Difficulty: 3)

90. The answer is B. Lactation consultant practice is based on scientific principles, current research, and published guidelines. The first step is to provide clinical evidence supporting or refuting this practice and discuss the evidence with your colleague. Option A would be appropriate later, if B and C do not result in a change of practice. D is inappropriate. (J. Legal; General Principles; Application; Difficulty: 4)

91. The answer is A. The Baby-Friendly Hospital Initiative is designed to protect breastfed babies from practices and policies that disrupt or interfere with breastfeeding. The 2006 Expanded and Integrated BFHI includes a module on the non-breastfeeding baby. (M. Public Health; General Principles; Knowledge; Difficulty: 4)

92. The answer is C. Mothers are reliable witnesses and reporters of their babies' conditions. Sudden disinterest in breastfeeding may indicate a significant problem in the baby. (G. Psychology; General Principles; Application; Difficulty: 3)

93. The answer is A. Mothers of multiples are more likely to attach to the unit before the individual children. (G. Psychology; General Principles; Knowledge; Difficulty: 4)

94. The answer is C. It is appropriate to discuss the potential side effects on milk supply with the mothers. The ethical principle in this case is the patients' right to autonomy over their health-care choices. (J. Legal; General Principles; Application; Difficulty: 5)

95. The answer is B. First, discuss the mother's accusations with the lactation consultant in question. If the mother's report is accurate, the lactation consultant is violating the IBLCE Code of Ethics and Standards of Practice, and a complaint should be lodged with IBLCE. (J. Legal; General Principles; Application; Difficulty: 3)

96. The answer is A. The concentration of drug in the milk is nearly always proportional to the level in maternal plasma. (F. Pharmacology; General Principles; Knowledge; Difficulty: 2)

97. The answer is C. Caffeine is the most likely to affect the baby because it is a central nervous system stimulant and highly lipid-soluble. Insulin is poorly absorbed orally; digoxin acts on muscle tissue and passes poorly into milk; warfarin has a large molecular weight and does not pass into milk. (F. Pharmacology; General Principles; Application; Difficulty: 2)

98. The answer is B. Maternal diabetes increases the risk of breast infections. (E. Pathology; General Principles; Knowledge; Difficulty: 2)

99. The answer is A. Exclusive breastfeeding means that the baby satisfies all nutrition and sucking at his mother's breast. Adding supplemental vitamins is not exclusive breastfeeding; neither is adding other fluids or pacifiers. (M. Public Health; General Principles; Knowledge; Difficulty: 5)

100. The answer is D. Alcohol in milk is directly related to levels in maternal serum and does not accumulate in milk. (F. Pharmacology; General Principles; Knowledge; Difficulty: 4)

101. The answer is A. Women over the age of 25 need the same amount of calcium regardless of breastfeeding or pregnancy status, and research suggests the same is true for women who are overlapping breastfeeding with pregnancy and tandem nursing moms. During pregnancy, even for malnourished mothers, extra calcium is excreted with the urine; instead the body acquires the needed calcium through intrinsic processes such as enhanced uptake. During the exclusive breastfeeding phase, bone mineral density typically dips and then begins to rebound once complementary foods are added to the baby's diet, and a study that included a tandem nursing mom showed the same results for her as for other breastfeeding moms. Research has shown that when breastfeeding and pregnancy overlap, the bones actually *increase* in bone mineral density. Dairy sources of calcium are the most bioavailable. (C. Biochemistry; Prenatal; Application; Difficulty: 5)

102. The answer is D. Current recommendations are for pregnant women of normal prepregnancy weight to gain 25–35 pounds (11.4–15.9 kg) during pregnancy. Underweight women and teenagers should gain even more weight to sustain their growing bodies and the developing fetus. (C. Biochemistry; Prenatal; Application; Difficulty: 3)

103. The answer is A. The first statement to the mother should be a positive statement. Afterward, a fuller explanation of induced lactation should take place, which might include any or all of the other choices. (G. Psychology; 1–3 months; Application; Difficulty: 2)

104. The answer is B. Breastfeeding at least 7 months reduces risk of urinary tract infections for up to 2 years, because of sIgA and lactoferrin in milk and because of human milk's anti-inflammatory and anti-infective properties. The difference seems to be more pronounced in girls because of genitourinary anatomy. (D. Immunology; > 12 months; Application; Difficulty: 5)

105. The answer is C. Domperidone (Motilium), metoclopramide (Reglan, Maxolon), and cimetidine (Tagamet) are sometimes used to increase milk supply. Of these, domperidone and metoclopramide have been studied most for effectiveness and safety. Beer raises prolactin levels when tested in men, but babies do not like the flavor of alcohol in milk and breastfeed less when milk alcohol levels are elevated. (F. Pharmacology; Prematurity; Application; Difficulty: 3)

106. The answer is C. There are a myriad of potential breastfeeding problems associated with epidural anesthesia. (F. Pharmacology; Labor/Birth; Application; Difficulty: 2)

107. The answer is D. The lymphatic system drains from the breast tissue; it does not supply components of milk manufacture. (A. Anatomy; General Principles; Knowledge; Difficulty: 2)

108. The answer is C. Homeopathic remedies have the least potential effect on the infant. Homeopathic remedies are extremely diluted preparations. (F. Pharmacology; 15–28 days; Knowledge; Difficulty: 4)

109. The answer is B. Painful stimulation is not appropriate and may even cause the baby to shut down further. Skin-to-skin comforting is the first strategy, followed by massage and other gentle stimulating strategies. (L. Techniques; 1–2 days; Application; Difficulty: 4)

110. The answer is C. Docosahexaenoic acid is a long-chain fatty acid that is found in the fatty portion of milk, not the whey portion. (C. Biochemistry; General Principles; Knowledge; Difficulty: 2)

111. The answer is D. Environmental estrogens are a speculated factor in lactation abnormalities. The other three maternal factors are far more likely to result in low milk volume at 3 weeks postpartum. (B. Physiology; 15–28 days; Knowledge; Difficulty: 2)

112. The answer is B. According to the Pan American Health Organization and World Health Organization, vegetarian diets cannot meet nutrient needs at this age unless supplements or fortified products are used. The other statements are true. (C. Biochemistry; > 12 months; Knowledge; Difficulty: 3)

113. The answer is D. Lactation reduces the risk of adult-onset diabetes in a woman with gestational diabetes. The other statements are true. (E. Pathology; Labor/Birth; Knowledge; Difficulty: 5)

114. The answer is A. Breastfeeding the child in the second year is mutually pleasurable even when the majority of the child's calories come from other sources. (G. Psychology; > 12 months; Knowledge; Difficulty: 5)

115. The answer is C. Screening for environmental contaminants is not routinely performed, although occasional case-by-case screening for a particular substance has been done. Pasteurization is common but not done in all nations. (K. Equipment; General Principles; Knowledge; Difficulty: 3)

116. The answer is A. The mother's short-term restricted diet has little or no bearing on milk composition or milk volume. The other statements are accurate. (B. Physiology; 4–6 months; Application; Difficulty: 3)

117. The answer is C. Breastfeeding with its proper sucking is least related to urogenital development and is involved in development of the other systems listed. (B. Physiology; General Principles; Application; Difficulty: 5)

118. The answer is B. Colostrum is rich in anti-infective and anti-inflammatory properties. Its protective role appears to be even more important than its role in providing calories to the infant. Beta-endorphins in colostrum are natural pain relievers. (D. Immunology; 1–2 days; Knowledge; Difficulty: 5)

119. The answer is D. Most mothers will produce plenty of milk for several breastfed babies, despite higher risk of early birth-related problems. (B. Physiology; 15–28 days; Knowledge; Difficulty: 2)

120. The answer is D. Rooming-in enhances the mother–baby relationship and has no known detrimental effect on relationships with grandparents. (G. Psychology; Labor/Birth; Knowledge; Difficulty: 2)

121. The answer is D. The other areas may have extra mammary and/or nipple tissue, which are remnants of the galactic band. (A. Anatomy; Preconception; Knowledge; Difficulty: 3)

122. The answer is D. Bottle feeding has been shown to be stressful for preterm infants and increases the risks of premature weaning. (K. Equipment; Prematurity; Application; Difficulty: 5)

123. The answer is A. The first statement is condescending and disempowering. The others validate and support a mother's emotional state and behavior and are thus empowering. (G. Psychology; Prematurity; Application; Difficulty: 3)

124. The answer is A. Separate sleeping is a recent and unusual developmental pattern for babies. (H. Growth; 1–3 months; Knowledge; Difficulty: 5)

125. The answer is D. Bottle feeding is not associated with normal broad palate configurations. Artificially fed children are more likely to need orthodontia, have weakened masseter muscles, have more speech disorders, and have a narrower palate. (A. Anatomy; > 12 months; Knowledge; Difficulty: 5)

126. The answer is A. This mother's breasts are mildly hypoplastic or underdeveloped and asymmetrical. Both conditions have been linked to limited lactation capacity in some women. (A. Anatomy; Prenatal; Application; Difficulty: 4)

127. The answer is B. Putting the baby to breast will help the uterus expel the placenta and reduce bleeding. Skilled home birth attendants carry medications to aid uterine contractions for emergency situations. (B. Physiology; Labor/Birth; Application; Difficulty: 5)

128. The answer is B. Normal 4-month-old babies take an average of 2/3 of the available milk over the course of the day. Adding complementary foods is no longer recommended; neither are routine vitamin D supplements. The highest risk of SIDS is at 2–4 months. (C. Biochemistry; 4–6 months; Knowledge; Difficulty: 5)

129. The answer is B. The mother's body produces disease-specific antibodies that appear in milk shortly after exposure. These protect the child from the disease, either entirely or partially. There is no evidence that this viral infection is transmitted through mother's own milk, and the mother will be holding the baby skin to skin regardless of feeding method. The mother did not ask you about medications, so D is an inappropriate response. (D. Immunology; 4–6 months; Application; Difficulty: 2)

130. The answer is D. The white blanched area is a vasospasm of the nipple, usually triggered by cold air or trauma, also known as Renaud's phenomenon. Keeping the nipple warm, especially immediately after the baby finishes nursing, should help avoid triggering this painful circulatory condition. (E. Pathology; General Principles; Application; Difficulty: 3)

131. The answer is A. Research shows that locally injected lidocaine, as well as other medications used for labor pain relief, alter the newborn's spontaneous ability to crawl to the breast, explore the breast with hands, and latch effectively to the breast. (F. Pharmacology; Labor/Birth; Knowledge; Difficulty: 4)

132. The answer is C. Supporting what the mother is doing is the first thing to do or say in nearly every situation. This mother and her babies are completely normal and thriving. The next step might be to assure that she is in contact with other mothers who are breastfeeding twins or triplets. (G. Psychology; 3–14 days; Application; Difficulty: 3)

133. The answer is A. An infant can imitate the adult's facial expressions shortly after birth. This baby is 4 days old and clearly is imitating the woman's expression. (H. Growth; 4–6 months; Knowledge; Difficulty: 4)

134. The answer is C. Comparing the lines with the closed circles with the lines with the open circles, the closed-circle lines (representing skin-to-skin babies) represent higher temperature at all three places where the temperature was measured. (I. Research; General Principles; Application; Difficulty: 3)

135. The answer is D. This mother needs immediate medical evaluation. Any breast lesion that does not quickly respond to common treatment for common problems during breastfeeding could have an ominous cause. This lesion is nipple cancer (Paget's disease). (J. Legal; General Principles; Application; Difficulty: 2)

136. The answer is B. Tube-feeding devices were originally designed for situations where the baby has a good suck, and the mother provides food via the tube while building up her milk supply. (K. Equipment; 15–28 days; Application; Difficulty: 4)

137. The answer is B. Upright positions will help this baby to feed. This baby had velopharyngeal insufficiency, and milk dripped out of whichever nostril was lower during the feeding. (L. Techniques; 3–14 days; Application; Difficulty: 4)

138. The answer is D. This 4-month-old, exclusively breastfed boy is completely normal and has no physiological need for solid food until about 6 months or later. The growth standards published by the World Health Organization in 2006 are based on normal, healthy, optimally fed breastfed children from several nations, cultures, and ethnic groups. (M. Public Health; 4–6 months; Knowledge; Difficulty: 4)

139. The answer is C. This woman's large breasts are normal; she has accessory mammary tissue in both axilla. This photo was taken on day 4 postbirth. (A. Anatomy; 3–14 days; Knowledge; Difficulty: 5)

140. The answer is D. This mother had breast reduction surgery with significant tissue removal many years ago. The scars on the lateral surface of her breast, near her arm, are the only visible clues of this underlying condition. The baby is in an effective (but perhaps awkward) position for feeding and shows no signs of hypertonia. (B. Physiology; 15–28 days; Application; Difficulty: 4)

141. The answer is B. The baby's skin is slightly yellow, suggesting hyperbilirubinemia. Assuring frequent, effective breastfeeds is the most appropriate strategy to use at this point. (B. Physiology; 1–2 days; Application; Difficulty: 4)

142. The answer is B. As this child naturally explores his environment, he is exposed to many more pathogens. Some immune components of human milk increase over time. (D. Immunology; 4–6 months; Application; Difficulty: 4)

143. The answer is B. This mother has Paget's disease, a form of nipple cancer. She had sore nipples for several months, then noticed this lesion, which continued growing rapidly until a breast surgeon performed a mastectomy. The scar on her breast is from a tumor that was removed, probably the original site of the cancer. (E. Pathology; General Principles; Application; Difficulty: 5)

144. The answer is C. Milk collected on day 5 is composed of colostrum plus increasing levels of lactose; the yellow color is from the beta-carotene in colostrum. Milk collected during mastitis does not contain pus, and there is no indication that the mother has a breast infection. Yellow-colored milk can be caused by foods or drugs the mother has consumed. (F. Pharmacology; 3–14 days; Application; Difficulty: 4)

145. The answer is C. An empathetic response that clarifies the mother's feelings is the first step to establishing rapport in a counseling situation. After the mother's feelings are clearly identified, then solutions can be addressed. (G. Psychology; 7–12 months; Application; Difficulty: 3)

146. The answer is A. Breastfed babies are often willing to try a different feeding method when they are not ravenously hungry. (K. Equipment; 7–12 months; Application; Difficulty: 3)

147. The answer is A. This 4-month-old boy is normal in every way. The earlier NCHS growth reference charts were developed based on babies receiving mixed feeds, not exclusively breastfed infants. New standards based on the healthy, breastfed baby were published by WHO in 2006. (H. Growth; 4–6 months; Application; Difficulty: 5)

148. The answer is C. This is peau d'orange, or orange-peel texture of the skin, is associated with breast cancer, overstretched skin, edema, hair follicle stimulation, and other conditions. Breast cancer should be ruled out by a qualified medical provider. The other answers would be appropriate after ruling out a dangerous condition. (J. Legal; General Principles; Knowledge; Difficulty: 5)

149. The answer is B. This baby's cleft was complete, and his tongue is small and posteriorly placed and drops easily into his airway. He has great difficulty feeding by any method. The Haberman feeder puts pressure on the tongue and positions it more anteriorly in the baby's mouth. (K. Equipment; 3–14 days; Application; Difficulty: 4)

150. The answer is A. This baby's most urgent need is for food. Direct breastfeeding is almost always the first strategy. In this child's case, breastfeeding has not been going well, as evidenced by his failure to thrive. Providing mother's own expressed milk would be the next strategy, combined with skin-to-skin care for comfort. (L. Techniques; 3–14 days; Application; Difficulty: 5)

151. The answer is B. Small nipples work just fine for breastfeeding. This woman's breast is entirely normal. (A. Anatomy; Preconception; Application; Difficulty: 5)

152. The answer is D. The Lactation Amenorrhea Method offers the highest (at least 98%) protection against unplanned pregnancy and is the most compatible method with continued breastfeeding. (B. Physiology; 15–28 days; Application; Difficulty: 5)

153. The answer is C. Persistent spitting up in the otherwise normal exclusively breastfed baby is most likely an allergic or hypersensitivity response to a substance in the mother's diet. Cow's milk is a highly likely cause. And cow's-milk allergy may be responsible for up to 42% of gastroesophageal reflux in babies. (E. Pathology; 4–6 months; Knowledge; Difficulty: 4)

154. The answer is D. She was diagnosed with a bacterial infection of the nipple skin, most likely streptococcus transferred from the baby's mouth. The rash is exactly where the baby's mouth had come into contact with her areolar tissue. (D. Immunology; 4–6 months; Application; Difficulty: 5)

155. The answer is C. Expressing or pumping milk may be helpful if a breast abscess is so close to the nipple that the baby cannot effectively feed. The other conditions are compatible with continued breastfeeding. (E. Pathology; 1–3 months; Knowledge; Difficulty: 3)

156. The answer is D. Mothers talking to other mothers has been shown to be an effective strategy for supporting breastfeeding since at least the 1920s. (G. Psychology; Labor/Birth; Knowledge; Difficulty: 5)

157. The answer is D. Many, if not most, babies sleep better when close to their mothers or are carried on their mothers' bodies. This is normal behavior. (H. Growth; 4–6 months; Knowledge; Difficulty: 2)

158. The answer is B. Baby B's rate of weight gain was the fastest, as represented by the steeply increasing angle of slope of the graph. None of the other conclusions can be drawn from the data presented. (I. Research; 15–28 days; Application; Difficulty: 3)

159. The answer is B. A clear description of your observation is most appropriate. Option A is less clear, C is offering a diagnosis, and D includes the mother's subjective feelings ("painful"). (J. Legal; General Principles; Application; Difficulty: 5)

160. The answer is A. The pumping pattern should closely mimic the baby's feeding pattern of rapid cycling until the milk lets down, then about 40–60 cycles of alternating vacuum and release per minute during milk flow. (K. Equipment; 3–14 days; Application; Difficulty: 3)

161. The answer is C. Breastfeeding with complementary family foods is recommended by UNICEF and the World Health Organization for the child in her second 6 months of life. (M. Public Health; 7–12 months; Knowledge; Difficulty: 4)

162. The answer is D. This baby was born at 42 completed weeks of gestation, which is considered the late end of normal gestation. Peeling skin is one visual clue to a baby nearing postterm gestational age. Breastfeeding difficulties are associated with preterm and sometimes postterm birth. (A. Anatomy; Labor/Birth; Knowledge; Difficulty: 4)

163. The answer is B. Fat content in milk rises as the breast empties, so the proportion of fat from one breast is highest when the baby has fed several times from that breast. (B. Physiology; 15–28 days; Knowledge; Difficulty: 4)

164. The answer is D. Twenty-four-hour rooming-in from birth onward is Step 7 of the Ten Steps to Successful Breastfeeding (Baby-Friendly Hospital Initiative). (M. Public Health; Labor/Birth; Application; Difficulty: 4)

165. The answer is A. This 5-month-old, exclusively breastfed baby is entirely normal. The teething behavior suggests that she will soon be interested in family foods. (C. Biochemistry; 4–6 months; Application; Difficulty: 3)

166. The answer is D. This baby is 4 days old. The milk in the cup is slightly yellow, suggesting transitional milk. The baby's skin is slightly yellow, suggesting mild jaundice, which would be considered pathological if the baby were younger than 3–4 days. (H. Growth; 3–14 days; Application; Difficulty: 4)

167. The answer is C. Taking a thorough history of the dyad's food intake is the first step in identifying any possible allergic reactions to ingested food or allergens transferred via milk. This child's rash is an allergic reaction. (D. Immunology; 4–6 months; Application; Difficulty: 4)

168. The answer is C. This mother's breasts are full and taut with milk, which inhibits her baby from a good, deep latch. She should express or pump some milk to soften her breasts before trying to feed him again. (E. Pathology; 3–14 days; Application; Difficulty: 3)

169. The answer is B. This is an allergic rash, which began when the baby ingested cow's-milk-based infant formula at daycare. (D. Immunology; 7–12 months; Application; Difficulty: 5)

170. The answer is C. This baby is 4½ months old and is most likely going through a growth spurt. He is too young to need solid foods. Teething and illness are less common reasons for a sudden change in nursing patterns. (H. Growth; 1–3 months; Application; Difficulty: 4)

171. The answer is D. Pre-2000 growth curves published by the National Center for Health Statistics were not based on exclusively breastfed babies. Newer research has established that artificially fed babies are fatter (heavier) per unit of length compared to breastfed babies in the 3- to 6-month period. The baby pictured is 4 months old. (I. Research; 7–12 months; Application; Difficulty: 4)

172. The answer is B. The most likely cause of her nipple pain is off-center placement of the nipple in the pump flange. At one time, this was thought to increase milk yield. Off-center positioning or a too-narrow diameter flange can cause friction and pain and inhibit milk flow. (K. Equipment; 3–14 days; Application; Difficulty: 4)

173. The answer is A. Correcting positioning and latch is the most important strategy to increase nipple comfort during breastfeeding. In this mother's case, deeper attachment significantly reduced pain; treating the mild thrush infection removed the remaining discomfort. (L. Techniques; 1–2 days; Application; Difficulty: 5)

174. The answer is A. This mother's breast has no visible areola. She experienced no breast changes during pregnancy, and this breast did not produce any milk postbirth. Sometimes one unusual anatomical finding, such as the lack of pigmented areola, indicates other unusual or pathological conditions. (A. Anatomy; 3–14 days; Knowledge; Difficulty: 3)

175. The answer is B. Babies placed skin-to-skin will usually begin breastfeeding within the first hour. (M. Public Health; Labor/Birth; Knowledge; Difficulty: 4)

176. The answer is C. This 4-week-old baby has gained weight appropriately and is entirely normal. (B. Physiology; 15–28 days; Knowledge; Difficulty: 3)

177. The answer is C. The average 2- to 4-week-old baby's milk consumption is approximately 750–800 ml (25–26.5 oz) per day. The amount can vary widely among normal babies. (C. Biochemistry; 15–28 days; Application; Difficulty: 5)

178. The answer is B. The crack at the base of the nipple was caused by a bacterial infection of her nipple and occurred at the same time that her baby was diagnosed with a streptococcal infection of the throat. (D. Immunology; 4–6 months; Application; Difficulty: 5)

179. The answer is B. Observing a breastfeed is the first step in identifying the cause of painful nipples. (L. Techniques; 15–28 days; Application; Difficulty: 3)

180. The answer is A. Differences in breast size during lactation are normal and common. (A. Anatomy; 15–28 days; Application; Difficulty: 2)

181. The answer is D. This is an accessory nipple on the woman's upper, inner thigh. This woman found the sensitivity of the skin paralleled her menstrual cycles. (A. Anatomy; Preconception; Knowledge; Difficulty: 4)

182. The answer is A. Most babies continue waking at night for feeding throughout the first year of life and may get up to 1/3 of their calories at night. (H. Growth; 4–6 months; Application; Difficulty: 4)

183. The answer is C. This is the most accurate description of this baby's tongue. Unseen in the photo is the baby's very short, tight lingual frenulum. (J. Legal; 3–14 days; Application; Difficulty: 4)

184. The answer is D. Mothers with large breasts may enjoy the support of a well-fitting bra. There is no pathology shown in this picture. Her baby is nursing well on day 4 postbirth. (K. Equipment; 3–14 days; Application; Difficulty: 4)

185. The answer is C. Immediate skin-to-skin contact is an excellent strategy to calm and warm a baby in preparation for breastfeeding. (L. Techniques; 1–2 days; Application; Difficulty: 4)

186. The answer is B. Suggestions to correct or improve breastfeeding technique are generally not the first consideration when working with a healthy 6-month-old. Older babies can place themselves in creative postures and still breastfeed effectively. The other questions assume the normalcy of breastfeeding and provide emotional support while obtaining useful data. (G. Psychology; 4–6 months; Application; Difficulty: 4)

187. The answer is A. Frequency of sexual intercourse is unrelated to the LAM method. (B. Physiology; 1–3 months; Knowledge; Difficulty: 2)

188. The answer is A. Doula care (the continuous presence of a trained attendant through the entire labor) enhances the husband's (partner's) involvement in birth. Doula care also extends the duration of breastfeeding, shortens labor, reduces cesarean births, and results in less infant asphyxia. (G. Psychology; Labor/Birth; Knowledge; Difficulty: 2)

189. The answer is C. The nutritional quality of human milk does not diminish at 6 months. Social aspects of family mealtimes are an important developmental milestone. Some children of this age reach for family foods, which is a cue of readiness. Age alone is not an indication of the need for complementary food. (C. Biochemistry; 7–12 months; Knowledge; Difficulty: 4)

190. The answer is A. This child is obviously thriving—his growth is not faltering in the slightest. Avoidance of family foods appears to be not unusual in babies from allergic families. (H. Growth; 4–6 months; Application; Difficulty: 4)

191. The answer is C. This flat nipple has damage on the upper surface. The baby was tongue-tied. The combination of a flat nipple and a baby with poor tongue mobility caused the abrasion. It is unlikely that this much damage would occur on a soft and pliable nipple tip. (A. Anatomy; General Principles; Application; Difficulty: 3)

192. The answer is D. Most cultures protect and support the new mother for several weeks postbirth, which facilitates the mother's reentry into the community. (G. Psychology; Labor/Birth; Application; Difficulty: 2)

193. The answer is D. Biting during nursing is not likely to cause a wound in this position—it is more likely to cause a wound at the nipple-areola juncture. The other causes are quite possible. In this mother's case, the baby had a shallow latch that was quickly and easily corrected. (B. Physiology; 3–14 days; Application; Difficulty: 5)

194. The answer is C. This is least likely to be an abscess because there is no redness or discoloration. The bulge on this woman's areola at the 10:00 position was a galactocele and caused her no discomfort or difficulty during breastfeeding. (E. Pathology; 1–2 days; Knowledge; Difficulty: 5)

195. The answer is D. Breastfed twins often are best friends and copy each other's breastfeeding behaviors, although they can compete with one another for the breast and at the breast. Many 8-month-old, breastfed babies of this age wake at night, and twins are no exception. (G. Psychology; 7–12 months; Application; Difficulty: 2)

196. The answer is D. Thorough cleaning after each use and sterilization once a day is recommended by most pump manufacturers. (K. Equipment; 3–14 days; Knowledge; Difficulty: 5)

197. The answer is A. Kangaroo care, or skin-to-skin contact, preserves infant energy as well as the other results listed. It is especially beneficial for premature infants. (L. Techniques; 1–2 days; Knowledge; Difficulty: 3)

198. The answer is C. This technique is ineffective for expressing milk, but might be helpful for the other situations listed. (L. Techniques; 1–2 days; Knowledge; Difficulty: 4)

199. The answer is B. Infant formula may be administered to a breastfed baby if a medical reason is documented. Very few conditions of the mother or baby are considered acceptable medical reasons for supplementation. (M. Public Health; General Principles; Knowledge; Difficulty: 3)

200. The answer is D. Finger-feeding is a therapeutic method to help a baby get back to direct breast-feeding. After palate repair, a soft object (like the breast) is less likely to hurt or damage the repair site. (L. Techniques; 15–28 days; Application; Difficulty: 3)

EXAM B QUESTIONS

1. A well-balanced diet with sufficient calories accompanied by early and regular prenatal care significantly reduces the incidence of:

   a. infants with diabetes.
   b. low birth weight.
   c. maternal gestational diabetes.
   d. lactation failure.

2. A mother of 10-week-old twins calls. She says that all she does all day is feed babies and she can't take it anymore. She asks how she can introduce some artificial baby milk or infant cereal without weaning her babies from the breast. The first thing you should do is:

   a. Suggest she feed her infants simultaneously in order to save time.
   b. Tell her that offering other foods will decrease milk production.
   c. Ask if she has any help with household chores.
   d. Actively listen, and praise her for breastfeeding two babies.

3. Bacterial counts 1 hour after expression are lower than immediately after collection. The most likely explanation for this is:

   a. The cooler temperature in the container is unsuitable for the growth of bacteria.
   b. Macrophages in milk are actively phagocytic.
   c. Gangliosides in milk disrupt the cell walls of bacteria.
   d. Bifidus factor starves the bacteria of nutrients.

4. In the global context, the foremost benefit of using an open cup for feeding a preterm baby who cannot yet breastfeed is:

   a. It is inexpensive and readily available.
   b. There is a low risk of fluid aspiration.
   c. It fosters appropriate tongue motions.
   d. It is easy to clean.

5. Which statement describes the most reliable research tool?

   a. The tool has not broken in 5 years of continuous use.
   b. Using the tool produces the same results, even when used by different people at different times.
   c. The tool is quick to master and easy to use by multiple researchers.
   d. The tool was developed by well-known researchers at a large, prestigious university.

6. Which drug property is most likely to permit high passage into milk?

    a. high lipid solubility
    b. high pH
    c. large molecular weight
    d. high protein binding

7. Which of the following protective components of milk is destroyed by freezing?

    a. lysozyme
    b. lymphocytes
    c. secretory IgA
    d. lactoferrin

8. When doing a review of the literature for a research study, which sources are most important to include?

    a. review articles that analyze several studies
    b. textbooks that explain basic concepts
    c. a peer-reviewed journal report of research, written by the researcher
    d. lectures given at large conferences by well-known speakers

9. Which category of drug administered to the mother is usually contraindicated during breastfeeding?

    a. antimicrobial
    b. antihypertensive
    c. antineoplastic
    d. antidepressant

10. Compared to term milk, preterm milk is higher in which component?

    a. protein
    b. lactose
    c. phosphorus
    d. iron

11. Which of the following is permissible under the terms of the World Health Organization's International Code of Marketing of Breast-Milk Substitutes?

    a. gift packs containing samples and coupons for formula given to new mothers at hospital discharge

    b. detailed information on product composition provided to health workers

    c. advertisements for toddler formula on local television stations

    d. picture of a happy baby on the label of infant formula containers

12. The standard temperature and time for Holder pasteurization used in donor human milk banks is:

    a. 87°C for 10 minutes.

    b. 70°C for 25 minutes.

    c. 62.5°C for 30 minutes.

    d. 60°C for 60 minutes.

13. Fat levels in mother's milk are highest:

    a. when the milk-ejection reflex is strong.

    b. during the night.

    c. when the mother eats a high-fat diet.

    d. when the breast is relatively empty.

14. In order to minimize your legal risk when practicing as a lactation consultant, it is most important for you to:

    a. keep accurate financial records.

    b. obtain detailed information from the primary care provider(s).

    c. establish a respectful rapport with open communication.

    d. accept mothers' insurance payment plans.

15. When would a drug given to the mother most readily pass into the milk?

    a. when the mother is collecting milk for a premature baby

    b. in the first 4 days postbirth

    c. when the mother has a breast infection

    d. when the drug is given transdermally

16. A research report indicates that a sample of breastfed infants had no differences in illness rates than a comparable sample of artificially fed infants. While reading this report, what is the most important point to look for?

    a. the type of study used
    b. operational definitions
    c. the sample used
    d. the review of the literature

17. What is the average normal heart rate of a full-term infant?

    a. 80–100 beats per minute
    b. 100–120 beats per minute
    c. 120–160 beats per minute
    d. 160–200 beats per minute

18. A pregnant woman with many allergies asks about infant feeding. Your best response is:

    a. A baby is never allergic to his mother's milk, but he may be sensitive to foods in the mother's diet.
    b. Since many allergic tendencies are inherited, there is nothing you can do to reduce your baby's chances of being allergic.
    c. The hypoallergenic formulas will prevent any allergic reaction in your baby.
    d. Whether you breastfeed or not, you should delay solid foods until 6 months or later to help your baby avoid allergies.

19. What is the average percent of a drug administered to a lactating woman that actually reaches the breastfeeding baby?

    a. 0.01%
    b. 0.1%
    c. 1.0%
    d. 10%

20. A researcher is studying breastfeeding incidence in two neighboring community prenatal clinics. In one clinic, a new videotape is used to teach breastfeeding; the other continues to use an older videotape. At the follow-up, both clinics report similar increases in breastfeeding initiation. The most likely reason for this is:

    a. all instructional videotapes are equivalent.
    b. the Hawthorne effect.
    c. changing the videotape had no effect.
    d. the Nedelsky effect.

21. The grandmother of a 4-week-old, exclusively breastfed baby who has 5–6 profuse, yellow, loose stools every day is worried and asks for an explanation. The most likely cause for stools of this kind is:

    a. diarrhea.
    b. infection with an intestinal parasite.
    c. the mother recently ate bright yellow squash.
    d. normal stools.

22. Which property of maternal medications increases the amount of the drug that gets to the breast-feeding baby via breast milk?

    a. short half-life
    b. no active metabolites
    c. high oral absorption
    d. high gut destruction

23. A 4-year-old girl was hurt in an auto accident, and as part of her treatment, a chest tube was placed between her ribs below and distal to her right nipple. What is the most significant effect that this surgery might have on her ability to breastfeed?

    a. damage to the ductal structure
    b. damage to the blood vessels supplying the breast
    c. severed nerve pathways to the nipple
    d. cut blood vessels to the breast

24. A healthy, full-term newborn is found to have a total bilirubin level of 14.2 mg/dL (245 µmol/L) on the fourth day of life. The best recommendation is:

    a. Breastfeed the baby at least 10 times a day.
    b. Feed artificial baby milk after breastfeedings.
    c. Feed artificial baby milk for 24 hours; maintain supply through pumping.
    d. Tell the mother that this level of bilirubin is rarely a problem.

25. A 27-year-old woman will birth her first baby in about 3 weeks. She asks her health care provider if she will be able to breastfeed after having a breast reduction with her nipple auto-transplanted at the age of 19. The best thing he could say is:

    a. There will be no problem breastfeeding.
    b. It may be possible for the first 3 months.
    c. You may not be able to breastfeed.
    d. You should try and see what happens.

26. Which of the following statements best describes fetal nutrition?

    a. The umbilical cord delivers nutrients directly to the fetal gut.
    b. The fetus swallows and digests amniotic fluid.
    c. The fetus absorbs nutrients from the amniotic fluid through his skin.
    d. The fetus has no digestive enzymes of his own until after 40 weeks.

27. Which nutrient is most difficult for premature babies to digest?

    a. carbohydrate
    b. protein
    c. fats
    d. minerals

28. A breastfeeding mother has been diagnosed with postpartum depression. Her physician contacts you to discuss whether or not she should continue to breastfeed during drug treatment. Your best response is:

    a. There are several antidepressant medications that are considered compatible with breastfeeding.
    b. All medications used to treat mental illness are contraindicated during breastfeeding.
    c. Her baby is in great danger and should be kept away from her at all costs.
    d. The hormones of breastfeeding will exacerbate her illness.

29. You have been working with a mother who describes excruciating pain every time her baby's mouth touches her breast, even if he does not latch on and breastfeed. You have ruled out injury, infections, and other causes of nipple pain, and her nipples are not reddened or irritated. You should next consider whether the mother has:

    a. a history of any kind of abuse.
    b. no interest in breastfeeding.
    c. a low pain threshold.
    d. allergies.

30. You are asked to evaluate a baby's ability to breastfeed before discharge following an uncomplicated hospital birth 12 hours ago. The baby weighs 2700 grams, or 6 pounds. Which of the following characteristics of her sucking would lead you to suspect that this child was born slightly preterm (or near term)?

    a. moves smoothly from rooting behavior to latch-on
    b. sucks, swallows, and breathes in a coordinated rhythm
    c. sucks in short bursts with pauses
    d. begins by sucking rapidly, then slows to a steady rhythm

31. A mother of newborn twins asks whether to feed her babies separately or together. Your best response is:

    a. Let's see which works best for you.
    b. Separately is better so you can focus on one at a time.
    c. Together is better to save you time.
    d. Feed them together to get their feeding patterns synchronized.

32. For optimal breastfeeding, which best describes effective positioning at breast?

    a. The nipple is inside the baby's mouth.
    b. No areola is visible outside the perimeter of the baby's mouth.
    c. The baby's nose lightly touches the mother's breast.
    d. The baby's mouth is open to a wide (> 120-degree) angle.

33. A mother calls about her 5-month-old infant, worried that she is losing her milk because her breasts are soft and her infant no longer seems content for 2 hours after feedings. He cries frequently and puts his fists to his mouth 45 minutes after feeding. The most likely cause for the situation she describes is:

    a. Her infant is experiencing a normal growth and behavior pattern.
    b. Offering bottles is interfering with breast-milk production.
    c. Her baby is developing colic.
    d. Her body is adapting well to her baby's demand for milk.

34. A mother was given high doses of pain-relieving drugs during labor. When the baby's cord blood is tested for the presence of drugs, none is found. The most likely explanation is:

    a. Pain-relieving drugs are lipid soluble and concentrate in the infant brain.
    b. Pain-relieving drugs do not cross the placenta.
    c. The mother's body metabolizes most drugs before birth.
    d. Pain-relieving drugs have a very short half-life.

35. At 14 days postbirth, a mother tells you that she has bright red vaginal bleeding and that her baby (birthweight 9 lbs, 2 oz/4.139 kg) seems constantly hungry. The most likely explanation for this is:

    a. a large-for-gestational-age baby.
    b. an early return of menses.
    c. a uterine infection.
    d. a retained placental fragment.

36. A breastfeeding mother fractured her pelvis and right leg in a car accident. She is in traction and taking pain medications. Her exclusively breastfed, 3-month-old baby has never taken a bottle. The most helpful action to support this family is:

    a. Get her a breast pump so she does not become engorged.
    b. Encourage her husband to teach the baby to take milk from a spoon or cup.
    c. Help her position the baby for nursing in a way that does not disturb her injuries.
    d. Obtain a prescription for birth control pills to dry up her milk.

37. A baby's tongue is pressing a mother's nipple against the baby's hard palate. Which cranial nerve was most responsible for this tongue movement?

    a. spinal accessory
    b. vagus
    c. hypoglossal
    d. trigeminal

38. During breastfeeding, where is the infant's tongue usually placed?

    a. resting behind the alveolar ridge
    b. covering the alveolar ridge
    c. spread flat across the floor of the mouth
    d. extended past the lower lip

39. A mother is concerned because her 3-week-old, exclusively breastfed baby suddenly became very fussy in the evenings. Her breastfeeding pattern did not change, and the baby is otherwise healthy. Which recently added item in her diet is most likely to be related to her baby's reaction?

    a. lemonade
    b. herbal tea
    c. green vegetables
    d. vitamin supplements

40. Which component of human milks is most variable?

    a. proteins
    b. lipids
    c. carbohydrates
    d. minerals

41. A mother comes to you for help with breastfeeding her 3-week-old baby, stating, "He just doesn't seem to be able to get it right." When you observe the baby breastfeeding, you note that the baby has a highly erratic suck-swallow pattern and that he never develops a good rhythmic suckling action. Which of the following is most likely to explain his sucking behavior?

   a. Many babies do not establish effective suckling patterns until 4–6 weeks after birth.
   b. The baby's head is still quite molded.
   c. The baby was born at 37 weeks gestation.
   d. The baby has cerebral palsy.

42. When during gestation does the mammary ridge form?

   a. 4–5 weeks
   b. 14–15 weeks
   c. 24–25 weeks
   d. 34–35 weeks

43. Which breast structure contains muscle fibers?

   a. lactiferous sinuses
   b. nipple-areola complex
   c. Montgomery tubercles
   d. lobules

44. A 16-year-old mother delivered her first baby by cesarean section and sustained significant blood loss requiring a blood transfusion. Four days later, her milk has not yet "come in." The most likely reason for delay in onset of copious milk synthesis is:

   a. young age.
   b. cesarean delivery.
   c. first lactation cycle.
   d. significant blood loss.

45. After an unmedicated labor and birth, how soon is a baby most likely to be able and ready to breastfeed?

   a. within the first 5 minutes
   b. within the first hour
   c. at approximately 6 hours
   d. by 12 hours

46. Which of the following citations is a primary reference or source?

    a. DeCoopman, JM. *Pacifier Use in Breastfed Infants: Review and Recommendations* [masters' thesis]. Ann Arbor: University of Michigan; 1996.
    b. Als H, Lester BM, Tronick E, Brazelton TB. Manual for the assessment of preterm infants' behavior (AFPB). In: Fitzgerald JE, Lester BM, Jogman MW, eds. *Theory and Research in Behavioral Pediatrics.* Vol. 1. New York: Plenum; 1982:64-133.
    c. Fildes V. *Breasts, Bottles and Babies: A History of Infant Feeding.* Edinburgh: Edinburgh University Press; 1986.
    d. Aarts C, Hornell A, Kylberg E, et al. Breastfeeding patterns in relation to thumb sucking and pacifier use. *Pediatrics.* 1999;104(4).

47. A mother complains that her baby cries constantly. She has been feeding her baby on a strict schedule found in a popular parenting book. Your best response to her is:

    a. It is acceptable to limit your baby's feeds to 10 minutes per breast.
    b. You can give a pacifier to help your baby extend the time between feeds.
    c. Babies do best when there are no restrictions on length or frequency of breastfeeds.
    d. Giving water between feeds will get your baby onto a more regular feeding schedule.

48. A mother complains of raw, inflamed skin on both areolas. Her infant is teething, has recently started solid foods, and is taking an antibiotic for strep throat. The most likely cause of this areolar irritation is:

    a. an allergic reaction to a food the baby consumed.
    b. an allergic reaction to the medication being given to her infant.
    c. psoriasis that was exacerbated by the infant's saliva.
    d. a bacterial infection of the nipple skin.

49. A mother is uncertain about providing her own milk for her preterm baby and has been told that her milk helps nerve development. Which sensory system is most compromised by the absence of human milk?

    a. olfactory
    b. auditory
    c. taste
    d. visual

50. A full-term baby 13 hours old has not yet been to breast. Your first choice to feed this baby is:

    a. curved-tip syringe.
    b. open cup.
    c. bottle with preemie nipple (teat).
    d. putting the baby to breast.

51. Which mother would have the highest risk of drug passage into milk?

    a. Sue, whose baby was born at 26 weeks' gestation and is now 3 weeks old
    b. Mary, who breastfeeds 5 times a day and supplements with infant formula
    c. Irene, who had a cesarean birth 2 days ago
    d. Claudia, whose 5-month-old twins are exclusively breastfed

52. Researchers have found that inguinal hernia and some other disorders of the urogenital tract are less common in breastfed babies. Which of the following components has the most significant role in tissue maturation of the infant?

    a. epidermal growth factor
    b. nerve growth factor
    c. secretory IgA
    d. lactoferrin

53. Which of the following approaches will be most helpful in assisting a breastfeeding mother who has a hearing impairment?

    a. Speak to her more slowly.
    b. Talk directly to her interpreter.
    c. Make frequent eye contact with her.
    d. Help her observe the baby's visual cues.

54. Within the first minute or two of beginning a breastfeed, a 2-week-old infant gulps, coughs and chokes, then releases the breast. This incident most likely describes:

    a. an infant with decreased oral tone.
    b. poor coordination of sucking, swallowing, and breathing.
    c. a strong milk-ejection reflex.
    d. gastroesophageal reflux.

55. Which description best describes the configuration of milk ducts in the lactating breast?

    a. deep in the breast, like the core of an apple
    b. branching beginning posterior to the areolar margin
    c. bulbous, pea-shaped swellings near the areolar margin
    d. superficial and easy to compress

56. A mother calls on day 12 to obtain a breast pump to increase her milk supply. She had an emergency cesarean, did not breastfeed or pump for the first 3 days, and has been pumping 3-4 times a day since then. She has not been able to get the baby to latch and feed effectively. Which of the following is most likely to increase the rate of milk synthesis?

    a. drinking 1/4 cup of fenugreek tea 3 times a day
    b. thoroughly draining the breasts every 2–3 hours by nursing, pumping, and/or expressing
    c. putting the baby to breast every 2–3 hours to stimulate the breasts even if the baby does not feed well
    d. a prescription of metoclopramide to increase prolactin

57. If a mother cannot provide her milk to her baby, the World Health Organization recommends that the next best food for her baby is:

    a. soy-based formula
    b. cow's-milk-based formula
    c. pasteurized donor human milk
    d. milk of another woman

58. At what developmental age is self-feeding most likely to begin?

    a. 3–4 months
    b. 6–7 months
    c. 9–10 months
    d. 12+ months

59. Guidelines from the U.S. Centers for Disease Control and Prevention state that health care workers should wear gloves when assisting breastfeeding mothers in which of the following situations?

    a. touching a mother's breast
    b. positioning a baby at breast
    c. helping a mother pump her milk
    d. processing donor human milk

60. Which of the following citations is a primary reference or source?

    a. Anderson GC. Current knowledge about skin-to-skin (kangaroo) care for preterm infants: Review of the literature. *J Perinatol.* 1991;XI:216–226.

    b. Als H, Lester BM, Tronick E, Brazelton TB. Manual for the assessment of preterm infants' behavior (AFPB). In: Fitzgerald JE, Lester BM, Jogman MW, eds. *Theory and Research in Behavioral Pediatrics.* Vol. 1. New York: Plenum; 1982:64–133.

    c. Ludington-Hoe SM, Golant SK. *Kangaroo Care: The Best You Can Do to Help Your Preterm Infant.* New York: Bantam Books; 1993.

    d. Ludington-Hoe SM, Hadeed AJ, Anderson GC. Physiologic responses to skin-to-skin contact in hospitalized premature infants. *J Perinatol.* XI,(1):19–24.

61. Which of the following is considered fair use of published written material according to international copyright laws?

    a. downloading or photocopying one copy of a published research article for your personal use

    b. making copies of a research article for all participants in your for-profit breastfeeding course

    c. using pictures downloaded from the Internet in your presentations or lectures

    d. making lecture handouts that include reproductions of copyrighted images that you purchased

62. Which of the infant's host defense systems are most effective at birth?

    a. ability to cough

    b. low pH of the stomach contents

    c. innate defensins in the baby's skin and vernix

    d. complement system and phagocytes

63. A mother was given 40 mg of a drug with a half-life of 4 hours. How much of the drug is left in her system after 4 half-lives have elapsed?

    a. 20 mg

    b. 10 mg

    c. 5 mg

    d. 2.5 mg

64. Which of the following is an example of a qualitative research design?

    a. What are mothers' experiences of breastfeeding after cesarean birth?

    b. How many mothers in Norway gave birth by cesarean section in 2003?

    c. Is there a relationship between cesarean birth and infant suck dysfunction?

    d. What percent of babies are helped by lactation consultant contact 3 days after a cesarean birth?

65. A cultural attitude that emphasizes the sexual nature of breasts is most likely associated with:

    a. harassment for breastfeeding in public.
    b. increased breast augmentation surgery.
    c. mothers enjoying the attention created by larger breasts during lactation.
    d. conflicts in custody disputes involving breastfeeding babies.

66. Cholecystokinin, which is released by sucking, has which of the following effects?

    a. arousal
    b. satiety
    c. agitation
    d. depression

67. Which drug property results in more transfer of the drug into mother's milk?

    a. milk-plasma ratio < 1.0
    b. molecular weight > 500
    c. high protein binding
    d. lipid solubility

68. Additional body contact, as occurs when the mother uses a soft tie-on type carrier, is most likely to have which of the following effects?

    a. decreased total crying
    b. increased dependency
    c. delayed walking
    d. more night waking

69. What is thought to be the primary function of the Montgomery glands?

    a. pigmented marker for visual targeting
    b. to lubricate the skin of the areola
    c. to secrete antibiotic substances
    d. changes elasticity of areola skin

70. Sudden onset of painless bright red bleeding from the nipple of a mother during the first week postpartum indicates the probable presence of:

    a. breast cancer.
    b. fibrocystic disease.
    c. intraductal papilloma.
    d. nipple tissue breakdown.

71. Which nodes collect most of the lymph drainage from the lactating breast?

    a. axillary nodes
    b. intermammary nodes
    c. subclavicular nodes
    d. mesenteric nodes

72. A mother is collecting milk for her ill, premature baby. Which is the best container for her milk?

    a. open plastic cups or bottles
    b. soft plastic polyethylene ("nurser") bags
    c. large containers holding several feeds
    d. glass containers with airtight lids

73. A mother asks why she can express an ounce of milk even after her baby finishes feeding. The most likely explanation for this is:

    a. The baby is not feeding effectively.
    b. Babies normally do not take all of the milk available at a given feeding.
    c. She has an oversupply of milk.
    d. Her baby does not like the taste of her milk.

74. Which nutritional recommendation is most relevant to a breastfeeding mother?

    a. Drink a large glass of water whenever you breastfeed.
    b. Avoid spicy or gas-producing foods.
    c. Increase your caloric intake to make enough milk.
    d. Follow your usual dietary practices.

75. Which of these statements best describes the mucosal defense system?

    a. A microbe is taken up by the mother's B cells and passed to M cells.
    b. Helper T cells break down the pathogens.
    c. The mother's secretory immune system provides targeted protection.
    d. The infant's mucosal membranes provide passive immunity.

76. A pregnant woman contracted chickenpox (Varicella) a short time ago. The lesions are now completely crusted over, and she is in labor. The most appropriate action to take when she gives birth is:

    a. Separate her from the baby until she is noninfectious.
    b. Allow her to hold but not breastfeed her baby.
    c. Separate her from the baby, but feed her expressed milk to the baby.
    d. Help her breastfeed immediately after birth with 24-hour rooming in.

77. A mother's lack of eye contact and little talking or caressing of her infant should alert you to the possibility of:

    a. a neurologically impaired infant.
    b. a neurologically impaired mother.
    c. a developmentally delayed infant.
    d. a clinically depressed mother.

78. A mother with a 5-day-old infant repeatedly requests rules for how many times a day she should feed her baby. This behavior is typical of which stage of maternal role acquisition?

    a. anticipatory
    b. formal
    c. informal
    d. personal

79. The mother of a 5-month-old breastfeeding baby is most likely to observe that the baby:

    a. plays with the mother's other nipple while breastfeeding.
    b. closes her eyes during breastfeeding.
    c. is easily distracted while nursing.
    d. does not awaken to breastfeed at night.

80. Which of the following is a result of pasteurizing donor human milk?

    a. concentration of lipids
    b. reduction in lactose
    c. no change in secretory IgA
    d. destruction of lactoferrin

81. A 4-month-old, exclusively breastfed baby feeds about 8–10 times per day with 1–2 feeds at night. His mother is concerned that she cannot make enough milk because her neighbor had to increase the amount of formula for her baby at 4 months. Your best response to her is:

    a. Your baby's feeding pattern indicates that he is ready for solids.
    b. Your baby's milk needs are stable for at least another 2 months.
    c. Your baby is clustering much of his milk intake at night, which is normal.
    d. Your baby will take more milk from your breasts if he needs more.

82. A laboring woman has received several bags of intravenous fluids during her labor. Her baby is now several hours old and is having trouble latching onto her breast. The most likely explanation for this is:

    a. Her breasts are edematous from the IV fluids.
    b. The labor affected the baby's ability to suck.
    c. Her milk tastes unpleasant because of the fluids given.
    d. The fluids diluted the colostrum available, and the baby is frustrated.

83. Which breast structure contains the cells that secrete milk?

    a. lactiferous ducts
    b. lobules
    c. alveoli
    d. nipple

84. The mother of a premature baby needs to express milk for her baby. She has relatively small breasts. Which expressing pattern is most likely to result in abundant supply?

    a. 6 times a day for 30 minutes per breast
    b. every 3–4 hours for 10 minutes per breast
    c. every 2–3 hours until the milk flow ceases
    d. every 1–2 hours during the day and once at night

85. At what gestational age does the swallowing reflex first appear?

    a. 16 weeks
    b. 22 weeks
    c. 28 weeks
    d. 32 weeks

86. An exclusively breastfed baby's risk of food allergies is:

    a. decreased, because few food allergens pass through mother's milk.
    b. decreased, because mother's milk makes passage of allergenic proteins through baby's gut less likely.
    c. increased, because allergens pass readily through mother's milk.
    d. increased, because mother's milk increases the permeability of the baby's gut.

87. An effective technique for hand expression of milk is:

    a. compressing the breast behind the areola, then sliding the fingers toward the nipple.

    b. pinching the base of the nipple.

    c. pressing deeply at the nipple-areolar juncture.

    d. positioning the fingers at the edge of the areola, pressing inward, and rolling toward the nipple.

88. A breastfeeding mother 6 weeks postbirth tells you, "None of your suggestions have worked, and I'm at the end of my rope. I'm a complete failure as a mom!" Which is the most likely condition affecting the mother?

    a. bipolar disorder

    b. anxiety disorder

    c. postpartum depression

    d. maternal deprivation syndrome

89. A mother of a fussy, gassy baby has been drinking 10 glasses of cow's milk per day on her doctor's recommendation. Your first action would be:

    a. Encourage her to follow her doctor's dietary advice.

    b. Take a thorough history, including allergy and food sensitivity in the family.

    c. Tell her that 6–8 glasses of any liquid is adequate during lactation.

    d. Tell her that consumption of dairy products is not related to her baby's symptoms.

90. A 2-day-old baby feeds from one breast for about 25 minutes, then falls asleep and releases the breast. A few minutes later, he wakes and feeds on the second breast for about 10 minutes, then falls asleep and releases the breast. The most likely explanation for this behavior is:

    a. The mother does not yet have enough milk to satisfy the baby.

    b. The baby is not latched deeply onto the breast.

    c. The baby is sleepy and poorly coordinated as a result of labor medications.

    d. This is a normal pattern for this age baby.

91. Which hormone in the milk is most responsible for anti-inflammation activity?

    a. prolactin

    b. prostaglandins

    c. oxytocin

    d. relaxin

92. Some brands of artificial baby milk produced in the 1980s lacked one essential mineral, causing brain damage and learning disabilities in the children who received this product exclusively. Absence of which of the minerals listed would have that effect?

a. sodium
b. chloride
c. potassium
d. calcium

93. An 8-day-old infant has been at breast constantly since birth. His mother complains of nipple pain and states that her baby makes a clicking sound and loses his grasp of her nipple frequently during the feed. You have corrected her latch-on technique. Your next action should be:

a. Provide her with a sterile nipple shield.
b. Instruct her to use several different breastfeeding positions.
c. Instruct her in suck training to correct the baby's sucking.
d. Refer her to a health professional qualified to evaluate for tongue-tie.

The next section of questions is constructed with a NEGATIVE STEM format. Be prepared to do a mental shift to think in negative terms, and read the stem and responses especially carefully before answering. Instead of selecting the one correct answer from incorrect responses, there is one *incorrect* answer among 3 correct responses. You are to pick the one "wrong" answer.

94. A mother calls you, frustrated because her 3-week-old baby's preference for nursing at the right breast is so strong that she is unable to get him to nurse on her left side. What is the **LEAST LIKELY** explanation for this baby's nursing behavior?

a. There is a subtle positioning difference in the mother's hold on her left side.
b. The baby has a cephalohematoma on his right side.
c. The mother has an undetected breast cancer in her left breast.
d. The baby's right clavicle is fractured.

95. During a routine examination in her second trimester of pregnancy, a doctor discovers that a woman has nonprotractile nipples. All of the following increase the probability that she will successfully breastfeed **EXCEPT**:

a. wearing breast shells for increasing amounts of time per day for a few weeks of her pregnancy.
b. appropriate positioning and latch-on techniques.
c. breastfeeding the baby during the first hour after birth.
d. nonpharmaceutical pain relief strategies for labor and birth.

96. Medical uses for donor human milk include all of the following conditions **EXCEPT**:

    a. postsurgical nutrition.
    b. skin treatment of burns.
    c. solid organ transplants.
    d. allergies and feeding intolerance.

97. Safe motherhood initiatives include breastfeeding because it protects women's health in all of the following ways **EXCEPT**:

    a. reduced postpartum bleeding.
    b. reduced risk of reproductive cancers.
    c. reduced postpartum fertility.
    d. reduced libido during breastfeeding.

98. A mother who is becoming ill with influenza should continue breastfeeding her 5-month-old, exclusively breastfed child for all of the following reasons **EXCEPT**:

    a. Her milk will quickly obtain specific antibodies to reduce the chance that her child will get this infection.
    b. Her milk contains white cells that will help her baby fight this infection.
    c. Lactation speeds up her own production of antibodies so her illness will be less severe.
    d. She will recover quicker without the additional burden of preparing artificial feeds.

99. Which is the **LEAST LIKELY** reason a 1-month-old child breastfeeds 4–8 times every day, including 1–2 times at night?

    a. The mother is pressuring the child to gratify her own desires.
    b. The child is recovering from gastroenteritis.
    c. The child is allergic to many foods.
    d. The mother is recovering from a hospital stay where the child could not visit.

100. Which of the following is **NOT** an example of mutual interdependency during breastfeeding?

    a. The baby's gut closure occurs around the time he is ready for solid foods.
    b. The mother's milk contains environmental chemicals, triggering the baby's immune system.
    c. Skin contact during breastfeeding helps regulate the baby's temperature.
    d. Sucking at breast triggers release of gut hormones in the mother and the baby.

101. The World Health Organization's International Code of Marketing of Breast-Milk Substitutes applies to all of the following products **EXCEPT**:

    a. breast pumps.
    b. infant formula.
    c. feeding bottles and teats.
    d. weaning foods.

102. The existing policy on the maternity unit at your hospital is to supplement all breastfeeding babies with 1 oz (30 cc) glucose water by bottle after every breastfeed. Which strategy is **LEAST LIKELY** to be effective in changing this policy?

    a. Include pediatricians, nursing staff, and neonatalogists on the policy planning committee.
    b. Distribute copies of research articles from peer-reviewed journals on the subject.
    c. Plan a series of in-service meetings for all affected staff to carefully educate them on the risks and benefits of supplementing breastfeeding babies.
    d. Develop the new policy with a small core group, then tell the staff that they must follow the new policy.

103. A woman had an emergency hysterectomy at 37 weeks' gestation. Which of the following statements is **LEAST** relevant to her ability to breastfeed?

    a. The mother may have difficulty establishing a full milk supply if she experienced excessive blood loss.
    b. The mother will be unable to produce milk if her ovaries were removed along with her uterus.
    c. The baby may nurse poorly due to the effects of the mother's anesthetics.
    d. The baby's first nursing may be delayed for several hours.

104. Which component of human milk is **LEAST** important in preventing neonatal septicemia?

    a. lysozyme in colostrum
    b. secretory IgA antibodies
    c. oligosaccharide receptor analogues
    d. lactoferrin protein

105. A mother is planning for surgery to repair her 5-month-old child's cleft palate. Your suggestions would include all of the following **EXCEPT**:

    a. Wean your baby at least a week before the surgery.
    b. Prepare to stay with your baby around the clock.
    c. Practice expressing milk in case the baby cannot nurse directly.
    d. Expect your baby to nurse very frequently afterward for a while.

106. A 3-week-old, exclusively breastfed baby with a strong family history of allergy has a severe reaction the first time he is fed with a cow's-milk-based formula. The **LEAST LIKELY** explanation for this is:

a. The baby was sensitized by intact cow's-milk protein that passed into the mother's milk.
b. The baby was given a bottle of formula in the hospital nursery.
c. The mother consumed large amounts of dairy products during pregnancy.
d. The allergic reaction was more likely due to the latex in the bottle nipple than the cow's milk.

107. Separating mothers and babies shortly after birth has all of the following consequences **EXCEPT**:

a. increased rates of infection.
b. improved rest for mother.
c. increase in infant stress hormones.
d. difficulty initiating breastfeeding.

108. Which of the following statements about the effect of human milk on the child's immune system is **FALSE**?

a. Human milk stimulates the baby to begin making his own sIgA and other antibodies.
b. Exclusively breastfed babies have a better response to immunizations.
c. Mother's own milk provides passive immunity between placentally acquired immunity and autonomous immune protection.
d. The breastfed baby has a higher risk of infection because he relies on his mother's immune protection during breastfeeding.

109. The WHO/UNICEF Ten Steps to Successful Breastfeeding (Baby-Friendly Hospital Initiative) prohibits the use of all of the following devices **EXCEPT**:

a. artificial teats (nipples).
b. pacifiers (dummies, soothers).
c. breast pumps.
d. feeding bottles.

110. Lactoferrin in human milk has all of the following functions **EXCEPT**:

a. nutrition.
b. nerve myelinization.
c. iron transport.
d. acting as an anti-inflammatory agent.

111. Pacifier (dummy, soother) use is associated with all of the following **EXCEPT**:

    a. improved dental development.
    b. increase in ear infections.
    c. increase in oral thrush.
    d. shorter duration of breastfeeding.

112. When a baby cannot breastfeed, advantages of using a small cup or spoon include all of the following **EXCEPT**:

    a. It is inexpensive and readily available.
    b. Suck response may diminish.
    c. It avoids bottle/teat use.
    d. It is easy to clean.

113. A mother asks you to help her write a birth plan that will optimize her success with breastfeeding. Her plan should include all of the following **EXCEPT**:

    a. the place of birth where she feels safest.
    b. her choice of companions and family members.
    c. access to furniture, hot tub, and equipment that encourages motion and posture changes.
    d. a professional attendant who will direct her actions during labor.

114. Women who do not breastfeed their babies are at higher risk for all of the following conditions related to reproduction **EXCEPT**:

    a. postpartum hemorrhage.
    b. delayed return to prepregnancy weight.
    c. menstrual irregularities and pain.
    d. closely spaced pregnancies.

115. A 34-week-old, premature infant is being discharged to his parents' care. Breastfeeding discharge teaching should include all of the following **EXCEPT**:

    a. He should be fed in a position that supports his head, neck, and shoulders.
    b. His sucking bursts are regular and rhythmic.
    c. Any supplements to direct breastfeeding should be mother's own expressed milk.
    d. He needs to be fed at least every 2–3 hours around the clock.

116. A newborn baby, 6 hours old, is awake and alert but having trouble breastfeeding. Which of the following is the **LEAST LIKELY** cause of his difficulty?

    a. His mother received antibiotic treatment for Group B streptococcus during labor.
    b. His mother was given epidural anesthesia 4 hours before delivery.
    c. His mother received narcotic analgesia immediately prior to delivery.
    d. His mother's labor was stimulated by pitocin (oxytocin), which was given intravenously.

117. All of the following developmental processes are interrupted by premature birth **EXCEPT**:

    a. bone mineralization.
    b. gut maturation.
    c. deposition of fat.
    d. hearing and taste.

118. Which fetal presenting position is the **LEAST LIKELY** to affect the baby's ability to breastfeed?

    a. left occiput anterior (LOA)
    b. right occiput posterior (ROP)
    c. left mentum anterior (LMA)
    d. right sacrum posterior (RSP)

119. Breastfeeding as an oral function of the baby involves all of the following **EXCEPT**:

    a. sense of taste and smell of milk.
    b. oral gratification as described by Freud.
    c. tactile sensation of the breast filling the infant's mouth.
    d. inability of the infant to control the shape of the breast.

120. Which statement is **FALSE** about experimental research designs?

    a. Subjects receive the intervention; controls do not.
    b. The dependent variable is manipulated to see what happens to the subjects.
    c. The independent variable is manipulated to test the hypothesis.
    d. Confounding variables will affect the results of the experiment.

121. A pregnant woman has heard that letting epidural anesthesia wear off prior to delivery will avoid anesthesia-related breastfeeding problems. You should tell her all of the following **EXCEPT**:

   a. Drugs can take much longer to clear the baby's system, so there is still possible breastfeeding risk with this approach.
   b. The combination of drugs used in epidural anesthesia makes it difficult to determine which medications cause breastfeeding problems.
   c. Epidural anesthesia has minimal or no effect on the baby regardless of how long before delivery it is administered.
   d. Epidural anesthesia increases the likelihood of other birth interventions that can affect breastfeeding.

122. Which is the **LEAST IMPORTANT** reason to use skin-to-skin (kangaroo mother care) contact for premature babies?

   a. Mothers are more inclined to breastfeed and produce more milk.
   b. Babies breastfeed from a younger gestational age and more frequently.
   c. Babies can be discharged to home earlier and more fully breastfeeding.
   d. The facility has a shortage of incubators (isolettes).

123. Implementation of the Baby-Friendly Hospital Initiative has been demonstrated to have all **EXCEPT** which one of the following outcomes?

   a. decreased rates of infant abandonment during the hospital stay
   b. decreased risk of upper respiratory tract infection in the first year of life
   c. increased rates of breastfeeding initiation, duration, and exclusivity
   d. decreased risk of gastrointestinal infection in the first year of life

124. A student in your prenatal class asks about the impact of labor-pain-relieving medications on the baby. Your responses should include all of the following **EXCEPT**:

   a. Narcotic analgesics can depress the baby's breathing and sucking.
   b. Epidural anesthesia has no effect on the baby.
   c. The effect of labor drugs on the baby is dose-related.
   d. Tranquilizers potentiate the action of other drugs.

125. A mother's breast is very hard and painful. All of the following interventions are appropriate **EXCEPT**:

   a. Document her history leading up to this situation.
   b. Wearing gloves, assess the degree of milk stasis in the breast tissue.
   c. Clean the incision and surrounding skin with an antiseptic solution.
   d. Gently teach or assist in expressing milk from the injured breast.

The following questions require the candidate to view a photograph to answer the question. The pictures (images) for these questions are on the CD in this book. Be sure to check the reference number of the image against the number of the question you are attempting to answer.

126. This picture was taken immediately after a feed ended. Which statement most likely describes the preceding feed?

    a. The baby had a shallow latch.
    b. The baby was deeply latched.
    c. The baby effectively transferred milk.
    d. The baby fed well, then self-detached.

127. This mother has a 2-week-old baby who has difficulty attaching to her smaller breast, has been fussy after feeds, and has not regained birth weight. She claims that she does not have enough milk. The most likely cause of this situation is:

    a. The mother is not feeding her baby frequently enough.
    b. The smaller breast has insufficient glandular tissue.
    c. The baby is attached incorrectly to the breast.
    d. The baby is sensitive to an allergen in his mother's milk.

128. Breast shells would be most helpful for this mother to:

    a. evert her nipples.
    b. protect the damaged skin from clothing.
    c. protect the nipple tip from the baby's palate.
    d. reduce areolar edema.

129. This full-term baby is 36 hours old. The most likely condition requiring this treatment is:

    a. exclusive, effective breastfeeding.
    b. ABO incompatibility.
    c. breast-milk jaundice.
    d. hypoglycemia.

130. This child's imitative behavior suggests which of the following?

    a. latent homosexuality
    b. normal behavior modeling
    c. deviant behavior
    d. precocious sexuality

131. A child of the age shown is most likely to be developmentally ready to:

    a. crawl and attempt to stand alone.
    b. wean from the breast.
    c. sleep through the night alone.
    d. separate easily from his mother.

132. When a breastfeeding baby has this condition, the first thing you would do is:

    a. Treat the baby and mother's breast for a fungal infection.
    b. Check the child for other manifestations of allergic responses.
    c. Advise the mother to change the baby's diaper more frequently.
    d. Have the mother apply a cortisone ointment on the rash.

133. This mother just finished pumping her milk. The most likely explanation for the condition pictured is:

    a. nipple thrush.
    b. the pump flange was too small in diameter.
    c. Reynaud's phenomenon.
    d. the pump has everted her nipples.

134. This baby has been at breast about 20 minutes. What is your best recommendation to this mother?

    a. Insert your finger to break the suction, then remove him.
    b. Pull his buttocks in closer to you for a better latch.
    c. Watch his sucking slow down as he prepares to self-detach.
    d. Tickle his feet to wake him so he can finish the feed.

135. This baby is having trouble feeding. Which suggestion is most likely to improve the situation?

    a. The mother should support her breast with her left hand.
    b. Pull the baby's hips and legs in closer to the mom's body.
    c. Place a pillow under the baby's body.
    d. Have the mother change to a horizontal position.

136. What is the most likely reason this baby cannot make a good seal on the mother's breast?

    a. The tongue is trough-shaped.
    b. The tongue is too thick.
    c. The baby has a small mouth opening.
    d. The lingual frenulum is short and tight.

137. Why would you want to discourage this practice in the first few hours postbirth?

   a. The grandmother might drop the baby or fail to support its head sufficiently.
   b. The clothing used to wrap the baby may be unclean or unsterile, risking an infection.
   c. It's more important that the baby's father and grandfather be the first to hold the baby.
   d. The grandmother's bacterial flora is foreign to the baby and prevents colonization with the mother's flora.

138. Which of the following is most likely to be found in the mouth of this mother's baby?

   a. dried milk on the tongue
   b. normal tongue
   c. oral thrush (*Candida*)
   d. strep throat

139. The first thing that the lactation consultant should do for this mother's nipple condition is:

   a. Arrange for the skin to be cultured for possible bacterial infection.
   b. Wash off the white substance to examine the underlying skin.
   c. Position the baby deeper onto the breast to prevent friction on the nipple tip.
   d. Instruct the mother to massage expressed milk into the nipple tip.

140. This baby is being breastfed with a silicone nipple shield, jaw support, and a straddle position at breast. The underlying condition that is being helped by these strategies is most likely:

   a. hypertonia
   b. hypotonia
   c. ataxia
   d. hypoglycemia

141. Which behavioral state is illustrated by the infant in this picture?

   a. active alert
   b. quiet alert
   c. light sleep
   d. drowsy

142. The most likely result of this mother's dietary practices would be:

   a. Her milk will contain more vitamin A.
   b. Her milk supply will increase.
   c. The baby's breath may smell like cantaloupe.
   d. The baby will reject the cantaloupe-flavored milk.

143. This mother has been using a piece of equipment to help resolve her breastfeeding problem. Which is the most likely product that she used?

    a. nipple shields
    b. breast shells
    c. bottle teat placed over her nipple
    d. breast pump

144. This baby attaches to the breast, feeds steadily and comfortably for about 17 minutes, then releases the breast. Which of the following suggestions is most appropriate for the mother?

    a. Use your other hand to support your breast during feeds.
    b. Bring your arm closer to your baby's neck.
    c. No suggestions.
    d. Pull your baby's legs closer to you.

145. What is the most likely cause of the condition pictured?

    a. acidic urine from human milk feedings
    b. yeast infection (*Candida*)
    c. allergic reaction to cow's-milk protein passing through the mother's milk
    d. sensitivity to chemicals in disposable diapers

146. You are caring for this mother and baby. The baby is 4 hours old and has breastfed well shortly after birth. Upon entering this mother's room, the first thing you should do is:

    a. Attempt to wake the baby for another feeding.
    b. Check the baby's blood glucose by doing a heel stick.
    c. Quietly observe the mother and baby but do not intervene.
    d. Have the mother put the baby in a crib next to the bed.

147. Why is this position for birth beneficial for the newborn's health?

    a. The grandmother can be the first to view the baby, thus enhancing bonding.
    b. The attendant cannot pull on the newborn's head, thus avoiding head and neck trauma.
    c. The mother can lift the baby out of her body herself, thus empowering her.
    d. The baby is exposed to its mother's normal gut flora in her feces, thus colonizing with beneficial bacteria.

148. Which statement best describes the reason this baby would begin reaching for table (family) food?

    a. The baby is developmentally ready for solid (family) food.
    b. The mother's milk supply is no longer adequate.
    c. The baby is just imitating and will not be ready for family foods for some time.
    d. The baby is jealous because everyone else is eating real food.

149. This pregnant mother calls and complains of tender nipples and lower milk supply. Your best response is:

    a. It's best if you start weaning your daughter; she's nursed long enough already.
    b. See your doctor about the sudden-onset nipple pain; it might be thrush.
    c. Drink fenugreek tea to increase your milk supply.
    d. What you're experiencing is common for women who are pregnant and still breastfeeding. How do you feel about continuing to breastfeed?

150. The most important action to take in helping this mother breastfeed is:

    a. Have her wear a nipple shield during feedings.
    b. Hand express milk before feeds to soften the large nipple area.
    c. Help the baby latch on to the breast deeply.
    d. Apply an antifungal preparation to the nipples after every feed.

151. This baby feeds for 30–45 minutes at each breast, each feeding, in the exact position shown in this picture. The most likely cause of this behavior is:

    a. normal behavior.
    b. disorganized sucking.
    c. the mother has low milk supply.
    d. delayed clearing of labor drugs.

152. The mother of this infant is most likely to complain of:

    a. difficulty getting her baby to latch on.
    b. stinging, burning nipples.
    c. vaginal discharge.
    d. plugged ducts.

153. Which of these practices most supports the baby's actions shown in the photograph?

    a. not washing off the amniotic fluid from the baby's hands
    b. bathing the mother immediately so her perspiration does not offend the baby
    c. giving narcotics by epidural during the labor so the mother is pain free at this stage
    d. suctioning the baby to clear his airway of mucus

154. Which hormone is especially high in this mother–baby dyad immediately postbirth?

  a. adrenalin
  b. oxytocin
  c. estrogen
  d. prolactin

155. What is the most likely cause of the condition shown?

  a. bacterial infection
  b. allergic reaction from laundry soap
  c. friction damage from baby's tongue
  d. mother's fair skin

156. How soon after birth should this activity take place for a birth facility to comply with BFHI guidelines?

  a. after the baby has been transitioned in the newborn nursery
  b. after the baby has been examined by a physician or midwife
  c. within the first hour after birth, before other procedures are done
  d. after the baby has been bathed, weighed, and measured

157. The breastfeeding equipment shown in this photograph is most likely being used for:

  a. provision of sufficient calories while increasing the milk supply.
  b. training the baby at the breast to suck correctly and effectively.
  c. ensuring adequate caloric intake because this baby is too small to obtain enough nourishment.
  d. aiding this baby to attach correctly to the breast and continue sucking.

158. To minimize physiologic stress to the infant from this procedure, the best strategy would be:

  a. Warm the room to prevent the infant from becoming chilled.
  b. Clamp the cord while the baby is resting skin to skin on the mother's body.
  c. Have the mother's partner or helper hold the baby while the cord is clamped.
  d. Ask the mother to breastfeed the baby while the baby is examined.

159. Which actions are most likely to support the baby breastfeeding?

  a. Lift the mother's breast into the baby's mouth.
  b. Ask the mother to sit up and bring her baby to breast.
  c. Support the baby while he crawls to the mother's breast.
  d. Have the mother compress her breast and tickle the baby's lips.

160. At this stage of lactation, which of the following components of human milk is most increased over newborn-period levels?

    a. lactoferrin
    b. lactose
    c. whey
    d. casein

161. The mother of this baby complains of stinging, burning pain in her nipples. The recommendation most likely to resolve her pain is:

    a. Breastfeed for frequent, short periods of time.
    b. Wear nipple shields during breastfeeding for 1 week.
    c. Get antifungal medication for you and your baby.
    d. Boil all the baby's pacifiers.

162. What is the most likely condition pictured?

    a. *Candida* infection at the base of the nipple
    b. large, fibrous nipple
    c. nipple edema from excessive pumping
    d. scars from breast reduction surgery

163. At which age is this breastfeeding behavior most likely to occur?

    a. 5–6 months
    b. 7–12 months
    c. 12–18 months
    d. 18–24 months

164. Which of the following is the most likely cause of the condition pictured?

    a. cold temperature in the room
    b. supplements of cow's-milk-based formula
    c. supplements of rice cereal
    d. the baby recently had a tetanus immunization

165. This mother of a 3-month-old began feeling pinpoint pain on her nipple tip 2 days ago. The pain is most likely due to:

    a. mastitis.
    b. a plugged nipple pore.
    c. a bacterial infection.
    d. a friction blister.

166. The most appropriate advice you can give this mother on feeding patterns is:

a. Your milk supply is very high, so use only one breast per feed.
b. Start on the fuller breast for about 10 minutes, then switch to the other.
c. Let the baby nurse on the first breast until he releases the breast on his own.
d. Switch sides several times during a feed to make sure both sides get stimulated.

167. This baby was born about 10 minutes ago. What is the first thing you would say to this mother?

a. You and your baby look so comfortable and happy!
b. When she's ready, I can help you get started with breastfeeding.
c. We'll give the baby a bath before you try breastfeeding.
d. Aren't you going to let your partner hold the baby, too?

168. Which immunofactor in human milk is at its highest level at this point in time?

a. sIgA
b. lactose
c. lysozyme
d. complement

169. This mother's baby is 8 days old. The most likely cause of the condition pictured is:

a. normal breastfeeding.
b. the baby is tongue-tied.
c. the baby is not latching deeply.
d. the baby is biting during feeds.

170. What is the name of the string-like structure under this baby's tongue?

a. labial frenulum
b. incisive papilla
c. lingual frenulum
d. mucus membrane

171. This mother complains of sudden-onset sore nipples. The first action you would take is:

a. Ask whether her baby has teeth.
b. Have the mother roll the baby inward toward her, so the baby's entire front side is facing hers.
c. Have the mother pull the baby's legs in closer to her.
d. Ask whether she has taken an antibiotic recently.

172. This baby is 1 day old. In this picture, what are the white structures in its mouth?

a. Epstein's pearls
b. natal teeth
c. incisive papilla
d. sucking blisters

173. This child's mother tried unsuccessfully to breastfeed, and her child now has difficulty eating. The most likely reason is that this child has:

a. anklyoglossia.
b. macroglossia.
c. microglossia.
d. micrognathia.

174. A woman requests information on allowing her children to take this action together. Your best response is:

a. The children look very cute when they are asleep.
b. The infant is at some danger from overlying, so make sure they sleep where you can observe them.
c. Children should learn to sleep in their own beds. The toddler certainly belongs in a crib.
d. Siblings sleeping together is common around the world. There is no risk to this practice.

175. This condition has persisted for 2+ months. What is the most helpful action you could take for this mother?

a. Thoroughly examine the baby's nursing technique at breast.
b. Refer her to a dermatologist for further evaluation.
c. Provide her with moist wound-healing preparations.
d. Recommend she pump or express and feed the baby with a device.

176. Which of the following is the most common breastfeeding behavior of a child at this age?

a. biting at the end of feeds
b. nursing strike
c. easily distracted while nursing
d. playfulness and vocalization during feeds

177. What could you do to decrease this baby's risk of SIDS?

    a. Move the mattress away from the unused fireplace.
    b. Put the baby in a crib.
    c. Give the baby a pacifier.
    d. Roll the baby onto her back.

178. Which visual element of this baby's latch is most likely to indicate a problem?

    a. deep puckering at the naso-labial crease
    b. eyes closed
    c. chin driven into the breast
    d. nose barely touching the breast

179. This mother is getting irritated with her child's nursing habits. The child is afraid of strangers, cries when left with a caregiver, and wakes several times at night. The most likely reason for this behavior pattern is:

    a. delayed development of autonomy caused by breastfeeding.
    b. the mother clinging to her child and discouraging autonomy.
    c. common and normal behavior in the second 6 months of life.
    d. the mother's inability to set limits for the child's behavior.

180. This baby's mother complains of clicking and smacking during breastfeeds. The most likely explanation is:

    a. high domed palate prevents deep latch.
    b. tongue-tie prevents deep attachment.
    c. tongue shape causes intermittent loss of seal.
    d. buccal fat pads are interfering with tongue movement.

181. At this postdelivery stage, which statement is most likely?

    a. Too many visitors can interfere with feeding.
    b. The mother is getting ready to go back to work.
    c. The baby can't consume all the milk that the mother is making.
    d. The baby is sleeping 6–8 hours at night.

The next section of questions is constructed with a NEGATIVE STEM format. Be prepared to do a mental shift to think in negative terms, and read the stem and responses especially carefully before answering. Continue to refer to the photos on the CD.

182. The condition pictured appeared on day 4 postpartum. The mother might be experiencing a similar phenomenon in any of the following locations **EXCEPT**:

    a. near the umbilicus
    b. upper, inner arm
    c. groin
    d. outer thigh

183. This mother is 4 days postpartum. All of the following recommendations are appropriate **EXCEPT**:

    a. Apply cool cabbage compresses to the lump in your right armpit.
    b. Feed your baby at least every 2–3 hours; more often if he cues.
    c. Apply hot compresses to help milk flow in your left breast.
    d. Use cool compresses after feeds if breasts feel full.

184. Which is the **LEAST** appropriate treatment for this condition?

    a. antifungal therapy
    b. continued breastfeeding
    c. breast binder for the mother
    d. antibiotic therapy

185. Of the following conditions, which is **LEAST LIKELY** to result in this pattern of growth?

    a. Down syndrome
    b. exclusive breastfeeding
    c. tongue-tied baby
    d. cystic fibrosis

186. After examining this woman's breasts, you would do all of the following **EXCEPT**:

    a. Instruct her on better cleaning procedures for her breast pump.
    b. Provide her with a nipple shield to wear during feeds.
    c. Request that the primary care provider culture the baby's mouth.
    d. Recommend that she wean immediately.

187. The behavior shown in this picture is **LEAST LIKELY** to be:

    a. distress at separation from his mother.
    b. an indication of pain.
    c. the infant's attempt to manipulate his mother.
    d. stressful to the baby's physiology.

188. This exclusively breastfed baby suddenly begins nursing every 1–2 hours around the clock. The mother is worried that her milk supply has dried up. Your responses would include all of the following **EXCEPT**:

    a. Milk supply often dips at this age, so you should begin supplementing.
    b. This sounds like a typical growth spurt, which is common at this age.
    c. Babies often nurse in that pattern even when they nurse as well as your baby does.
    d. It's reassuring to see your baby gaining weight even when he seems to need to nurse that often.

189. Appropriate treatments for this condition include all of the following **EXCEPT**:

    a. cabbage leaf compresses.
    b. hot compresses.
    c. cold compresses.
    d. gentle massage.

190. When this condition is seen in a breastfeeding infant, all of the following recommendations are appropriate **EXCEPT**:

    a. simultaneous treatment of the baby and mother's breast.
    b. treat only the baby's mouth with an antifungal medication, unless the mother has signs of infection.
    c. check the mother's nipples for signs or symptoms of infection.
    d. assume that mother's nipples, all infant sucking objects, and possibly other infant areas are infected until proven otherwise.

191. Which of the following behaviors is **LEAST LIKELY** to occur in the breastfeeding child of this age?

    a. The mother and child have a code word for breastfeeding.
    b. The child can postpone nursing for short periods.
    c. Nighttime breastfeeding increases the child's risk of dental caries.
    d. The child receives substantial immune protection from breastfeeding.

192. Documentation of this woman's breasts might include all of the following **EXCEPT**:

    a. Her breasts are asymmetric with a pinkish nipple/areola complex.

    b. Her right beast is very small; her left breast is moderate size and saggy.

    c. Both breasts have scant palpable glandular tissue.

    d. Her right breast has insufficient glandular tissue for lactation.

193. What is the **LEAST LIKELY** cause of the condition shown?

    a. Paget's disease

    b. plugged nipple pore

    c. persistent wound from the baby's tongue thrust

    d. nipple thrush (*Candida*)

194. This breastfeeding mother says that this condition appeared when her baby was about 4 months old. Which is the **LEAST LIKELY** cause of the condition shown?

    a. atopic dermatitis

    b. fungal infection

    c. eczema

    d. psoriasis

195. All of the following are appropriate actions for this mother's situation **EXCEPT**:

    a. Advise her to stop breastfeeding on this breast.

    b. Assist her to express milk from this breast thoroughly every few hours.

    c. Encourage her to rest and continue breastfeeding on the other breast.

    d. Support her taking any prescribed antibiotics.

196. Common breastfeeding behaviors of babies at this age include all of the following **EXCEPT**:

    a. smiling up at their moms during feeds.

    b. biting or clamping down at the end of a feed.

    c. distractibility.

    d. feeding mostly with eyes closed.

197. You would recommend this technique for all of the following **EXCEPT**:

    a. for a premature baby.

    b. for a separation of the mother and baby for any reason.

    c. for a mother taking a contraindicated medication.

    d. if the mother has a history of sexual abuse.

198. To help prevent rickets in this child, you would recommend all of the following **EXCEPT**:

    a. Expose the child's face to sunlight for 20 minutes every day.

    b. The mother should take a vitamin D supplement.

    c. The mother should expose her face and head to sunlight for 2 hours a week.

    d. Give the child a vitamin D supplement regardless of symptoms.

199. This mother complains of sharp nipple pain. Your suggestions should include all of the following **EXCEPT**:

    a. apply purified lanolin to the irritated area.

    b. wear a silicone nipple shield during feeds.

    c. wear breast shells between feeds.

    d. bring the baby deeply onto the breast.

200. What is the **LEAST LIKELY** reason this grandmother would engage in the behavior shown?

    a. competition with the baby's mother

    b. soothe the baby while mother finishes a nap

    c. medical condition requires baby to maintain an upright posture

    d. genuine affection for her grandchild

EXAM B ANSWERS

The parenthetical material at the end of each answer includes the discipline and time period ("general principles" will be noted for questions that don't pertain to one time period), indicates whether the question pertains to knowledge or application, and specifies the degree of difficulty.

1. The answer is B. A good maternal diet during pregnancy significantly reduces the incidence of low-birth-weight infants. Diet may have a relationship to the development of gestational diabetes. Maternal diet does not directly affect A or D. (M. Public Health; Prenatal; Knowledge; Difficulty: 3)

2. The answer is D. Active listening is the first action because the mother is obviously emotionally upset. Understanding, addressing, and exploring feelings are key to counseling the breastfeeding mother. (G. Psychology; 1–3 months; Application; Difficulty: 4)

3. The answer is B. Macrophages and possibly neutrophils and T-lymphocytes actively kill microbes by phagocytosis. (D. Immunology; General Principles; Knowledge; Difficulty: 5)

4. The answer is D. Spoons and open cups are easier to clean than other feeding devices. (K. Equipment; Prematurity; Application; Difficulty: 4)

5. The answer is B. Reliability of a test instrument means that the instrument produces consistent results regardless of user, time of use, use over a duration of time, and when applied to different subjects. (I. Research; General Principles; Knowledge; Difficulty: 2)

6. The answer is A. High lipid solubility would increase drug transfer into milk. The other factors would inhibit passage into milk. (F. Pharmacology; General Principles; Application; Difficulty: 2)

7. The answer is B. Freezing destroys living white cells such as T- and B-lymphocytes. The other components are not significantly affected by freezing. (B. Biochemistry; General Principles; Knowledge; Difficulty: 5)

8. The answer is C. Original research (primary references) is the most important type of source to include in a literature review. Texts and review articles may help you locate primary references on a subject. Lectures also may direct you to primary references. (I. Research; General Principles; Application; Difficulty: 4)

9. The answer is C. Antineoplastics, often called chemotherapy agents, are used in treating malignant tumors. Breastfeeding is usually contraindicated because of the potential risk to the infant. (F. Pharmacology; General Principles; Knowledge; Difficulty: 4)

10. The answer is A. Preterm milk is higher in protein and similar to term milk in lactose, phosphorus, iron, and most other components. (B. Biochemistry; Prematurity; Knowledge; Difficulty: 2)

11. The answer is B. The Code specifies that information on artificial feeding provided to health workers should be scientific and accurate. Detailed, accurate information on product composition, provided to health workers, is appropriate marketing of products within the scope of the Code. (M. Public Health; General Principles; Knowledge; Difficulty: 2)

12. The answer is C. Holder pasteurization by donor human milk banks raises milk to 62.5°C for 30 minutes. (K. Equipment; General Principles; Knowledge; Difficulty: 5)

13. The answer is D. Research in Australia has found that the relative fullness of the breast accounts for about 70% of the fat variation in milk. (B. Biochemistry; General Principles; Knowledge; Difficulty: 4)

14. The answer is C. The most effective protection against legal actions is establishing a mutually respectful relationship and rapport. (J. Legal; General Principles; Knowledge; Difficulty: 4)

15. The answer is B. Drugs more readily pass into milk in the first few days postbirth because the junctures between mammary secretory cells are open at this point, permitting passage of medications and other substances into the alveolar lumen. (F. Pharmacology; 1–2 days; Knowledge; Difficulty: 4)

16. The answer is B. Operational definitions, or how the authors define the term "breastfeeding," are critical. (I. Research; General Principles; Application; Difficulty: 3)

17. The answer is C. A normal newborn heart rate is 120–160 beats per minute. Tachycardia (fast heart rate) or bradycardia (slow heart rate) can interfere with the baby's ability to breastfeed. (A. Anatomy; 1–2 days; Knowledge; Difficulty: 5)

18. The answer is A. Exclusive breastfeeding for about 6 months is the best strategy to reduce the baby's risk. The mother's avoidance of known allergens during pregnancy may also reduce the baby's risks of allergy. It is more important that the mother exclusively breastfeed for about 6 months than other actions she should be considering at this time. Delaying solid foods does not address the baby's more likely early exposure to cow's milk and soy proteins, which are very common allergens in humans. (D. Immunology; Prenatal; Knowledge; Difficulty: 3)

19. The answer is C. About 1% of most medications given to a lactating woman actually gets to her breastfed baby. (F. Pharmacology; General Principles; Knowledge; Difficulty: 3)

20. The answer is B. The Hawthorne effect means that observing a population for a specific behavior change often produces the desired change, independent of the intervention being studied. (I. Research; Prenatal; Application; Difficulty: 2)

21. The answer is D. Stools of exclusively breastfed babies in the first month are exactly as described. (B. Physiology; 15–28 days; Application; Difficulty: 3)

22. The answer is C. Drugs that are highly absorbable via oral ingestion more easily transfer to breast milk. The other properties reduce the amount that may get to the baby. (F. Pharmacology; General Principles; Knowledge; Difficulty: 3)

23. The answer is C. Severing nerve pathways would be the worst consequence to lactation. (A. Anatomy; Prenatal; Application; Difficulty: 5)

24. The answer is A. It is always appropriate to make sure the baby is feeding well as the first strategy. While that level of bilirubin is rarely a problem for a healthy, full-term newborn, the lactation consultant should always make sure the baby is effectively feeding as a top priority. (B. Physiology; 3–14 days; Application; Difficulty: 3)

25. The answer is D. No assumptions can be made about her ability to breastfeed after breast surgery, although she should be followed closely in the first week postbirth because surgery can disrupt ducts and nerve pathways needed for adequate milk synthesis. (B. Physiology; Prenatal; Application; Difficulty: 3)

26. The answer is B. Amniotic fluid provides protein and other nutrients to the fetus in addition to nutrients present in the cord blood vessels. (B. Biochemistry; Prenatal; Knowledge; Difficulty: 3)

27. The answer is C. Fats are most difficult for preterm babies to digest. Human milk fat is released simultaneously with digestive enzymes, making it optimal for preterm babies. (B. Biochemistry; Prematurity; Knowledge; Difficulty: 4)

28. The answer is A. There are several antidepressant medications considered compatible with breast-feeding. Continuing to breastfeed may help her recover from her illness. (F. Pharmacology; 1–2 days; Application; Difficulty: 4)

29. The answer is A. Extreme nipple pain in the absence of visual symptoms may indicate a deeper problem such as prior history of abuse. (E. Pathology; 1–2 days; Knowledge; Difficulty: 5)

30. The answer is C. Short sucking bursts with pauses is an indicator of immaturity. The other patterns are indicators of a mature infant. (A. Anatomy; 1–2 days; Application; Difficulty: 2)

31. The answer is A. Each mother–baby system will develop unique feeding patterns. The lactation consultant supports any and all patterns that meet the mother's and babies' needs. (G. Psychology; 1–2 days; Application; Difficulty: 5)

32. The answer is D. A wide gape is the most important visible feature of effective positioning and latch. All of the nipple and a portion of the areola should be inside the infant's mouth, but not necessarily all of it, depending on the areola diameter. The nose may lightly touch the breast, or be close to it, but not buried in the breast. (A. Anatomy; 1–2 days; Application; Difficulty: 2)

33. The answer is A. Her infant is experiencing a normal growth and behavior pattern and possibly a sudden increase in appetite. Initial breast edema is resolved, and the breasts are becoming calibrated to produce enough milk for her baby without feeding overfull. The behavior she describes is a normal pattern for breastfed babies. (B. Physiology; 1–3 months; Application; Difficulty: 4)

34. The answer is A. Pain-relieving drugs work on the central nervous system and therefore are highly lipid soluble and sequester in the infant brain. The other answers are incorrect. (F. Pharmacology; Labor/birth; Application; Difficulty: 3)

35. The answer is D. Bright red lochia at 14 days with signs of low milk supply suggest that retained placental fragments are suppressing the onset of lactogenesis II. (B. Physiology; 3–14 days; Application; Difficulty: 3)

36. The answer is C. The only limiting factor to breastfeeding is the mother's injuries. Compatible pain medications are available. She and her baby still need each other while she recovers. (E. Pathology; 15–28 days; Application; Difficulty: 4)

37. The answer is C. The hypoglossal nerve (CN XII) is the primary motor nerve of the tongue. The other nerves listed are involved in suck-swallow-breathe but play a lesser role in tongue movement. (A. Anatomy; General Principles; Application; Difficulty: 5)

38. The answer is B. The tongue usually extends past the lower gum ridge (alveolar ridge) and is cupped around the breast. It may also extend past the lower lip. (A. Anatomy; General Principles; Application; Difficulty: 4)

39. The answer is B. Herbal teas may contain substances that exert a pharmacological effect on the baby. (F. Pharmacology; 15–28 days; Application; Difficulty: 4)

40. The answer is B. Lipids are the most variable of the components listed. The proportion of fat in milk increases as the breast empties, and there is a slight variation in fatty acid profiles with maternal diet. The others are very stable across women, over the course of a day, and over the duration of breastfeeding. (B. Biochemistry; General Principles; Knowledge; Difficulty: 3)

41. The answer is B. Persistent cranial molding can interfere with nervous system functioning in the early weeks, which can interfere with the suck-swallow pattern. (E. Pathology; 15–28 days; Application; Difficulty: 3)

42. The answer is A. The mammary ridge forms at 4–5 weeks' gestation. (A. Anatomy; Preconception; Knowledge; Difficulty: 3)

43. The answer is B. Smooth muscle fibers are found in the nipple-areola complex. (A. Anatomy; General Principles; Knowledge; Difficulty: 3)

44. The answer is D. Severe blood loss can cause pituitary shock (Sheehan's syndrome), which blocks prolactin responses needed for lactogenesis III. (E. Pathology; 3–14 days; Knowledge; Difficulty: 5)

45. The answer is B. The Baby-Friendly Hospital Initiative Step 4 states, "Place babies in skin-to-skin contact with their mothers immediately following birth for at least an hour and encourage mothers to recognize when their babies are ready to breastfeed, offering help if needed." Some babies are at breast and nursing well in the first 5 minutes; many unmedicated babies are nursing well by 30 minutes, while some babies take about an hour to accomplish their first feed. The baby should be placed on the mother's breast immediately after birth and assistance offered as needed. (B. Physiology; 1–2 days; Application; Difficulty: 4)

46. The answer is D. A research article published in a peer-reviewed professional journal is a primary reference. A is a review, which is a secondary reference. B is a chapter in a book, which is a secondary or tertiary source. C is a book, interpreting other sources in its recommendations. (I. Research; General Principles; Application; Difficulty: 4)

47. The answer is C. Babies feed for varying lengths and at varying intervals according to their hunger, emotional needs, growth and developmental stages, and other physiological factors. Placing restrictions on length or frequency or offering substitutes disrupts the breastfeeding relationship and interferes with fulfillment of infant needs. (B. Physiology; 15–28 days; Application; Difficulty: 2)

48. The answer is D. She was diagnosed a bacterial infection of the nipple skin, most likely streptococcus transferred from the baby's mouth. The rash is exactly where the baby's mouth had come in contact with the areolar tissue. A and B are possibly correct, but less likely. (E. Pathology; 4–6 months; Application; Difficulty: 5)

49. The answer is D. The visual system is the last sensory system to develop during gestation, therefore the most affected by preterm nutrition. Human milk makes a significant difference in visual development of the preterm infant, partly because of fatty acid profiles. (A. Anatomy; Prematurity; Knowledge; Difficulty: 2)

50. The answer is D. Direct breastfeeding should be tried first. Devices should only be considered when direct breastfeeding is impossible. (K. Equipment; 1–2 days; Application; Difficulty: 3)

51. The answer is C. The risk of drug passage into milk is highest in the early postpartum period when the junctures between the mammary secretory epithelial cells (lactocyctes) are open. After the first week or so, the tight junctures between cells inhibit most drugs from passing into milk. (F. Pharmacology; 1–2 days; Application; Difficulty: 4)

52. The answer is A. Epidermal growth factor plays a major role in gut maturation. Lactoferrin also promotes tissue maturation. (B. Biochemistry; General Principles; Knowledge; Difficulty: 5)

53. The answer is D. Mothers with hearing (auditory) impairments are generally very familiar with visual and tactile communication. Breastfeeding may be easier for her than artificial feeding. (G. Psychology; 1–2 days; Application; Difficulty: 4)

54. The answer is B. By 2 weeks, most term infants should be able to handle the mother's milk-ejection reflex. If the baby cannot coordinate sucking and swallowing with breathing, he may choke and gasp for breath as the milk releases. Occasionally, a normal baby may still have difficulty handling a mother's strong milk-ejection reflex. (E. Pathology; 15–28 days; Application; Difficulty: 3)

55. The answer is D. Ultrasound research confirms that milk ducts are easily compressed, do not display typical sinuses, and are superficial to the breast surface. (A. Anatomy; General Principles; Knowledge; Difficulty: 4)

56. The answer is B. Thorough removal milk will increase the *rate* of milk synthesis. Stimulation without removal is not effective because milk stasis slows the rate of milk synthesis. Galactagogues are not well researched. Metoclopramide will increase prolactin, but needs to be combined with adequate milk removal. (B. Physiology; 3–14 days; Application; Difficulty: 5)

57. The answer is D. The question lists the foods from least priority to highest according to WHO recommendations. (M. Public Health; General Principles; Knowledge; Difficulty: 4)

58. The answer is B. Babies start being able to self-feed around 6 months. Offering a variety of family foods that the child can pick up and explore is appropriate. (H. Growth; 4–6 months; Knowledge; Difficulty: 4)

59. The answer is D. The U.S. Centers for Disease Control does not require health care workers to wear gloves when assisting breastfeeding except in high-exposure situations such as donor milk banking. (J. Legal; General Principles; Knowledge; Difficulty: 5)

60. The answer is D. A research article published in a peer-reviewed professional journal is a primary reference. A is a review article, which is a secondary reference. B is a chapter in a book, which is a secondary or tertiary source. C is a book for parents, interpreting other sources in its recommendations. (I. Research; Prematurity; Application; Difficulty: 4)

61. The answer is A. Making or downloading one copy of a copyrighted work for personal use is considered fair use. Making multiple copies without permission from the copyright holder violates copyright laws. Pictures and images posted on Internet sites are protected by international copyright laws. You may use legitimately purchased images in your presentations with proper attribution, but further distributing these images without specific permission, as in printed handouts, is not considered fair use. (J. Legal; General Principles; Application; Difficulty: 3)

62. The answer is C. Innate defenses on the baby's skin and in the vernix provide a measure of protection to the newborn. The other systems are not fully mature at birth. Breast milk compensates for and enhances the development of other host defense systems. (D. Immunology; General Principles; Knowledge; Difficulty: 5)

63. The answer is D. One half-life is the time it takes for half of the drug to be metabolized. In the first half-life, 20 mg would be metabolized, leaving 20 mg. After the second half-life, half of the remaining 20 mg would be metabolized, leaving 10 mg. After the third half-life, 5 mg would be left. After 4 half-lives, 2.5 mg of the drug would remain. (F. Pharmacology; General Principles; Application; Difficulty: 4)

64. The answer is A. Studying experiences of an event is a qualitative research method. The other responses are quantitative designs: B is descriptive, C is correlational, and D is experimental research. (E. Pathology; General Principles; Knowledge; Difficulty: 4)

65. The answer is A. Cultures that sexualize the breast are often the most resistant to women using their breasts to feed their infants anywhere and everywhere. (G. Psychology; General Principles; Knowledge; Difficulty: 5)

66. The answer is B. The release of cholecystokinin causes satiety and relaxation. (B. Physiology; General Principles; Knowledge; Difficulty: 2)

67. The answer is D. Lipid solubility facilitates transfer of drugs into the mother's milk. The other factors inhibit drug transfer to milk. (F. Pharmacology; General Principles; Knowledge; Difficulty: 4)

68. The answer is A. Increased carrying when the baby is not fussy as well as when he is fussy reduces total crying per day. (K. Equipment; General Principles; Knowledge; Difficulty: 2)

69. The answer is B. The Montgomery glands are sebaceous glands which produce oil to lubricate the nipple and areolar skin and may have other functions. (A. Anatomy; General Principles; Application; Difficulty: 4)

70. The answer is C. Intraductal papilloma is the most likely cause of painless bright red bleeding in the early postpartum period. (E. Pathology; 1–2 days; Knowledge; Difficulty: 4)

71. The answer is A. The axillary nodes collect most of the lymph fluid; the intermammary and subclavicular nodes collect some lymph from the breast. The mesenteric nodes are in the abdomen. (A. Anatomy; General Principles; Knowledge; Difficulty: 4)

72. The answer is D. Glass is a recommended storage container for mother's own milk. Hard plastic (polycarbonate or polypropylene) containers with lids are acceptable. (K. Equipment; General Principles; Knowledge; Difficulty: 2)

73. The answer is B. Babies consume about 2/3 of the available milk in a breast during any given feeding. (B. Physiology; 15–28 days; Application; Difficulty: 3)

74. The answer is D. Mothers' dietary practices have very little effect on lactation. Following good dietary practices is important for the breastfeeding mother's general health, yet has little relevance to milk volume or composition.. (B. Biochemistry; General Principles; Application; Difficulty: 5)

75. The answer is C. The mother's secretory immune system provides targeted protection through the entero-mammary and broncho-mammary pathways. (D. Immunology; General Principles; Knowledge; Difficulty: 5)

76. The answer is D. Chickenpox is no longer contagious when all the lesions are completely crusted over. The mother can breastfeed normally. (E. Pathology; Labor/birth; Application; Difficulty: 5)

77. The answer is D. A mother's lack of eye contact and little talking or caressing of her infant may be signs of postpartum depression. The lactation consultant should report these signs to the mother's primary care provider immediately. (E. Pathology; 1–2 days; Knowledge; Difficulty: 4)

78. The answer is B. During the formal stage, mothers seek consistent, concrete rules to govern their actions. (G. Psychology; 3–14 days; Knowledge; Difficulty: 4)

79. The answer is C. Distractibility is a common behavioral characteristic in the 4- to 6-month age. (H. Growth; 4–6 months; Knowledge; Difficulty: 3)

80. The answer is C. SIgA is stable to heat treatment and freezing. (K. Equipment; General Principles; Knowledge; Difficulty: 5)

81. The answer is D. Babies deliberately leave some milk in the breasts, consuming about 2/3 of the available milk volume at a given feed. Milk volumes consumed are relatively stable from the first week or so until at least 6 months. The normal range varies widely. Artificially fed babies may need more milk as they get older because the nutrients are less available for growth. (B. Physiology; 4–6 months; Application; Difficulty: 4)

82. The answer is A. Overhydration during labor may cause breast, nipple, and areolar edema, making latch-on difficult for the baby. To date, little research has investigated this issue. (B. Physiology; Labor/birth; Application; Difficulty: 5)

83. The answer is C. The alveoli contain secretory cells that produce milk. (A. Anatomy; General Principles; Knowledge; Difficulty: 3)

84. The answer is C. Small breasts usually have less storage capacity than larger breasts, so frequent expression triggers a high rate of milk synthesis. The rate of synthesis is highest when the breasts are emptiest, so expressing until the flow ceases will also maximize the rate of milk synthesis. (B. Physiology; Prematurity; Application; Difficulty: 4)

85. The answer is A. The infant is able to swallow from about 16 weeks and develops an immature suck pattern at around 26 weeks' gestational age. (H. Growth; Prematurity; Knowledge; Difficulty: 4)

86. The answer is B. Breast milk optimizes the environment in the baby's gut. Allergens may be present in breast milk and may create problems for a sensitive baby, but the risk of allergies is significantly reduced through breastfeeding. (D. Immunology; 4–6 months; Application; Difficulty: 4)

87. The answer is D. The rolling action presses milk out of the milk ducts sinuses toward the nipple. Little milk is stored in the ducts, but of the techniques listed, this is likely the most effective method for hand expressing. (K. Equipment; General Principles; Application; Difficulty: 3)

88. The answer is C. Unresolved stress from the birth can trigger or exacerbate postpartum depression. She needs to see her primary care provider immediately for thorough evaluation, diagnosis, and treatment. (G. Psychology; 1–3 months; Knowledge; Difficulty: 4)

89. The answer is B. Taking a thorough history is top priority when solving a breastfeeding problem. The baby may be having an allergic reaction to the large amount of milk consumed by the mother. (E. Pathology; 1–3 months; Application; Difficulty: 3)

90. The answer is D. This is a normal pattern on day 2. The baby's appetite, interest, and ability to feed will determine whether one or both breasts are taken at a given feeding. This pattern would be described as a paired breastfeed. (B. Physiology; 1–2 days; Application; Difficulty: 5)

91. The answer is B. Prostaglandins in the milk have anti-inflammatory properties that protect all tissues, especially the infant gut. (B. Biochemistry; General Principles; Knowledge; Difficulty: 4)

92. The answer is B. Manufacturers omitted chloride in a mistaken effort to impact adult cardiac disease by changing infant intake of salt. Chloride is an essential nutrient for human brain development. (E. Pathology; General Principles; Knowledge; Difficulty: 5)

93. The answer is D. The baby described is tongue-tied. Frenotomy (incision of the lingual frenulum) is an appropriate and effective treatment, especially when ordinary lactation techniques have not been helpful. The next action for the lactation consultant is to put the mother in contact with a professional who is qualified to evaluate and treat this anatomic condition of the infant. (J. Legal; 3–14 days; Application; Difficulty: 5)

94. The answer is C. Undetected breast cancer is very unlikely this early postbirth. Any birth injury may be painful for the baby. Placing the sore side higher than the normal side may reduce pain, resulting in the baby's strong preference for the more comfortable position. Breasts differ in configuration and flow, and one side may be much easier for the baby to manage in the early weeks. (E. Pathology; 15–28 days; Application; Difficulty: 2)

95. The answer is A. Breast shells have not been found to be effective for correcting nonprotractile nipples. The other statements are all appropriate. (K. Equipment; Prenatal; Application; Difficulty: 2)

96. The answer is B. As of this writing, donor milk has not been prescribed for skin treatment of burns. (D. Immunology; General Principles; Knowledge; Difficulty: 5)

97. The answer is D. Libido is not addressed in safe mother hood initiatives. Libido is not necessarily lower during breastfeeding. (M. Public Health; General Principles; Knowledge; Difficulty: 2)

98. The answer is C. It is currently unknown whether lactation boosts the mother's own immune system. Antibodies and white cells that she produces quickly get into her milk and protect the baby, and a mother who is sick certainly does not benefit from the additional work of preparing artificial feeds and coping with probable sudden milk stasis. (E. Pathology; 4–6 months; Application; Difficulty: 2)

99. The answer is A. Breastfeeding cannot be forced on a child at any age. The child who does not want to breastfeed will either bite or refuse to latch on. The other reasons are all common reasons for continued breastfeeding well into the second year of the child's life. (G. Psychology; >12 months; Application; Difficulty: 2)

100. The answer is B. Environmental chemicals that may appear in the mother's milk have no documented effect on the baby or its immune system. Mother's milk helps build the baby's immune system. The other choices are true. (H. Growth; General Principles; Knowledge; Difficulty: 2)

101. The answer is A. Breast pumps are not currently covered by the International Code. However, feeding bottles (baby bottles) not used as collection containers attached to breast pumps are included in the scope of the Code. (M. Public Health; General Principles; Knowledge; Difficulty: 2)

102. The answer is D. Involving all pertinent staff, planning sufficient education, and providing substantial evidence of the safety and effectiveness of the new policy are all successful strategies for changing policies. Forcing new policies on staff is likely to result in open and covert resistance. (M. Public Health; 1–2 days; Application; Difficulty: 2)

103. The answer is B. Ovarian function postbirth is not related to lactation. The other statements are relevant. (B. Physiology; Prematurity; Application; Difficulty: 2)

104. The answer is A. Lysozyme is probably the least important, even though it may play a role. The other responses are major factors in protecting against neonatal septicemia. (E. Pathology; Prematurity; Knowledge; Difficulty: 4)

105. The answer is A. Hospitalization is usually a traumatic experience for the child, and the emotional comfort from breastfeeding is especially important at that time. (L. Techniques; 4–6 months; Application; Difficulty: 2)

106. The answer is D. Although sudden, severe latex allergies are possible, the reaction is more likely to be caused by an ingested allergen, especially cow's-milk protein. All of the other choices are possible sources or routes of sensitization. (D. Immunology; 15–28 days; Application; Difficulty: 2)

107. The answer is B. Research shows mothers rest better when mothers and babies are kept together following birth. (G. Psychology; 1–2 days; Knowledge; Difficulty: 2)

108. The answer is D. Breastfeeding triggers and enhances maturation of the baby's own immune system. (B. Physiology; General Principles; Application; Difficulty: 5)

109. The answer is C. The Baby-Friendly Hospital Initiative, Step 9 is "Give no artificial teats or pacifiers (also called dummies or soothers) to breastfeeding infants." This step also includes prohibition of feeding bottles. Bottles that are attached to breast pumps are not addressed. (M. Public Health; 1–2 days; Knowledge; Difficulty: 2)

110. The answer is B. Lactoferrin has no known function relative to nerve myelinization or growth. It is a major protein source and iron transport agent, and it reduces/prevents inflammation. (B. Biochemistry; General Principles; Knowledge; Difficulty: 5)

111. The answer is A. Some allege that orthodontic-shaped pacifiers improve dentition, but research reveals more orthodontic problems in children who use pacifiers. (K. Equipment; 15–28 days; Knowledge; Difficulty: 2)

112. The answer is B. Cup feeding for an extended time may reduce the baby's sucking urge. (B. Physiology; Prematurity; Application; Difficulty: 2)

113. The answer is D. The laboring woman is disempowered when others direct her actions during labor. All of the other items increase her empowerment. The take-charge attitude of the attendant puts her into a passive role, which has been shown to interfere with breastfeeding. (G. Psychology; Prenatal; Application; Difficulty: 2)

114. The answer is C. Menstrual irregularities and pain are not known to be related to whether the woman breastfed her children. (D. Immunology; Preconception; Knowledge; Difficulty: 2)

115. The answer is B. Premature babies often exhibit an irregular and arrhythmic sucking pattern that improves as they mature. All the other statements are accurate and appropriate. (B. Physiology; Prematurity; Application; Difficulty: 2)

116. The answer is A. Antibiotic drugs have no documented affect on the fetus or newborn's ability to breastfeed. The other choices are more likely to contribute to breastfeeding difficulties. (F. Pharmacology; General Principles; Application; Difficulty: 2)

117. The answer is D. Hearing and taste develop early in gestation. All the other processes are compromised by preterm birth. (B. Physiology; Prematurity; Knowledge; Difficulty: 2)

118. The answer is A. Left occiput anterior (LOA) is the most common fetal presentation and least likely to cause birth trauma that could affect the baby's ability to breastfeed. Posterior presentations are less common; mentum and sacrum presentations are rare. (A. Anatomy; Prenatal; Application; Difficulty: 2)

119. The answer is D. The oral experience of breastfeeding is pleasurable and normal. The infant controls and molds the shape of the breast in its mouth. (H. Growth; General Principles; Application; Difficulty: 2)

120. The answer is B. The dependent variable is the result of the manipulation, not the part of the experiment that is changed. The other three statements about experimental research designs are true. (I. Research; General Principles; Knowledge; Difficulty: 2)

121. The answer is C. All labor drugs cross the placenta, including those administered in the epidural space. The effect on the baby's ability to breastfeed appears to be dose-related. (F. Pharmacology; Labor/birth; Application; Difficulty: 5)

122. The answer is D. Although a shortage of equipment led to the development of kangaroo mother care, research now supports the other reasons as far more important. (L. Techniques; Prematurity; Application; Difficulty: 4)

123. The answer is B. Evidence of lower risk of respiratory infections following implementation of BFHI policies is the weakest of the conditions listed. (M. Public Health; General Principles; Knowledge; Difficulty: 3)

124. The answer is B. Epidural analgesia and narcotics cross the placenta and have documented effects on the baby's motor and neurobehavioral scores. (F. Pharmacology; Labor/birth; Application; Difficulty: 2)

125. The answer is C. Wound cleaning is not a standard part of lactation consultant practice. The other actions are appropriate. (J. Legal; 7–12 months; Application; Difficulty: 3)

126. The answer is A. The peaked shape with barely visible damage in the center of the nipple tip is most often associated with either a poor (shallow) latch or a baby with a sucking problem. In this case, the baby was tongue-tied. Rarely would a deeply latched baby cause this severe nipple distortion. When a baby is poorly latched or has a suck deficit, effective milk transfer and self-detachment are less likely. (E. Pathology; 4–6 months; Application; Difficulty: 4)

127. The answer is B. The smaller breast has characteristics of insufficient glandular tissue. (A. Anatomy; 15–28 days; Application; Difficulty: 4)

128. The answer is B. Breast shells with wide backs will protect the injured skin from the rubbing of her bra or clothing. (K. Equipment; 3–14 days; Application; Difficulty: 3)

129. The answer is B. ABO incompatibility is a cause of early-onset jaundice. Breast-milk jaundice becomes apparent or continues to rise after the 3rd day, and bilirubin levels may peak at any time from the 7th to the 10th day, or even as late as the 15th day. Effective, exclusive breastfeeding does not result in high enough levels of bilirubin to warrant treatment with light therapy. Hypoglycemia is not treated in this manner. (E. Pathology; 3–14 days; Application; Difficulty: 4)

130. The answer is B. Young children imitating breastfeeding with a doll is a common and normal occurrence in most cultures worldwide. (G. Psychology; Preconception; Application; Difficulty: 2)

131. The answer is A. The developmental milestones characteristic of the 7- to 12-month age include separation anxiety, sleep changes, especially increased night waking, and decreased (not increased) likelihood of self-weaning. (H. Growth; 7–12 months; Application; Difficulty: 4)

132. The answer is B. This rash on the baby's thigh is one manifestation of allergic responses (atopic disease). A lactation consultant may not make a diagnosis or prescribe, so A and D are inappropriate responses. (J. Legal; General Principles; Application; Difficulty: 5)

133. The answer is B. The pump flange was too small in diameter for this mother's relatively large, fibrous nipples. (K. Equipment; 1–2 days; Application; Difficulty: 4)

134. The answer is C. This baby is nearing the end of the feed on this breast and should be allowed to self-detach at his own pace. He is correctly positioned. (L. Techniques; 15–28 days; Application; Difficulty: 4)

135. The answer is B. The baby's head is too extended relative to his trunk, so pulling the legs closer to the mother will better align the hip and shoulders. Supporting the breast will not correct the infant's position. The horizontal position and use of a pillow are not likely to help. (L. Techniques; 15–28 days; Application; Difficulty: 2)

136. The answer is D. The baby's lingual frenulum is short and tight, attached at the tongue tip and on the bottom (alveolar) gum ridge. This prevents the tongue from creating a good seal at breast. (A. Anatomy; 3–14 days; Application; Difficulty: 4)

137. The answer is D. Colonization with the mother's flora sets up the optimal microbial environment for the newborn. When anyone else holds the baby, there is a greater risk of colonization with less-friendly organisms. (D. Immunology; Labor/birth; Application; Difficulty: 3)

138. The answer is C. The shiny, reddened color of this mother's nipple and areola is typical of thrush (*Candida*) infection. Her baby's mouth is likely to show white plaques that do not rub off and are typical of oral thrush/fungal (*Candida*) infections. (D. Immunology; 15–28 days; Application; Difficulty: 4)

139. The answer is A. This is a bacterial infection of the nipple, therefore the lactation consultant should arrange for a medical provider to properly diagnose the infection. Washing with water and positioning the baby more deeply onto the breast are reasonable actions after medical diagnosis is in progress. Massaging expressed milk into the nipple is inappropriate because there is no benefit, and it could exacerbate the infection. (J. Legal; General Principles; Application; Difficulty: 4)

140. The answer is C. This baby's hypotonia (low muscle tone) is caused by Prader Willi syndrome. The nipple shield (barely visible), jaw support, and upright straddle position are all techniques that can assist a baby with low tone to maximize milk obtained directly at breast. (E. Pathology; 1–3 months; Application; Difficulty: 2)

141. The answer is B. In the quiet alert state, the baby's eyes are open, arms extended and relaxed, hands loosely open. The baby's expression is calm and relaxed. (H. Growth; 15–28 days; Knowledge; Difficulty: 4)

142. The answer is C. Mothers' milk contains traces of flavors present in the mother's food choices, which helps the baby learn and enjoy family food preferences. Shortly after this picture was taken, the baby's breath smelled faintly of cantaloupe. (B. Biochemistry; 3–14 days; Application; Difficulty: 3)

143. The answer is B. The indentation visible on the areolar skin was caused by a breast shell placed over her nipple to allow air drying of the wound. (K. Equipment; 3–14 days; Application; Difficulty: 4)

144. The answer is C. This baby is adequately attached and positioned for feeding, and the pattern is normal in length and comfortable for both mother and baby. While A, B, and D would be appropriate if the feeding pattern was uncomfortable or ineffective, suggesting too many technique changes could undermine the mother's confidence in breastfeeding. (L. Techniques; 15–28 days; Application; Difficulty: 2)

145. The answer is C. The reddened skin is only found on the genitalia and anal opening, suggesting an allergic response. Yeast infections are characterized by blisters or papules. Acidic urine does not result from human milk feedings, and chemical sensitivities would likely appear under the entire diaper area. This baby was in fact allergic to dairy products ingested by her mother. (D. Immunology; 15–28 days; Application; Difficulty: 3)

146. The answer is C. This mother and baby are content, safe, and warm. Keeping the mother and baby in skin-to-skin contact is ideal for stabilizing the baby's systems. Preserving the mother–baby relationship is a primary responsibility of the lactation consultant. Continue observing the dyad; the baby will likely wake to feed soon. (G. Psychology; Labor/birth; Application; Difficulty: 2)

147. The answer is D. The newborn is born sterile. Exposure to its mother's feces colonizes the infant with her beneficial gut bacteria, which helps avoid colonization with harmful pathogens from the environment. (D. Immunology; Labor/birth; Knowledge; Difficulty: 5)

148. The answer is A. Many babies show signs of developmental readiness around 6 months of age, such as reaching for family foods. Exclusive breastfeeding is recommended for at least 6 months. (H. Growth; 7–12 months; Application; Difficulty: 4)

149. The answer is D. The lactation consultant should help the mother clarify the mother's feelings about continuing to breastfeed and support her decision. The other responses are not appropriate. (G. Psychology; 15–28 days; Application; Difficulty: 3)

150. The answer is C. Assuring proper positioning and latch is always the first action. This mother's bifurcated nipple was fully functional, and the baby fed from this breast easily and effectively. (L. Techniques; 1–2 days; Application; Difficulty: 4)

151. The answer is B. A common sign of disorganized sucking is the baby feeds for extended periods with its eyes closed. Feeding for 30–45 minutes per breast is not normal behavior for this healthy 3-week-old. The mother's milk supply cannot be ascertained by infant feeding behavior, and the effect of most labor drugs would have diminished by now. (B. Physiology; 15–28 days; Application; Difficulty: 5)

152. The answer is B. This baby has oral thrush, which easily transfers to mother's nipples. Although a mother may have a vaginal *Candida* infection, it is most likely that she will have symptoms of thrush on her nipples. (D. Immunology; 1–3 months; Application; Difficulty: 3)

153. The answer is A. The baby finds his way to the breast partly by smell. Placing the unwashed baby on his mother's unwashed body facilitates the baby's ability to self-attach to the breast. The other practices listed would interfere with this natural process. This baby is smelling his hands as he crawls to the breast. (B. Physiology; Labor/birth; Knowledge; Difficulty: 3)

154. The answer is B. Oxytocin is especially high in the immediate postbirth period, which helps mother and baby develop trust in one another. (B. Physiology; Labor/birth; Knowledge; Difficulty: 4)

155. The answer is C. This is mechanical (friction) damage from a tongue-tied baby. A and B do not cause open wounds. D is an old myth, not consistent with current knowledge and research evidence. (E. Pathology; 1–2 days; Application; Difficulty: 2)

156. The answer is C. The newborn should be placed at breast immediately postbirth, and assisted (if needed) to begin breastfeeding within the first hour. The BFHI and other policies suggest that all non–life-saving procedures be delayed until after the first effective breastfeed. (M. Public Health; Labor/birth; Application; Difficulty: 2)

157. The answer is A. Nursing supplementers were designed to provide food at breast for an adopted baby so that the baby's sucking will help stimulate the mother's breast to make milk. There is no research evidence that feeding tube devices accomplish any of the other outcomes. (K. Equipment; 1–3 months; Application; Difficulty: 4)

158. The answer is B. Skin-to-skin contact is calming and soothing for the infant. Most procedures can be done while the baby is resting skin to skin on the mother's body. In theory, the mother might be breastfeeding during this procedure. However, holding the baby skin to skin would be more realistic and not depend on the infant's readiness to feed. (B. Physiology; Labor/birth; Application; Difficulty: 5)

159. The answer is C. This baby is capable of crawling to the breast unassisted. Self-attachment suggests that the baby has completed the required behavioral sequencing and will suck normally and effectively. There is no indication that any of the other actions are necessary or even appropriate. (L. Techniques; Labor/birth; Application; Difficulty: 5)

160. The answer is D. Casein in milk increases in proportion to whey over time. Lactose and lactoferrin increase slightly over time. (B. Biochemistry; 7–12 months; Knowledge; Difficulty: 4)

161. The answer is C. The baby's mouth is infected with thrush (*Candida*), which is a fungus. Mother and baby need to be treated simultaneously with an antifungal agent. (E. Pathology; 3–14 days; Application; Difficulty: 5)

162. The answer is B. This is a large, fibrous nipple with no abnormal conditions. (A. Anatomy; 3–14 days; Knowledge; Difficulty: 4)

163. The answer is B. "Gymnastic" nursing, pincer grasp and self-feeding, and increased mobility are typical of the 7- to 12-month-old baby. (H. Growth; 7–12 months; Knowledge; Difficulty: 5)

164. The answer is B. This was diagnosed as eczema, an allergic reaction which began soon after this baby was given supplements of cow's-milk-based formula. Rice cereal is a less common allergen. It is unlikely that cold temperature or a tetanus immunization triggered this response. (D. Immunology; 15–28 days; Application; Difficulty: 3)

165. The answer is B. This is a plugged nipple pore, also known as a "bleb" or "white spot." These are thought to be due to plugs of milk that solidify at the opening of a milk duct on the nipple skin. (E. Pathology; 1–3 months; Application; Difficulty: 3)

166. The answer is C. Allowing the baby to set the pace of feeds is most appropriate. This mother has very large breasts, and the baby may even want to feed more than one time from one breast before switching sides. (L. Techniques; 3–14 days; Application; Difficulty: 4)

167. The answer is A. Supporting the mother is always the first response, especially when she is as happy as the mother in the photo. Choice B would be appropriate after you've complimented the mother. The other two responses are not appropriate. (G. Psychology; Labor/birth; Application; Difficulty: 3)

168. The answer is A. Secretory IgA in milk/colostrum is 10 times higher on the first postpartum day than at any other time during lactation. Lactose is low at this time because lactose is low in colostrum. (D. Immunology; Labor/birth; Application; Difficulty: 4)

169. The answer is B. This nipple wound was caused by a baby with tongue-tie (short and/or tight lingual frenulum). Normal breastfeeding does not cause this kind of wound; shallow latch is unlikely to cause this much damage in just 8 days, and an 8-day-old is unlikely to be biting during feeds. (E. Pathology; 3–14 days; Knowledge; Difficulty: 3)

170. The answer is C. The string-like structure connecting the tongue to the floor of the mouth is the lingual frenulum (or frenum). The labial frenulum is on the upper (maxillary) gum ridge. The incisive papilla are behind the upper gum ridge, and mucus membrane covers most of the inside of the baby's mouth. (A. Anatomy; General Principles; Knowledge; Difficulty: 4)

171. The answer is B. The most likely explanation for sudden onset soreness is poor positioning, causing pulling or tugging on the nipple skin. The first intervention would be correcting positioning and latch. The other choices are possibilities after poor positioning has been ruled out. (L. Techniques; 4–6 months; Application; Difficulty: 5)

172. The answer is B. The white structures in this newborn's mouth are natal teeth. (A. Anatomy; 1–2 days; Knowledge; Difficulty: 3)

173. The answer is A. This child is tongue-tied, often referred to as ankyloglossia. The lingual frenulum is short and/or tight. Without full normal tongue mobility, breastfeeding and eating (and other activities involving movement of the tongue) are compromised. (A. Anatomy; >12 months; Knowledge; Difficulty: 3)

174. The answer is B. Although siblings sleeping together is a practice found in many cultures, new research on sudden unexpected deaths in infancy (SUDI) suggests that infants under 6 months are at some risk of suffocation from bed partners who are relatively unaware of the infant's presence, such as young siblings. Babies should sleep in proximity to an attentive adult. (G. Psychology; 1–3 months; Application; Difficulty: 4)

175. The answer is A. Always evaluate the baby's breastfeeding technique first. This mother's baby was tongue-tied, and friction from his tongue was causing the persistent nipple wound. (L. Techniques; 3–14 days; Application; Difficulty: 4)

176. The answer is D. The over-1-year-old nursing child often plays and explores mother's body during breastfeeding sessions. (H. Growth; >12 months; Application; Difficulty: 5)

177. The answer is D. Supine sleeping is the safest position for sleeping, especially if the baby is sleeping alone. This firm, flat mattress on the floor is not a risk, nor is the proximity of the unused fireplace. The child is sleeping in proximity to her mother, who is not shown working in the same room. Pacifier use to prevent SIDS is a controversial recommendation that is not fully supported by research, and often interferes with breastfeeding. (E. Pathology; 1–3 months; Application; Difficulty: 4)

178. The answer is A. Deep puckering suggests poor tongue position or motion. In this case, the baby was tongue-tied. Feeding with the eyes closed is a lesser indicator of a problem. The chin and nose are well positioned. (L. Techniques; 3–14 days; Application; Difficulty: 3)

179. The answer is C. These are typical and normal behaviors of breastfeeding children in the 7- to 12-month period. (H. Growth; 7–12 months; Application; Difficulty: 3)

180. The answer is C. This baby's tongue shape is unusual. This baby's other oral anatomic structures are normal. (A. Anatomy; 1–3 months; Application; Difficulty: 3)

181. The answer is C. Many mothers have more milk than their baby needs in the first 2 weeks. Supply gradually adjusts to baby's needs over the first 6 weeks or so. (B. Physiology; 3–14 days; Application; Difficulty: 4)

182. The answer is D. Accessory mammary tissue may be found along the milk lines that run from the upper inner arm to the inguinal region. Accessory mammary tissue develops during fetal development. (A. Anatomy; 3–14 days; Application; Difficulty: 4)

183. The answer is C. There is no research supporting the use of hot compresses to relieve milk stasis or edema. This woman's chief complaint is the accessory breast tissue in her armpit; her breasts are neither overfull nor swollen, and the baby is nursing well. (E. Pathology; 3–14 days; Application; Difficulty: 2)

184. The answer is C. Breast binders have not been found to be safe or effective for inflammatory conditions of the lactating breast. (L. Techniques; 3–14 days; Application; Difficulty: 5)

185. The answer is B. Appropriate exclusive breastfeeding is unlikely to cause this pattern. The other conditions could result in growth compromise as charted. (H. Growth; 7–12 months; Knowledge; Difficulty: 5)

186. The answer is D. This was diagnosed as a bacterial infection of the nipple skin. Immediate weaning is not appropriate, because the baby has already been exposed and may even have caused the infection. A nipple shield may provide some comfort, providing it is thoroughly cleaned between uses. Choices A and C are also appropriate. (E. Pathology; 15–28 days; Application; Difficulty: 3)

187. The answer is C. Babies cue or signal for their needs to be met. Crying is a late sign of hunger; and it is also a sign that the baby has exhausted all other resources in getting his needs met. (H. Growth; 3–14 days; Application; Difficulty: 2)

188. The answer is A. This child is about 8 months old, an age during which children go through a period of separation anxiety and may want to breastfeed much more frequently for a while. Other babies normally and naturally nurse in that pattern. It is very unlikely that this mother's supply is reduced because the baby in the photo is obviously thriving. (G. Psychology; 7–12 months; Application; Difficulty: 2)

189. The answer is B. This mother's breast is engorged—a combination of edema and milk stasis. Hot compresses can make edema worse and have no documented advantage in correcting milk stasis. (E. Pathology; 3–14 days; Application; Difficulty: 5)

190. The answer is B. Mother-baby cross infection is likely when the baby has an oral infection. Assume that the mother's nipples are also infected with the same organism, as well as other infant body parts and any/all sucking objects. (D. Immunology; 1–3 months; Application; Difficulty: 2)

191. The answer is C. There is no evidence of increased dental caries from nighttime breastfeeding in the second year of life. The child who nurses past 12 months of age receives substantial immune protection, nutrition, and psychological benefits from breastfeeding (E. Pathology; >12 months; Application; Difficulty: 3)

192. The answer is D. Determination of sufficient or insufficient glandular tissue for lactation cannot be determined by physical examination alone. This woman breastfed two children for over 2 years each. (J. Legal; General Principles; Application; Difficulty: 5)

193. The answer is A. Paget's disease is a type of nipple cancer and the least likely cause of the small wound shown. The lesion is an unhealed wound caused by the baby's poor suck due to a short frenulum that was uncorrected for 2 months. (E. Pathology; 1–3 months; Knowledge; Difficulty: 5)

194. The answer is B. Fungal infections on the lactating breast are typically not localized to one small area. The other conditions are more likely, and the lactation consultant should be collaborating with her medical care provider for a thorough diagnosis. (E. Pathology; 4–6 months; Knowledge; Difficulty: 3)

195. The answer is A. Weaning from the affected breast following abscess formation or treatment is rarely necessary. All the other actions are appropriate. (E. Pathology; 1–3 months; Application; Difficulty: 2)

196. The answer is D. Four to 6-month-old babies are very interactive with their mothers during breast-feeding, including making intense eye contact. (H. Growth; 4-6 months; Application; Difficulty: 2)

197. The answer is D. A mother with a history of sexual abuse should first be encouraged to breastfeed. Only if direct breastfeeding is rejected should pumping be suggested. The other reasons for pumping are appropriate. (K. Equipment; 3–14 days; Application; Difficulty: 2)

198. The answer is D. Routine supplementation of all breastfed babies is not justified by the prevailing research. Supplementation should be based on history and a case-by-case basis. (B. Biochemistry; 4–6 months; Application; Difficulty: 2)

199. The answer is B. A silicone nipple shield is the least helpful of the above suggestions. The sore spot on her nipple tip is very tiny, and most often better positioning and latch will remedy the problem. (K. Equipment; 3–14 days; Application; Difficulty: 2)

200. The answer is A. Competition with the baby's own mother is highly unlikely. This picture shows the author carrying her perfectly normal, wonderful, gorgeous, and brilliant granddaughter at about 4 weeks of age. (G. Psychology; 15–28 days; Knowledge; Difficulty: 2)

PART 3 Additional Resources

CLINICAL (FIELD) EXERCISES

Clinical (field) exercises help the lactation consultant candidate experience the full depth and breadth of breastfeeding in real-life situations. They add a practical, dynamic, and multidimensional aspect to the course material. The IBLCE examination is highly based on practical help for real-life situations, and an early analysis of courses and candidates' results suggests that doing and writing up various clinical exercises are related to higher scores on the exam. Merely doing the exercises is helpful. Analyzing and writing up what you learned are even better. The write-up could be an analytical references research paper, or it could take a more artistic form such as a poem, song, collage, or drawing. Doing a write-up is an excellent way of analyzing, synthesizing, and understanding the topic that is being investigated.

If your experience in lactation is primarily in one chronological state of breastfeeding or one topic area (early postpartum, mother-to-mother breastfeeding groups, prenatal education), it is helpful to spend considerable time on unfamiliar areas or topics than on familiar ones.

SHADOWING/OBSERVATION GUIDELINES

1. Before the observation

   a. Seek permission from the facility, the lactation consultant (LC) or health professional, the support group leader, and especially the mother/client(s) being observed.
   b. The facility or LC may welcome you but the mother may feel uncomfortable with your presence. If the mother is even the slightest bit uncomfortable, do not continue with that observation.

2. During the observation

   a. Your role is an observer and guest, not a group leader or therapist—even if you are a professional observing a peer. Refrain from engaging in the client-LC interaction unless invited to do so by the mother and the professional.
   b. Address the mother and baby by name if you do briefly engage. Do not treat the mother as a patient or lab animal. Also, remember that it is rude to discuss a third party in their presence.
   c. Refrain from exhibiting negative body language in the presence of your sponsor and the mother.
   d. Obey any local protocols (wearing scrubs, etc.).
   e. Take thorough notes on what you have observed.
   f. Thank the mother for her willingness to allow you to observe.
   g. Do not observe when you are ill, stressed, or are unprepared to give the experience your full attention.

3. After the observation

    a. Arrange time after the observation period to meet with the LC for feedback and discussion.

    b. If you have observed something that you disagree with, tactfully request information on the LC's rationale. It is easy to offend if you have an attitude that you know better than the LC. The LC's information and actions were likely most appropriate for that circumstance regardless of what the books say or what your previous experience dictates.

    c. Finally, thank the LC in writing. Let her know how she has facilitated your education and about the positive things you experienced and saw. Everyone likes a pat on the back for a job well done. Be genuine; do not fabricate. You can always find something to compliment!

CLINICAL EXERCISES

Overview of Lactation Consultation

1. Interview three or more practicing LCs in a variety of settings. Ask the LCs how they bring the concepts of protection, support, and promotion into their work; their philosophy of care; how they integrate therapy into their practice; and how they view their role.

2. Write an analysis of the breastfeeding content in your own academic or professional training. Compare this to your personal experience with breastfeeding and information learned from informal sources. Include your feelings about how your formal training affected your personal experiences with breastfeeding. Describe how both kinds of learning have been helpful or harmful in your clinical practice.

Exercises by Discipline

The following exercises are related to the 13 disciplines included in the 2000 Exam Blueprint. Each exercise is intended to broaden or deepen the candidate's understanding of the body of knowledge in that discipline. One exercise may overlap more than one discipline or chronological stage, which will additionally benefit the candidate.

    A. Maternal and Infant Anatomy

        a. Compare new ultrasound studies of the lactating breast by Donna Ramsay Geddes and other authors with at least three books or references published prior to 2004. Describe differences in structure and function and the implication of these differences on breastfeeding management, techniques, and education of parents. Prepare a bibliography of breast structure and function.

b. Read at least three research articles or a textbook on the infant mouth, which could include articles on palate shape, tongue and other structures, size and jaw configuration, maturity, anomalies and/or defects. Discuss the influence on breastfeeding of at least three different aspects of infant oral anatomy.

B. Maternal and Infant Normal Physiology and Endocrinology

a. Using the concept of autocrine control of milk supply, assist three or more women to increase their milk supply. For each, record your strategies; the results in milk volume and how quickly the supply changed; and the mother's feelings and experiences using the strategies. Provide at least five current references.

b. Interview three women who are using the lactational amenorrhea method (LAM) of family planning. Include feeding patterns, night feeding arrangements, reasons the mothers are using this method, drawbacks or obstacles they encountered, return of menstruation, and effect of this method on other health behaviors in their families.

c. Design a management protocol that enables both a mother to relactate and an adoptive mother to induce lactation. Give rationales and references for your management plan. If possible, design your plan for a specific mother you have met.

C. Maternal and Infant Normal Nutrition and Biochemistry

a. Examine at least three different sources for recommendations on complementary feeding of breastfed babies. Include the age recommended for starting solids, the order and texture of foods presented, and mother–baby interactions involved in feeding. Compare these recommendations with Pan American Health Organization's "Guiding Principles for Complementary Feeding of the Breastfed Child."

b. Prepare a presentation on milk biochemistry, using at least three references and including the following points: (1) Compare the protein, fat, immune factors, and vitamin content of colostrum, preterm milk, mature milk, and milk produced after 12 months of lactation. (2) Discuss the influence of fatty acids in human milk in relation to brain development. (3) Explain the effect of maternal diet on the fat, protein, carbohydrates, minerals, and fat-soluble and water-soluble vitamins in her milk.

c. Describe in detail how the biochemistry of human milk supports the optimum growth of the human infant during 6 months of exclusive breastfeeding and continued breastfeeding for at least 24 months as recommended by the Global Strategy for Infant and Young Child Feeding.

d. Observe five babies at breast for two consecutive complete feeding episodes. The babies should be of different ages. Estimate the total volume of milk obtained based on quality and quantity of feeding. Weigh the babies prefeed and postfeed on a digital or gram-sensitive scale to verify your estimates.

D. Maternal and Infant Immunology and Infectious Disease

a. Interview at least three mothers whose children have allergies. Describe the strategies and resources used by the mothers to confirm and manage the allergens that affect each child and any modifications made by each mother and rest of her family. Prepare a list of common allergic triggers and reactions in children under 12 months old, using your interviews and published books and research on allergies to support your lists.

    b. Select 1–3 immune components in human milk and research the function of those components thoroughly. Describe any variations in these components over time, as well as during heating or freezing and storage.

    c. Select 1–3 long-term health issues that are affected by breastfeeding. Investigate support groups, Internet sites, and educational resources on those issues to see how much information on breastfeeding is (or is not) included in easily available resources. Contact one organization dedicated to a long-term health issue affected by breastfeeding and find out how breastfeeding could be inserted into their educational and support programs.

    d. Describe in detail at least five uses for expressed mothers' milk or banked, pasteurized human milk for babies with serious illnesses, metabolic deficiencies, or other pathological conditions.

E. Maternal and Infant Pathology

    a. Write a descriptive essay of the lactation consultant's role in providing care for the mother affected by a pathological breast condition. Include care plan instructions (problem description, goal for intervention, strategies for intervention, considerations for follow-up, etc.) for at least three specific mothers with a pathological breast condition.

    b. Observe at least three breastfeeding problems in a variety of contexts. For each, write at least a 1-page brief summary of the problem and how the problem should or could have been prevented or handled at a lower level of intervention. Include a discussion of any conflict with other professionals in any aspect of the situation, whether by omission or commission.

    c. Interview three mothers whose babies were premature or ill at birth, requiring longer-than-usual hospitalizations for the newborns. Explore how breastfeeding was affected by each baby's condition, and how each mother managed to maintain lactation and assist the baby to breastfeed directly during their baby's hospitalization.

    d. Interview three mothers whose babies had sucking or feeding problems after full-term births. For each baby, address the problem's impact on breastfeeding, as well as the impact of breastfeeding on the baby and/or the problem.

    e. Conduct a literature review on one of the following conditions: nipple and oral thrush; congenital abnormality or structural defect; or endocrine irregularity in the mother or infant. Interview at least one mother whose baby has that condition. Prepare an information sheet on that condition using at least three current references.

    f. Read several professional organizations' position papers and policies on jaundice and hypoglycemia. Compare these resources to at least five research articles on these topics, and discuss the differences and any contradictions.

    g. Tour a neonatal intensive care init at a hospital other than where you work. Ask the following questions: What is your policy on breastfeeding? Which babies are most likely to be breastfed? What is your policy on giving expressed breastmilk to babies? What are your criteria for determining which milk is usable or unusable? How do mothers obtain breast pumps and attachment kits? What is the recommended pumping regimen? At what point do mothers begin to breastfeed their babies? What kind of breastfeeding support is provided for breastfeeding families? Under what circumstances do you not recommend breastfeeding? Write up your impressions and compare the answers to current research.

    h. Contact a new mother with a handicapping condition or chronic illness. Interview her concerning the impact of her condition on pregnancy, birth, breastfeeding, and caring for her baby. Analyze her responses and identify key areas of support that she received or failed to receive from family, professionals, or the community. Prepare a list of resources for professionals and/or parents about that condition, including a bibliography of references that address that condition and its impact on lactation.

F. Maternal and Infant Pharmacology and Toxicology

    a. Write a case study of two breastfeeding women taking a prescription drug. Include signs and symptoms of illness; date of onset; duration of symptoms; interventions (if any); drug—including dose, mode of delivery, and frequency taken; prescribed by whom; any instructions given to the mother by her physician, nurse, or counselor; passage of drug into milk; implications for the baby; and alternatives.

    b. Pick at least five of the following medications: aspirin, pseudoephedrine, technetium 99, medroxyprogesterone acetate, cimetedine, paroxetine, ciprofloxacin, triamcinolone, cephalexin, fluconazole, and metronidazole. Using at least two references, discuss the compatibility of the drug to breastfeeding.

    c. Investigate the history of galactagogues and lactation suppressants, including folk remedies and cultural beliefs, prescription drugs, and herbs. Describe any research available on the safety and effectiveness of at least one preparation.

    d. Observe at least one complete hospital-based labor and birth episode. Focus on the mother's knowledge and use of nondrug and pharmacologic pain-relief techniques and coping techniques and their effect on mother and baby. Provide at least three references on any drugs used during the labor and their impact on any aspect of breastfeeding. Describe the status of breastfeeding one week after birth.

G. Psychology, Sociology, and Anthropology

    a. Interview 3–5 women who have experienced childbirthing experiences different from what they expected, or negative experiences. You may include yourself as one of the mothers. Ask them what they didn't like, what they would have done differently, what they wanted others to have done differently, and how this experience affected their sense of self as a parent and their relationship with their child. Caution: Be an active listener. Do not attempt to justify or rationalize the behavior of others. Stay focused on the mother's feelings.

    b. Complete La Leche League's human relations enrichment programmed text/manual *or* attend at least Level I of La Leche League International's Communication Skills Enrichment program. Practice the active listening skills at work and at home for at least a week or two. Describe others' general responses to you when you use these techniques.

    c. Ask three breastfeeding mothers to record feeding frequency and duration of all feeds for three consecutive days. Select infants of different ages. Compare the patterns of the mother–baby pairs to popular parenting books. Discuss with the mothers why they did or did not read or follow these books' advice.

    d. Attend a full 4-meeting series of La Leche League or other organized mother-support group. Observe the communications and group dynamics techniques in use at the meetings, and analyze the apparent effects of those techniques.

e. Interview a mother who breastfed or is breastfeeding twins, triplets, or quadruplets. Include in your interview the following questions: When did you first learn you were having twins? How did you feel? How did your family react to the news? What is the easiest part about breastfeeding twins? The hardest part? What would you want another mother expecting twins to know? What are the unique features of mothering and breastfeeding more than one baby at a time?

f. If you have breastfed, write an essay describing your thoughts on being pregnant; attitudes about labor and birth; feelings about being a mother, and the impact of the attitudes of your immediate family on your becoming a mother. Focus on what surprised you emotionally. If you have not breastfed, interview two mothers concerning the above topics, and write an essay on their comments and your reactions to their discussion of their feelings.

H. Growth Parameters and Developmental Milestones

a. Attend two different meetings of La Leche League, the Australian Breastfeeding Association, or another breastfeeding mother-support group. Observe variations in mother-infant breastfeeding interactions related to individual differences in infant behavior, infant age, and maternal response. Listen to the comments and concerns that mothers raise during the meeting and during breaks. Write up your observations, and compare them to what you've heard in your professional role.

b. Go to a local shopping mall, park, or other public place and watch at least 10 mothers and babies under the age of 3 years interacting. Estimate the age of each child based on its behavior, then verify the child's age by asking the mother. At least half the sample should include breastfeeding dyads.

c. Carefully examine the 2006 WHO Growth Standards and compare them with older growth monitoring documents, including anthropometric data, why the selection sites were chosen, and how the mothers and families were supported. Investigate how the new data are being used in your community.

I. Interpretation of Research

a. Write a critique of a research report (article) related to any aspect of breastfeeding from a recent (within 2 years) primary source. Consider submitting this critique to a journal or other source.

b. Write a review of a videotape, book, or teaching aid pertinent to any aspect of breastfeeding. Follow the rules for reviews from a professional journal. Consider submitting it to a professional journal for publication.

J. Ethical and Legal Issues

a. Review at least three lactation consultant assessment forms, which can be from the same or varied clinical settings. Write an analysis of the strengths and weaknesses of each and any changes you would make, *or* design a set of assessment and reporting forms for use in your setting, and have them reviewed by someone else.

b. For each of the following scenarios, decide whether the behavior is ethical or not, give a thorough rationale for your decision, and include any relevant references to support your point of view.

  i. Scenario 1: The LC sees every patient of the doctor for whom she works. When asked by the doctor's patients what to take to the hospital to facilitate the breastfeeding experience, the LC sells them a package of breastfeeding aids (shells, lanolin, manual breast pump, bra pads, a book). The LC keeps 100% of the profit.

  ii. Scenario 2: The LC teaches all the breastfeeding and childbirth classes in XYZ hospital. Mrs. A attends the childbirth class and later calls the LC for help. She needs more help than can be provided by phone. The LC arranges a home visit and charges the mother for this service. There is no other breastfeeding care provider in this community.

  iii. Scenario 3: The LC is working with Baby B, who has an obvious short frenulum, which severely inhibits breastfeeding. The doctors in this community refuse to acknowledge the need for treatment for short frenulum, and they recommend cessation of breastfeeding if it causes a problem. The LC tells Baby B's mother about a dentist in the neighboring community who can diagnose and treat the short frenulum; the LC does not ask permission from the primary care physician to make the referral.

  iv. Scenario 4: You, the LC at ABC hospital, have been tasked with providing in-service education on breastfeeding to the entire professional staff—doctors, nurses, etc. You have been offered funds from two sources: Abbott-Ross Laboratories and Proctor & Gamble. Your supervisor tells you to use the Abbott funds to pay for the in-service sessions because the representative recently purchased a new photocopier for the unit.

c. Prepare an annotated bibliography of ethical and legal aspects of breastfeeding with primary and secondary references.

K. Breastfeeding Equipment and Technology

  a. Examine and measure several infant feeding devices (teats, pacifiers, tubes) and/or devices used inside the infant mouth (nipple shields, bulb syringes, gavage tubes). Compare the length, diameter, and flexibility (texture) of these devices and the dimensions of the infant mouth at three different ages (premature; first month; and after 6 months of age) and discuss the implications to breastfeeding.

  b. Follow an international board-certified lactation consultant on hospital rounds for an entire shift, for a total of at least 6 hours. Complete an observation form on at least two mothers. Discuss with the LC what you observed including all equipment used by mothers or babies observed during that period.

  c. Test at least 10 devices for assisting breastfeeding. Milk-removal devices can be tested using a vacuum gauge or balloons. If you prefer, interview at least 10 women who have used several different kinds of equipment to assist in breastfeeding. Discuss the advantages and drawbacks of these devices or techniques including cost, comfort, and the effect on the mother–baby relationship. Include your philosophy of the use of equipment in lactation consultant practice.

L. Techniques

    a. Assist five women in attaching their babies to breast in at least two different positions. Include at least two babies over two weeks old. Document pre-and post-intervention outcomes (what changed as a result of improved technique).

    b. Observe at least three different breastfeeding care providers helping a mother resolve a breastfeeding problem. Using a standard charting method or format, describe the circumstances of their interactions. Identify the strengths and weaknesses of the providers' care plan, including anything you would have done differently, with a rationale.

    c. Perform breast exams and nipple assessments of 10 different women in different stages of lactation. Include prenatal, lactating, and postweaning breasts. Record your findings on a form, and write a narrative description of each, including the implication of each situation on the breastfeeding dyad.

    d. Interview at least three LCs who work in different practice settings. Compare and contrast their role, commenting on the similarities and differences.

M. Public Health

    a. Do at least two of the following: (1) Compile at least five laws protecting breastfeeding, and reiterate the protections for breastfeeding. (2) Prepare testimony designed to convince your local legislators to protect breastfeeding in your community, including a statement of the forum in which this testimony would be delivered. (3) Design an action plan that details breastfeeding protection strategies for your workplace.

    b. Using the UNICEF/WHO joint statement or BFHI self-evaluation criteria, evaluate some aspect of your work setting for friendliness to breastfeeding. Devise at least two short-term and long-term strategies for improving breastfeeding management that you personally can implement where you work.

    c. Contact the employee benefits representative at your work site and obtain policies about maternity and paternity leave; breastfeeding; children on premises; nursing breaks permitted; breaks permitted for any other reason, including other health impairments; any complaints that have been lodged related to child care, breastfeeding, or maternity issues; any plans for new policies. If you are not employed or if you are self-employed, contact any local business or any employees' union and ask the same questions. Prepare a bibliography of local, national, and international documents and policies relevant to maternity protection.

    d. Create a directory of breastfeeding resources in your community, including warm lines, equipment depots, breastfeeding care providers and support groups, etc.

    e. Establish a breastfeeding coalition, consortium, or network in your community. Hold at least one meeting and write up what your goals are to promote, support, and protect breastfeeding in your community in the next year.

    f. Interview someone who has worked at the national or state level in some aspect of breastfeeding promotion. Discuss how they became involved, what obstacles or resistance they have encountered, what progress they have seen, and their vision for the future.

CHRONOLOGICAL PERIODS

For each period addressed by the IBLCE exam blueprint, interview at least two women about any one aspect of breastfeeding. The aspect could be normal breastfeeding behavior or patterns, problems they've heard about or encountered, what they already know, sources of information, etc. Compare the differences in responses across the chronological periods. Summarize a theme or core issue for each chronological period.

BIBLIOGRAPHY

Abate P, Varlinskaya EI, Cheslock SJ, Spear NE, Molina JC. Neonatal activation of alcohol-related pre-natal memories: impact on the first suckling response. *Alcohol Clin Exp Res.* 2002;26(10):1512-1522.

Abiona TC, Onayade AA, Ijadunola KT, Obiajunwa PO, Aina OI, Thairu LN. Acceptability, feasibility and affordability of infant feeding options for HIV-infected women: a qualitative study in south-west Nigeria. *Matern Child Nutr.* 2006;2(3):135-44.

Ahluwalia IB, Morrow B, Hsia J. Why do women stop breastfeeding? Findings from the pregnancy risk assessment and monitoring system. *Pediatrics* 2005;116(6):1408-1412.

Aidam BA, Perez-Escamilla R, Lartey A. Lactation counseling increases exclusive breast-feeding rates in Ghana. *J Nutr.* 2005;135(7):1691-1695.

Akkuzu G, Taskin L. Impacts of breast-care techniques on prevention of possible postpartum nipple problems. *Prof Care Mother Child* 2000;10(2):38-41.

Aljazaf K, Hale TW, Ilett KF, et al. Pseudoephedrine: effects on milk production in women and esti-mation of infant exposure via breastmilk. *Br J Clin Pharmacol.* 2003;56(1):18-24.

American Academy of Pediatrics, Committee on Fetus and Newborn, American College of Obstetricians and Gynecology, Committee on Obstetric Practice. The Apgar score. *Pediatrics* 2006;117(4):1444-1447.

Amir L, Garland S. Painful nipples in nursing mothers. *Aust Fam Physician* 2003;32(10):776; author reply 777.

Amir L. Test your knowledge. Nipple pain in breastfeeding. *Aust Fam Physician* 2004;33(1-2):44-45.

Amir LH, Forster D, McLachlan H, Lumley J. Incidence of breast abscess in lactating women: report from an Australian cohort. *BJOG* 2004;111(12):1378-1381.

Amir LH, Garland SM, Lumley J. A case-control study of mastitis: nasal carriage of Staphylococcus aureus. *BMC Fam Pract.* 2006;7:57.

Amir LH, James JP, Beatty J. Review of tongue-tie release at a tertiary maternity hospital. *J Paediatr Child Health* 2005;41(5-6):243-245.

Amir LH, Lumley J, Garland SM. A failed RCT to determine if antibiotics prevent mastitis: cracked nipples colonized with Staphylococcus aureus: a randomized treatment trial [ISRCTN65289389]. *BMC Pregnancy Childbirth* 2004;4(1):19.

Amir LH, Lumley J. The treatment of Staphylococcus aureus infected sore nipples: a randomized comparative study. *J Hum Lact.* 2001;17(2):115-117.

Amir LH. Breast pain in lactating women—mastitis or something else? *Aust Fam Physician* 2003;32(3):141-145.

Amir LH. Candida and the lactating breast; predisposing factors. *J Hum Lact.* 1991;7(4):177-181.

Anand KJ, Runeson B, Jacobson B. Gastric suction at birth associated with long-term risk for func-tional intestinal disorders in later life. *J Pediatr.* 2004;144(4):449-454.

Anderson AK, Damio G, Himmelgreen DA, Peng YK, Segura-Perez S, Perez-Escamilla R. Social capi-tal, acculturation, and breastfeeding initiation among Puerto Rican women in the United States. *J Hum Lact.* 2004;20(1):39-45.

Anderson AK, Damio G, Young S, Chapman DJ, Perez-Escamilla R. A randomized trial assessing the efficacy of peer counseling on exclusive breastfeeding in a predominantly Latina low-income community. *Arch Pediatr Adolesc Med.* 2005;159(9):836-841.

Anderson AK, Himmelgreen DA, Peng YK, Segura-Perez S, Perez-Escamilla R. Social capital and breastfeeding initiation among Puerto Rican women. *Adv Exp Med Biol.* 2004;554:283-286.

Anderson GC, Moore E, Hepworth J, Bergman N. Early skin-to-skin contact for mothers and their healthy newborn infants. *Cochrane Database Syst Rev.* 2003(2):CD003519.

Anderson GC. Risk in mother-infant separation postbirth. *Image J Nurs Sch.* 1989;21(4):196-199.

Anderson GH, Atkinson SA, Bryan MH. Energy and macronutrient content of human milk during early lactation from mothers giving birth prematurely and at term. *Am J Clin Nutr.* 1981;34(2):258-265.

Anderson JE, Held N, Wright K. Raynaud's phenomenon of the nipple: a treatable cause of painful breastfeeding. *Pediatrics* 2004;113(4):e360-e364.

Arifeen S, Black RE, Antelman G, Baqui A, Caulfield L, Becker S. Exclusive breastfeeding reduces acute respiratory infection and diarrhea deaths among infants in Dhaka slums. *Pediatrics* 2001;108(4):E67.

Arnold LDW. The ethics of donor human milk banking. *Breastfeeding Med.* 2006;1(1):3-13.

Baddock SA, Galland BC, Bolton DPG, Williams SM, Taylor BJ. Differences in infant and parent behaviors during routine bed sharing compared with cot sleeping in the home setting. *Pediatrics* 2006;117(5):1599-1607.

Bahl R, Frost C, Kirkwood BR, et al. Infant feeding patterns and risks of death and hospitalization in the first half of infancy: multicentre cohort study. *Bull World Health Organ.* 2005;83(6):418-426.

Baird J, Fisher D, Lucas P, Kleijnen J, Roberts H, Law C. Being big or growing fast: systematic review of size and growth in infancy and later obesity. *BMJ* 2006:bmj.38586.411273.E0.

Baker JL, Michaelsen KF, Rasmussen KM, Sorensen TI. Maternal prepregnant body mass index, duration of breastfeeding, and timing of complementary food introduction are associated with infant weight gain. *Am J Clin Nutr.* 2004;80(6):1579-1588.

Ball HL, Blair PS, Ward-Platt MP. "New" practice of bedsharing and risk of SIDS. *Lancet* 2004;363(9420):1558.

Ball HL, Ward Platt MP, Heslop E, Leech SJ, Brown KA. Randomised trial of infant sleep location on the postnatal ward. *Arch Dis Child.* 2006.

Ball HL. Breastfeeding, bed-sharing, and infant sleep. *Birth* 2003;30(3):181-188.

Ball HL. Triadic bed-sharing and infant temperature. *Child Care Health Dev.* 2002;28(suppl 1):55-58.

Ball TM, Wright AL. Health care costs of formula-feeding in the first year of life. *Pediatrics* 1999;103(4):870-876.

Ballard JL, Auer CE, Khoury JC. Ankyloglossia: assessment, incidence, and effect of frenuloplasty on the breastfeeding dyad. *Pediatrics.* 2002;110(5):e63.

Barankin B, Gross MS. Nipple and areolar eczema in the breastfeeding woman. *J Cutan Med Surg.* 2004;8(2):126-130.

Barnes NP, Roberts P. "Extrasystoles" during kangaroo care. *Pediatr Crit Care Med.* 2005;6(2):230.

Basile LA, Taylor SN, Wagner CL, Horst RL, Hollis BW. The effect of high-dose vitamin D supplementation on serum vitamin D levels and milk calcium concentration in lactating women and their infants. *Breastfeeding Med.* 2006;1(1):27-35.

Baumgarder DJ, Muehl P, Fischer M, Pribbenow B. Effect of labor epidural anesthesia on breast-feeding of healthy full-term newborns delivered vaginally. *J Am Board Fam Pract.* 2003;16(1):7-13.

Baumgarner NJ. *Mothering Your Nursing Toddler.* Revised ed. Shaumburg, IL: LaLeche League International; 2000.

Beal AC, Chou S-C, Palmer RH, Testa MA, Newman C, Ezhuthachan S. The changing face of race: risk factors for neonatal hyperbilirubinemia. *Pediatrics.* 2006;117(5):1618-1625.

Beal JA, Wood SH. Getting to know you: mothers' experiences of kangaroo care. *MCN Am J Matern Child Nurs.* 2005;30(5):338.

Beal JA, Wood SH. Implications of kangaroo care for growth and development in preterm infants. *MCN Am J Matern Child Nurs.* 2005;30(5):338.

Beaudry M, Dufour R, Marcoux S. Relation between infant feeding and infections during the first six months of life. *J Pediatr.* 1995;126:191-197.

Beck CT. The effects of postpartum depression on maternal-infant interaction: A meta-analysis. *Nurs Rev.* 1995;44:298-304.

Becquet R, Leroy V, Ekouevi DK, et al. Complementary feeding adequacy in relation to nutritional status among early weaned breastfed children who are born to HIV-infected mothers: ANRS 1201/1202 Ditrame Plus, Abidjan, Cote d'Ivoire. *Pediatrics.* 2006;117(4):e701-710.

Beilin Y, Bodian CA, Weiser J, et al. Effect of labor epidural analgesia with and without fentanyl on infant breast-feeding: a prospective, randomized, double-blind study. *Anesthesiology.* 2005;103(6):1211-1217.

Belenky MF, Clinchy BM, Goldberger NR, Tarule JM. *Women's Ways of Knowing.* New York: Basic Books; 1986.

Benis MM. Are pacifiers associated with early weaning from breastfeeding? *Adv Neonatal Care.* 2002;2(5):259-266.

Benn CS, Michaelsen KF. Does the effect of breast-feeding on atopic dermatitis depend on family history of allergy? *J Pediatr.* 2005;147(1):128-129; author reply 129.

Benson S. What is normal? A study of normal breastfeeding dyads during the first sixty hours of life. *Breastfeed Rev.* 2001;9(1):27-32.

Bergh AM, Arsalo I, Malan AF, Patrick M, Pattinson RC, Phillips N. Measuring implementation progress in kangaroo mother care. *Acta Paediatr.* 2005;94(8):1102-1108.

Bergman NJ, Linley LL, Fawcus SR. Randomized controlled trial of skin-to-skin contact from birth versus conventional incubator for physiological stabilization in 1200- to 2199-gram newborns. *Acta Paediatr.* 2004;93(6):779-785.

Berlin CM Jr, Kacew S, Lawrence R, LaKind JS, Campbell R. Criteria for chemical selection for programs on human milk surveillance and research for environmental chemicals. *J Toxicol Environ Health A.* 2002;65(22):1839-1851.

Berlin CM Jr, LaKind JS, Fenton SE, et al. Conclusions and recommendations of the expert panel: technical workshop on human milk surveillance and biomonitoring for environmental chemicals in the United States. *J Toxicol Environ Health A.* 2005;68(20):1825-1831.

Berlin CM Jr, LaKind JS, Sonawane BR, et al. Conclusions, research needs, and recommendations of the expert panel: technical workshop on human milk surveillance and research for environmental chemicals in the United States. *J Toxicol Environ Health A.* 2002;65(22):1929-1935.

Bhutani VK, Johnson L. Kernicterus in late preterm infants cared for as term healthy infants. *Semin Perinatol.* 2006;30(2):89-97.

Blair A, Cadwell K, Turner-Maffei C, Brimdyr K. The relationship between positioning, the breast-feeding dynamic, the latching process and pain in breastfeeding mothers with sore nipples. *Breastfeed Rev.* 2003;11(2):5-10.

Blair P, Ward Platt MP, Smith IJ, Fleming PJ. Sudden infant death syndrome and sleeping position in pre-term and low birthweight infants: an opportunity for targeted intervention. *Arch Dis Child.* 2005:adc.2004.070391.

Blair PS, Ball HL. The prevalence and characteristics associated with parent-infant bed-sharing in England. *Arch Dis Child.* 2004;89(12):1106-1110.

Blair PS, Platt MW, Smith IJ, Fleming PJ. Sudden infant death syndrome and sleeping position in pre-term and low birth weight infants: an opportunity for targeted intervention. *Arch Dis Child.* 2006;91(2):101-106.

Blair PS, Sidebotham P, Berry PJ, Evans M, Fleming PJ. Major epidemiological changes in sudden infant death syndrome: a 20-year population-based study in the UK. *Lancet.* 2006;367(9507):314-319.

Bland RM, Rollins NC, Solarsh G, Van den Broeck J, Coovadia HM. Maternal recall of exclusive breastfeeding duration. *Arch Dis Child.* 2003;88(9):778-783.

Block BM, Liu SS, Rowlingson AJ, Cowan AR, Cowan JA Jr, Wu CL. Efficacy of postoperative epidural analgesia: a meta-analysis. *JAMA.* 2003;290(18):2455-2463.

Bloom SL, Leveno KJ, Spong CY, et al. Decision-to-incision times and maternal and infant outcomes. *Obstet Gynecol.* 2006;108(1):6-11.

Blyth RJ, Creedy DK, Dennis C-L, et al. Breastfeeding duration in an Australian population: the influence of modifiable antenatal factors. *J Hum Lact.* 2004;20(1):30-38.

Bodner-Adler B, Bodner K, Kimberger O, et al. The effect of epidural analgesia on the occurrence of obstetric lacerations and on the neonatal outcome during spontaneous vaginal delivery. *Arch Gynecol Obstet.* 2002;267(2):81-84.

Bonuck KA, Trombley M, Freeman K, McKee D. Randomized, controlled trial of a prenatal and postnatal lactation consultant intervention on duration and intensity of breastfeeding up to 12 months. *Pediatrics.* 2005;116(6):1413-1426.

Borghi E, de Onis M, Garza C, et al. Construction of the World Health Organization child growth standards: selection of methods for attained growth curves. *Stat Med.* 2006;25(2):247-265.

Bornmann PG, Ross GL. Using the law of battery to protect and support breastfeeding. *J Hum Lact.* 2000;16(1):47-51.

Bottcher MF, Fredriksson J, Hellquist A, Jenmalm MC. Effects of breast milk from allergic and non-allergic mothers on mitogen- and allergen-induced cytokine production. *Pediatr Allergy Immunol.* 2003;14(1):27-34.

Bottcher MF, Jenmalm MC, Bjorksten B, Garofalo RP. Chemoattractant factors in breast milk from allergic and nonallergic mothers. *Pediatr Res.* 2000;47(5):592-597.

Bottcher MF, Jenmalm MC, Garofalo RP, Bjorksten B. Cytokines in breast milk from allergic and non-allergic mothers. *Pediatr Res.* 2000;47(1):157-162.

Bowen WH, Lawrence RA. Comparison of the cariogenicity of cola, honey, cow milk, human milk, and sucrose. *Pediatrics.* 2005;116(4):921 926.

Brandt KA, Andrews CM, Kvale J. Mother-infant interaction and breastfeeding outcome 6 weeks after birth. *J Obstet Gynecol Neonatal Nurs.* 1998;27(2):169-174.

Brandtzaeg P. The secretory immunoglobulin system: regulation and biological significance. Focusing on human mammary glands. *Adv Exp Med Biol.* 2002;503:1-16.

Bricker L, Lavender T. Parenteral opioids for labor pain relief: a systematic review. *Am J Obstet Gynecol.* 2002;186(5 suppl nature):S94-S109.

Britton JR, Britton HL, Gronwaldt V. Breastfeeding, sensitivity, and attachment. *Pediatrics.* 2006;118(5):e1436-e1443.

Brooke H, Gibson A, Tappin D, Brown H. Case-control study of sudden infant death syndrome in Scotland, 1992-5. *BMJ.* 1997;314(7093):1516-1520.

Brown KH, Akhtar NA, Robertson AD, Ahmed MG. Lactational capacity of marginally nourished mothers: relationships between maternal nutritional status and quantity and proximate composition of milk. *Pediatrics.* 1986;78(5):909-919.

Brown LP, Bair AH, Meier PP. Does federal funding for breastfeeding research target our national health objectives? *Pediatrics.* 2003;111(4 pt 1):e360-e364.

Brown SJ, Alexander J, Thomas P. Feeding outcome in breast-fed term babies supplemented by cup or bottle. *Midwifery.* 1999;15(2):92-96.

Bumgarner NJ. *Mothering Your Nursing Toddler.* Revised (3rd) ed. Schaumburg, IL: La Leche.

Burgess SW, Dakin CJ, O'Callaghan MJ. Breastfeeding does not increase the risk of asthma at 14 years. *Pediatrics.* 2006;117(4):e787-e792.

Bystrova K, Widstrom AM, Matthiesen AS, et al. Skin-to-skin contact may reduce negative consequences of "the stress of being born": a study on temperature in newborn infants, subjected to different ward routines in St. Petersburg. *Acta Paediatr.* 2003;92(3):320-326.

Cadwell K. *Growing the Breastfeeding Friendly Community.* Weston, MA: National Alliance for Breastfeeding Advocacy; 1996.

Caglar MK, Ozer I, Altugan FS. Risk factors for excess weight loss and hypernatremia in exclusively breast-fed infants. *Braz J Med Biol Res.* 2006;39(4):539-544.

Campos RG. Soothing pain-elicited distress in infants with swaddling and pacifiers. *Child Dev.* 1989;60(4):781-792.

Carbajal R, Veerapen S, Couderc S, Jugie M, Ville Y. Analgesic effect of breast feeding in term neonates: randomised controlled trial. *BMJ.* 2003;326(7379):13.

Carbajal R. Nonpharmacologic management of pain in neonates. *Arch Pediatr.* 2005;12(1):110-116.

Carmichael AR, Dixon JM. Is lactation mastitis and shooting breast pain experienced by women during lactation caused by *Candida albicans*? *Breast.* 2002;11(1):88-90.

Carpenter RG, Irgens LM, Blair PS, et al. Sudden unexplained infant death in 20 regions in Europe: case control study. *Lancet.* 2004;363(9404):185-191.

Casey CE, Neifert MR, Seacat JM, Neville MC. Nutrient intake by breast-fed infants during the first five days after birth. *Am J Dis Child.* 1986;140(9):933-936.

Casiday RE, Wright CM, Panter-Brick C, Parkinson KN. Do early infant feeding patterns relate to breast-feeding continuation and weight gain? Data from a longitudinal cohort study. *Eur J Clin Nutr.* 2004;58(9):1290-1296.

Castelo PM, Gaviao MB, Pereira LJ, Bonjardim LR. Relationship between oral parafunctional/nutritive sucking habits and temporomandibular joint dysfunction in primary dentition. *Int J Paediatr Dent.* 2005;15(1):29-36.

Caton D, Corry MP, Frigoletto FD, et al. The nature and management of labor pain: executive summary. *Am J Obstet Gynecol.* 2002;186(5 suppl nature):S1-S15.

Chamberlain LB, McMahon M, Philipp BL, Merewood A. Breast pump access in the inner city: a hospital-based initiative to provide breast pumps for low-income women. *J Hum Lact.* 2006;22(1):94-98.

Chamberlain LB, Merewood A, Malone KL, Cimo S, Philipp BL. Calls to an inner-city hospital breastfeeding telephone support line. *J Hum Lact.* 2005;21(1):53-58.

Chang ZM, Heaman MI. Epidural analgesia during labor and delivery: effects on the initiation and continuation of effective breastfeeding. *J Hum Lact.* 2005;21(3):305-314; quiz 315-319, 326.

Chantry CJ, Howard CR, Auinger P. Full breastfeeding duration and associated decrease in respiratory tract infection in US children. *Pediatrics.* 2006;117(2):425-432.

Chapman D, Damio G, Young S, Perez-Escamilla R. Association of degree and timing of exposure to breastfeeding peer counseling services with breastfeeding duration. *Adv Exp Med Biol.* 2004;554:303-306.

Chapman DJ, Damio G, Perez-Escamilla R. Differential response to breastfeeding peer counseling within a low-income, predominantly Latina population. *J Hum Lact.* 2004;20(4):389-396.

Chapman DJ, Damio G, Young S, Perez-Escamilla R. Effectiveness of breastfeeding peer counseling in a low-income, predominantly Latina population: a randomized controlled trial. *Arch Pediatr Adolesc Med.* 2004;158(9):897-902.

Chapman DJ, Perez-Escamilla R. Maternal perception of the onset of lactation is a valid, public health indicator of lactogenesis stage II. *J Nutr.* 2000;130(12):2972-2980.

Chapman DJ, Young S, Ferris AM, Perez-Escamilla R. Impact of breast pumping on lactogenesis stage II after cesarean delivery: a randomized clinical trial. *Pediatrics.* 2001;107(6):E94.

Charpak N, Ruiz JG, Zupan J, et al. Kangaroo mother care: 25 years after. *Acta Paediatr.* 2005;94(5):514-522.

Charpak N, Ruiz-Pelaez JG, Figueroa Z. Influence of feeding patterns and other factors on early somatic growth of healthy, preterm infants in home-based kangaroo mother care: a cohort study. *J Pediatr Gastroenterol Nutr.* 2005;41(4):430-437.

Chatterton RT Jr, Hill PD, Aldag JC, Hodges KR, Belknap SM, Zinaman MJ. Relation of plasma oxytocin and prolactin concentrations to milk production in mothers of preterm infants: influence of stress. *J Clin Endocrinol Metab.* 2000;85(10):3661-3668.

Chen A, Rogan WJ. Breastfeeding and the risk of postneonatal death in the United States. *Pediatrics.* 2004;113(5):e435-e439.

Chen CH, Chi CS. Maternal intention and actual behavior in infant feeding at one month postpartum. *Acta Paediatr Taiwan.* 2003;44(3):140-144.

Chen DC, Nommsen-Rivers L, Dewey KG, Lonnerdal B. Stress during labor and delivery and early lactation performance. *Am J Clin Nutr.* 1998;68(2):335-344.

Chiu SH, Anderson GC, Burkhammer MD. Newborn temperature during skin-to-skin breastfeeding in couples having breastfeeding difficulties. *Birth.* 2005;32(2):115-121.

Christensson K, Nilsson BA, Stock S, Matthiesen AS, Uvnas-Moberg K. Effect of nipple stimulation on uterine activity and on plasma levels of oxytocin in full term, healthy, pregnant women. *Acta Obstet Gynecol Scand.* 1989;68(3):205-210.

Christensson K, Siles C, Cabrera T, et al. Lower body temperatures in infants delivered by caesarean section than in vaginally delivered infants. *Acta Paediatr.* 1993;82(2):128-131.

Clifford TJ, Campbell MK, Speechley KN, Gorodzinsky F. Factors influencing full breastfeeding in a southwestern Ontario community: assessments at 1 week and at 6 months postpartum. *J Hum Lact.* 2006;22(3):292-304.

Cotterman KJ. Reverse pressure softening: a simple tool to prepare areola for easier latching during engorgement. *J Hum Lact.* 2004;20(2):227-237.

Coutsoudis A. Breastfeeding and the HIV positive mother: the debate continues. *Early Hum Dev.* 2005;81(1):87-93.

Cregan MD, DeMello TR, Hartmann PE. Pre-term delivery and breast expression: consequences for initiating lactation. *Adv Exp Med Biol.* 2000;478:427-428.

Cregan MD, DeMello TR, Kershaw D, McDougall K, Hartmann PE. Initiation of lactation in women after preterm delivery. *Acta Obstet Gynecol Scand.* 2002;81(9):870-877.

Cregan MD, Hartmann PE. Computerized breast measurement from conception to weaning: clinical implications. *J Hum Lact.* 1999;15(2):89-96.

Cregan MD, Mitoulas LR, Hartmann PE. Milk prolactin, feed volume and duration between feeds in women breastfeeding their full-term infants over a 24 h period. *Exp Physiol.* 2002;87(2):207-214.

Cregan MD, Mitoulas LR, Hartmann PE. Variation in prolactin consumption by fully breastfed infants. *Adv Exp Med Biol.* 2004;554:431-433.

Cristensson K, Siles C, Moreno L, et al. Temperature, metabolic adaptation and crying in healthy full-term newborns cared for skin-to-skin or in a cot. *Acta Pediatr.* 1992;81:488-493.

Crowell MK, Hill PD, Humenick SS. Relationship between obstetric analgesia and time of effective breast feeding. *J Nurse Midwifery.* 1994;39(3):150-156.

Cutler BD, Wright RF. The U.S. infant formula industry: is direct-to-consumer advertising unethical or inevitable? *Health Mark Q.* 2002;19(3):39-55.

da Silva OP, Knoppert DC, Angelini MM, Forret PA. Effect of domperidone on milk production in mothers of premature newborns: a randomized, double-blind, placebo-controlled trial. *CMAJ.* 2001;164(1):17-21.

Dahlgren UI, Hanson LA, Telemo E. Maturation of immunocompetence in breast-fed vs. formula-fed infants. *Adv Nutr Res.* 2001;10:311-325.

Daley HK, Kennedy CM. Meta analysis: effects of interventions on premature infants feeding. *J Perinat Neonatal Nurs.* 2000;14(3):62-77.

Daltveit AK, Irgens LM, Oyen N, Skjaerven R, Markestad T, Wennergren G. Circadian variations in sudden infant death syndrome: associations with maternal smoking, sleeping position and infections—the Nordic epidemiological SIDS study. *Acta Paediatr.* 2003;92(9):1007-1013.

Darzi MA, Chowdri NA, Bhat AN. Breast feeding or spoon feeding after cleft lip repair: a prospective, randomised study. *Br J Plast Surg.* 1996;49(1):24-26.

De Lathouwer S, Lionet C, Lansac J, Body G, Perrotin F. Predictive factors of early cessation of breastfeeding: a prospective study in a university hospital. *Eur J Obstet Gynecol Reprod Biol.* 2004;117(2):169-173.

DeCarvalho M, Robertson S, Merkatz R, Klaus M. Milk intake and frequency of feeding in breast fed infants. *Early Hum Dev.* 1982;7(2):155-163.

Degan VV, Puppin-Rontani RM. Prevalence of pacifier-sucking habits and successful methods to eliminate them—a preliminary study. *J Dent Child (Chic).* 2004;71(2):148-151.

Demerath EW, Schubert CM, Maynard LM, et al. Do changes in body mass index percentile reflect changes in body composition in children? Data from the Fels longitudinal study. *Pediatrics.* 2006;117(3):e487-e495.

Demissie K, Rhoads GG, Smulian JC, et al. Operative vaginal delivery and neonatal and infant adverse outcomes: population based retrospective analysis. *BMJ.* 2004;329(7456):24-29.

Dennis CL, Hodnett E, Gallop R, Chalmers B. The effect of peer support on breast-feeding duration among primiparous women: a randomized controlled trial. *CMAJ.* 2002;166(1):21-28.

Dewey KG, Nommsen-Rivers LA, Heinig MJ, Cohen RJ. Risk factors for suboptimal infant breast-feeding behavior, delayed onset of lactation, and excess neonatal weight loss. *Pediatrics.* 2003;112(3 pt 1):607-619.

Dewey KG. Maternal and fetal stress are associated with impaired lactogenesis in humans. *J Nutr.* 2001;131(11):3012S-3015S.

Di Daniele N, Carbonelli MG, Candeloro N, Iacopino L, De Lorenzo A, Andreoli A. Effect of supplementation of calcium and vitamin D on bone mineral density and bone mineral content in peri- and post-menopause women; a double-blind, randomized, controlled trial. *Pharmacol Res.* 2004;50(6):637-641.

DiGirolamo A, Thompson N, Martorell R, Fein S, Grummer-Strawn L. Intention or experience? Predictors of continued breastfeeding. *Health Educ Behav.* 2005;32(2):208-226.

DiGirolamo AM, Grummer-Strawn LM, Fein S. Maternity care practices: implications for breastfeeding. *Birth.* 2001;28(2):94-100.

DiGirolamo AM, Grummer-Strawn LM, Fein SB. Do perceived attitudes of physicians and hospital staff affect breastfeeding decisions? *Birth.* 2003;30(2):94-100.

Dodd V, Chalmers C. Comparing the use of hydrogel dressings to lanolin ointment with lactating mothers. *J Obstet Gynecol Neonatal Nurs.* 2003;32(4):486-494.

Dodd VL. Implications of kangaroo care for growth and development in preterm infants. *J Obstet Gynecol Neonatal Nurs.* 2005;34(2):218-232.

Dollberg S, Lahav S, Mimouni FB. A comparison of intakes of breast-fed and bottle-fed infants during the first two days of life. *J Am Coll Nutr.* 2001;20(3):209-211.

Dombrowski MA, Anderson GC, Santori C, Roller CG, Pagliotti F, Dowling DA. Kangaroo skin-to-skin care for premature twins and their adolescent parents. *MCN Am J Matern Child Nurs.* 2000;25(2):92-94.

Donath SM, Amir LH. Relationship between prenatal infant feeding intention and initiation and duration of breastfeeding: a cohort study. *Acta Paediatr.* 2003;92(3):352-356.

Donovan SM. Role of human milk components in gastrointestinal development: Current knowledge and future needs. *J Pediatr.* 2006;149(3 Suppl):S49-61.

Donovan W, Leavitt L, Taylor N. Maternal self-efficacy and experimentally manipulated infant difficulty effects on maternal sensory sensitivity: a signal detection analysis. *Dev Psychol.* 2005;41(5):784-798.

Dorosko SM. Vitamin A, mastitis, and mother-to-child transmission of HIV-1 through breast-feeding: current information and gaps in knowledge. *Nutr Rev.* 2005;63(10):332-346.

Dowling DA, Madigan E, Siripul P. The effect of fluid density and volume on the accuracy of test weighing in a simulated oral feeding situation. *Adv Neonatal Care.* 2004;4(3):158-165.

Dowling DA, Meier PP, DiFiore JM, Blatz M, Martin RJ. Cup-feeding for preterm infants: mechanics and safety. *J Hum Lact.* 2002;18(1):13-20; quiz 46-49, 72.

Downs FS. *Handbook of Research Methodology.* New York: American Journal of Nursing Company; 1988.

Drudy D, Mullane NR, Quinn T, Wall PG, Fanning S. *Enterobacter sakazakii:* an emerging pathogen in powdered infant formula. *Clin Infect Dis.* 2006;42(7):996-1002.

Dubois L, Girard M. Social determinants of initiation, duration and exclusivity of breastfeeding at the population level: the results of the Longitudinal Study of Child Development in Quebec (ELDEQ 1998-2002). *Can J Public Health.* 2003;94(4):300-305.

Duncan LL, Elder SB. Breastfeeding the infant with PKU. *J Hum Lact.* 1997;13:231-235.

Dundar NO, Anal O, Dundar B, Ozkan H, Caliskan S, Buyukgebiz A. Longitudinal investigation of the relationship between breast milk leptin levels and growth in breast-fed infants. *J Pediatr Endocrinol Metab.* 2005;18(2):181-187.

Dyson L, McCormick F, Renfrew MJ. Interventions for promoting the initiation of breastfeeding. *Cochrane Database Syst Rev.* 2005(2):CD001688.

Edhborg M, Matthiesen AS, Lundh W, Widstrom AM. Some early indicators for depressive symptoms and bonding 2 months postpartum—a study of new mothers and fathers. *Arch Women Ment Health.* 2005;8(4):221-231.

Edmond KM, Zandoh C, Quigley MA, Amenga-Etego S, Owusu-Agyei S, Kirkwood BR. Delayed breastfeeding initiation increases risk of neonatal mortality. *Pediatrics.* 2006;117(3):e380-e386.

Eidelman AI. The Talmud and human lactation: the cultural basis for increased frequency and duration of breastfeeding among orthodox Jewish women. *Breastfeeding Med.* 2006;1(1):36-40.

Eidelman, Al, Hoffmann NW, Kaitz M. Cognitive deficits in women after childbirth. *Obstet Gynecol.* 1993;81:764-767.

Ekstrom A, Matthiesen AS, Widstrom AM, Nissen E. Breastfeeding attitudes among counselling health professionals. *Scand J Public Health.* 2005;33(5):353-359.

Ekstrom A, Nissen E. A mother's feelings for her infant are strengthened by excellent breastfeeding counseling and continuity of care. *Pediatrics.* 2006;118(2):e309-e314.

Elias MF, Nicolson NA, Bora C, Johnston J. Sleep/wake patterns of breast-fed infants in the first 2 years of life. *Pediatrics.* 1986;77:322-329.

Ellis MH, Short JA, Heiner DC. Anaphylaxis after ingestion of a recently introduced hydrolyzed whey protein formula. *J Pediatr.* 1991;118:74-77.

Emanuel EJ, Emanuel LL. Four models of the physician-patient relationship. *JAMA.* 1992;267(16):2221-2226.

Emond AM, Drewett RF, Blair PS, Emmett PM. Postnatal factors associated with failure to thrive in term infants in the Avon Longitudinal Study of Parents and Children. *Arch Dis Child.* 2006.

England L, Brenner R, Bhaskar B, et al. Breastfeeding practices in a cohort of inner-city women: the role of contraindications. *BMC Public Health.* 2003;3:28.

Epperson CN, Jatlow PI, Czarkowski K, Anderson GM. Maternal fluoxetine treatment in the postpartum period: effects on platelet serotonin and plasma drug levels in breastfeeding mother-infant pairs. *Pediatrics.* 2003;112(5):e425.

Escobar GJ, Braveman PA, Ackerson L, et al. A randomized comparison of home visits and hospital-based group follow-up visits after early postpartum discharge. *Pediatrics.* 2001;108(3):719-727.

Faerk J, Skafte L, Petersen S, Peitersen B, Michaelsen KF. Macronutrients in milk from mothers delivering preterm. *Adv Exp Med Biol.* 2001;501:409-413.

Fairbank L, O'Meara S, Renfrew MJ, Woolridge M, Sowden AJ, Lister-Sharp D. A systematic review to evaluate the effectiveness of interventions to promote the initiation of breastfeeding. *Health Technol Assess.* 2000;4(25):1-171.

Fairbank L, O'Meara S, Sowden AJ, Renfrew MJ, Woolridge MM. Promoting the initiation of breast feeding. *Qual Health Care.* 2001;10(2):123-127.

Falceto OG, Giugliani ERJ, Fernandes CLC. Couples' relationships and breastfeeding: is there an Association? *J Hum Lact.* 2004;20(1):46-55.

Fetherston C. Mastitis in lactating women: physiology or pathology? *Breastfeed Rev.* 2001;9(1):5-12.

Fetherston C. Risk factors for lactation mastitis. *J Hum Lact.* 1998;14(2):101-109.

Fetherston CM, Lai CT, Mitoulas LR, Hartmann PE. Excretion of lactose in urine as a measure of increased permeability of the lactating breast during inflammation. *Acta Obstet Gynecol Scand.* 2006;85(1):20-25.

Fetherston CM, Lee CS, Hartmann PE. Mammary gland defense: the role of colostrum, milk and involution secretion. *Adv Nutr Res.* 2001;10:167-198.

Fewtrell M, Lucas P, Collier S, Lucas A. Randomized study comparing the efficacy of a novel manual breast pump with a mini-electric breast pump in mothers of term infants. *J Hum Lact.* 2001;17(2):126-131.

Fewtrell MS, Lucas P, Collier S, Singhal A, Ahluwalia JS, Lucas A. Randomized trial comparing the efficacy of a novel manual breast pump with a standard electric breast pump in mothers who delivered preterm infants. *Pediatrics.* 2001;107(6):1291-1297.

Fidler N, Sauerwald TU, Demmelmair H, Koletzko B. Fat content and fatty acid composition of fresh, pasteurized, or sterilized human milk. *Adv Exp Med Biol.* 2001;501:485-495.

Fildes V. *Breasts, Bottles and Babies: A History of Infant Feeding.* Edinburgh, Scotland: Edinburgh University Press; 1986.

Fildes V. *Wet Nursing: A History from Antiquity to the Present.* New York: Basil Blackwell; 1988.

Filteau S. The influence of mastitis on antibody transfer to infants through breast milk. *Vaccine.* 2003;21(24):3377-3781.

Fisler RE, Cohen A, Ringer SA, Lieberman E. Neonatal outcome after trial of labor compared with elective repeat cesarean section. *Birth.* 2003;30(2):83-88.

Fituch CC, Palkowetz KH, Goldman AS, Schanler RJ. Concentrations of IL-10 in preterm human milk and in milk from mothers of infants with necrotizing enterocolitis. *Acta Paediatr.* 2004;93(11):1496-1500.

Flacking R, Ewald U, Nyqvist KH, Starrin B. Trustful bonds: a key to "becoming a mother" and to reciprocal breastfeeding. Stories of mothers of very preterm infants at a neonatal unit. *Soc Sci Med.* 2006;62(1):70-80.

Fleming P, Tsogt B, Blair PS. Modifiable risk factors, sleep environment, developmental physiology and common polymorphisms: Understanding and preventing sudden infant deaths. *Early Hum Dev.* 2006;82(12):761-766.

Fleming PJ, Blair PS, Bacon C, et al. Environment of infants during sleep and risk of the sudden infant death syndrome: results of 1993-5 case-control study for confidential inquiry into stillbirths and deaths in infancy—confidential enquiry into stillbirths and deaths regional coordinators and researchers. *BMJ.* 1996;313(7051):191-195.

Fleming PJ, Blair PS, Pollard K, et al. Pacifier use and sudden infant death syndrome: results from the CESDI/SUDI case control study. *Arch Dis Child.* 1999;81(2):112-116.

Fleming PJ, Blair PS, Ward Platt M, Tripp J, Smith IJ. Sudden infant death syndrome and social deprivation: assessing epidemiological factors after post-matching for deprivation. *Paediatr Perinat Epidemiol.* 2003;17(3):272-280.

Fleming PJ, Blair PS. How reliable are SIDS rates? The importance of a standardised, multiprofessional approach to "diagnosis." *Arch Dis Child.* 2005;90(10):993-994.

Fleming PJ, Blair PS. Sudden unexpected deaths after discharge from the neonatal intensive care unit. *Semin Neonatol.* 2003;8(2):159-167.

Flores M, Filteau S. Effect of lactation counselling on subclinical mastitis among Bangladeshi women. *Ann Trop Paediatr.* 2002;22(1):85-88.

Francis-Morrill J, Heinig MJ, Pappagianis D, Dewey KG. Diagnostic value of signs and symptoms of mammary candidosis among lactating women. *J Hum Lact.* 2004;20(3):288-295; quiz 296-299.

Franco P, Seret N, Van Hees J-N, Scaillet S, Groswasser J, Kahn A. Influence of swaddling on sleep and arousal characteristics of healthy infants. *Pediatrics.* 2005;115(5):1307-1311.

Frank-Stromberg M, Olsen SJ. *Instruments for Clinical Health-Care Research.* 2nd ed. Sudbury, MA: Jones & Bartlett Publishers; 1997.

Fransson AL, Karlsson H, Nilsson K. Temperature variation in newborn babies: importance of physical contact with the mother. *Arch Dis Child Fetal Neonatal Ed.* 2005;90(6):F500-F504.

Frantz K. *Breastfeeding Product Guide.* Sunland, CA: Geddes Productions; 1994.

Fraval MMPR. A pilot study: osteopathic treatment of infants with a sucking dysfunction. *AAO J.* 1998;8(2):25-33.

Fredrickson D. Breastfeeding study design problems—health policy, epidemiologic and pediatric perspectives. In: Stuart-Macadam P, Dettwyler KA. *Breastfeeding: Biocultural Perspectives.* New York: Aldine De Gruyter; 1995.

Friedman NJ, Zeiger RS. The role of breast-feeding in the development of allergies and asthma. *J Allergy Clin Immunol.* 2005;115(6):1238-1248.

Frolich MA, Burchfield DJ, Euliano TY, Caton D. A single dose of fentanyl and midazolam prior to Cesarean section has no adverse neontal effects [In French]. *Can J Anaesth.* 2006;53(1):79-85.

Fujita M, Endoh Y, Saimon N, Yamaguchi S. Effect of massaging babies on mothers: pilot study on the changes in mood states and salivary cortisol level. *Complement Ther Clin Pract* 2006;12(3):181-185.

Furman L, Kennell J. Breastmilk and skin-to-skin kangaroo care for premature infants. Avoiding bonding failure. *Acta Paediatr.* 2000;89(11):1280-1283.

Furman L, Minich N, Hack M. Correlates of lactation in mothers of very low birth weight infants. *Pediatrics.* 2002;109(4):e57.

Furman L, Minich N. Efficiency of breastfeeding as compared to bottle-feeding in very low birth weight (VLBW < 1.5 kg) infants. *J Perinatol.* 2004;24(11):706-713.

Furman L, Wilson-Costello D, Friedman H, Taylor HG, Minich N, Hack M. The effect of neonatal maternal milk feeding on the neurodevelopmental outcome of very low birth weight infants. *J Dev Behav Pediatr.* 2004;25(4):247-253.

Gale Mobbs EJ. Human imprinting and breastfeeding—are the textbooks deficient? *Breastfeed Rev.* 1989;1(14):39-41.

Gartner LM, Morton J, Lawrence RA, et al. Breastfeeding and the use of human milk. *Pediatrics.* 2005;115(2):496-506.

Gerrard JA, Chudasama G. Screening to reduce HIV transmission from mother to baby. *Nurs Times.* 2003;99(35):44-45.

Goer H. *Obstetric Myths versus Research Realities: A Guide to the Medical Literature.* Westport, CT: Bergin & Garvey; 1995.

Goetzl L, Cohen A, Frigoletto F Jr, Ringer SA, Lang JM, Lieberman E. Maternal epidural use and neonatal sepsis evaluation in afebrile mothers. *Pediatrics.* 2001;108(5):1099-1102.

Goetzl L, Rivers J, Evans T, et al. Prophylactic acetaminophen does not prevent epidural fever in nulliparous women: a double-blind placebo-controlled trial. *J Perinatol.* 2004;24(8):471-475.

Goldfield EC, Richardson MJ, Lee KG, Margetts S. Coordination of sucking, swallowing, and breathing and oxygen saturation during early infant breast-feeding and bottle-feeding. *Pediatr Res.* 2006;60(4):450-455.

Goldman AS. The immunological system in human milk: the past—a pathway to the future. *Adv Nutr Res.* 2001;10:15-37.

Gorbe E, Kohalmi B, Gaal G, et al. The relationship between pacifier use, bottle feeding and breast feeding. *J Matern Fetal Neonatal Med.* 2002;12(2):127-131.

Grajeda R, Perez-Escamilla R. Stress during labor and delivery is associated with delayed onset of lactation among urban Guatemalan women. *J Nutr.* 2002;132(10):3055-3060.

Gravetter FJ, Wallnau LB. *Statistics for the Behavioral Sciences.* 3rd ed. St. Paul, MN: West Publishing; 1992.

Gray L, Miller LW, Philipp BL, Blass EM. Breastfeeding is analgesic in healthy newborns. *Pediatrics.* 2002;109(4):590-593.

Gray L, Watt L, Blass EM. Skin-to-skin contact is analgesic in healthy newborns. *Pediatrics.* 2000;105(1):e14.

Gray RH, Campbell OM, Apelo R, et al. Risk of ovulation during lactation. *Lancet.* 1990;335(8680):25-29.

Greenhalgh T. How to read a paper: assessing the methodological quality of published papers. *Br Med J.* 1997;315:305.

Greenhalgh T. How to read a paper: getting your bearing (deciding what the paper is about). *Br Med J.* 1997;315:243.

Greenhalgh T. How to read a paper: papers that go beyond numbers (qualitative research). *Br Med J.* 1997;315:740.

Greenhalgh T. How to read a paper: papers that summarize other papers (systematic reviews and meta-analyses). *Br Med J.* 1997;315:672.

Greenhalgh T. How to read a paper: statistics for the non-statistician II: significant relationships and their pitfalls. *Br Med J.* 1997;315:422.

Greenhalgh T. How to read a paper: the Medline database. *Br Med J.* 1997;315:180.

Greve LC, Wheeler MD, Green-Burgeson DK, Zorn EM. Breastfeeding in the management of the newborn with phenylketonuria: a practical approach to dietary therapy. *J Am Diet Assoc.* 1994;94:305-309.

Griffiths DM. Do tongue ties affect breastfeeding? *J Hum Lact.* 2004;20(4):409-414.

Griffiths RJ. Breast pads: their effectiveness and use by lactating women. *J Hum Lact.* 1993;9(1):19-26.

Groer M, Davis M, Casey K, Short B, Smith K, Groer S. Neuroendocrine and immune relationships in postpartum fatigue. *MCN Am J Matern Child Nurs.* 2005;30(2):133-138.

Groer M, Davis M, Steele K. Associations between human milk SIgA and maternal immune, infectious, endocrine, and stress variables. *J Hum Lact.* 2004;20(2):153-158; quiz 159-163.

Groer MW, Davis MW, Hemphill J. Postpartum stress: current concepts and the possible protective role of breastfeeding. *J Obstet Gynecol Neonatal Nurs.* 2002;31(4):411-417.

Groer MW, Davis MW. Cytokines, infections, stress, and dysphoric moods in breastfeeders and formula feeders. *J Obstet Gynecol Neonatal Nurs.* 2006;35(5):599-607.

Groer MW. Differences between exclusive breastfeeders, formula-feeders, and controls: a study of stress, mood, and endocrine variables. *Biol Res Nurs.* 2005;7(2):106-117.

Gromada KK, Spangler AK. Breastfeeding twins and higher-order multiples. *JOGNN.* 1998;27:441-449.

Gromada KK. Breastfeeding more than one: multiples and tandem breast-feeding. *NAACOG's (AWHONN's) Clin Issues Perina Women's Health Nurs.* 1992;3:656-666.

Gromada KK. Maternal-infants attachment: The first step toward individualizing twins. *MCN.* 1981;6:129-134.

Gromada KK. *Mothering Multiples: Breastfeeding and Care for Twins or More!* 2nd ed. Schaumburg, IL: La Leche League International; 1999.

Grummer-Strawn LM, Mei Z. Does breastfeeding protect against pediatric overweight? Analysis of longitudinal data from the Centers for Disease Control and Prevention pediatric nutrition surveillance system. *Pediatrics.* 2004;113(2):e81-e86.

Guillette EA, Conard C, Lares F, Aguilar MG, McLachlan J, Guillette LJ Jr. Altered breast development in young girls from an agricultural environment. *Environ Health Perspect.* 2006;114(3):471-475.

Haas DM, Howard CS, Christopher M, Rowan K, Broga MC, Corey T. Assessment of breastfeeding practices and reasons for success in a military community hospital. *J Hum Lact.* 2006;22(4):439-445.

Haider R, Ashworth A, Kabir I, Huttly SR. Effect of community-based peer counsellors on exclusive breastfeeding practices in Dhaka, Bangladesh: a randomised controlled trial [see commments]. *Lancet.* 2000;356(9242):1643-1647.

Haider R, Kabir I, Huttly SR, Ashworth A. Training peer counselors to promote and support exclusive breastfeeding in Bangladesh. *J Hum Lact.* 2002;18(1):7-12.

Haisma H, Coward WA, Albernaz E, et al. Breast milk and energy intake in exclusively, predominantly, and partially breast-fed infants. *Eur J Clin Nutr.* 2003;57(12):1633-1642.

Hale TW. Maternal medications during breastfeeding. *Clin Obstet Gynecol.* 2004;47(3):696-711.

Hale TW. *Medications and Mothers' Milk 2006.* Amarillo, TX: Hale Publishing, 2006.

Hale TW. Medications in breastfeeding mothers of preterm infants. *Pediatr Ann.* 2003;32(5):337-347.

Halken S. Prevention of allergic disease in childhood: clinical and epidemiological aspects of primary and secondary allergy prevention. *Pediatr Allergy Immunol.* 2004;15(suppl 16):4-5, 9-32.

Hall DM, Renfrew MJ. Tongue tie. *Arch Dis Child.* 2005;90(12):1211-1215.

Halpern SH, Ioscovich A. Epidural analgesia and breast-feeding. *Anesthesiology.* 2005;103(6):1111-1112.

Hansen WF, McAndrew S, Harris K, Zimmerman MB. Metoclopramide effect on breastfeeding the preterm infant: a randomized trial. *Obstet Gynecol.* 2005;105(2):383-389.

Hanson LA, Ceafalau L, Mattsby-Baltzer I, et al. The mammary gland–infant intestine immunologic dyad. *Adv Exp Med Biol.* 2000;478:65-76.

Hanson LA, Korotkova M, Haversen L, et al. Breast-feeding, a complex support system for the offspring. *Pediatr Int.* 2002;44(4):347-352.

Hanson LA, Korotkova M, Lundin S, et al. The transfer of immunity from mother to child. *Ann N Y Acad Sci.* 2003;987:199-206.

Hanson LA, Korotkova M, Telemo E. Breast-feeding, infant formulas, and the immune system. *Ann Allergy Asthma Immunol.* 2003;90(6 suppl 3):59-63.

Hanson LA, Korotkova M. The role of breastfeeding in prevention of neonatal infection. *Semin Neonatol.* 2002;7(4):275-281.

Hanson LA, Silfverdal SA, Korotkova M, et al. Immune system modulation by human milk. *Adv Exp Med Biol.* 2002;503:99-106.

Hanson LA. *Immunobiology of Human Milk: How Breastfeeding Protects Babies.* Amarillo, TX: Pharmasoft Publishing; 2004.

Hanson LA. Protective effects of breastfeeding against urinary tract infection. *Acta Paediatr.* 2004;93(2):154-156.

Hanson LA. The mother–offspring dyad and the immune system. *Acta Paediatr.* 2000;89(3):252-258.

Harder T, Bergmann R, Kallischnigg G, Plagemann A. Duration of breastfeeding and risk of overweight: a meta-analysis. *Am J Epidemiol.* 2005;162(5):397-403.

Harner HM, McCarter-Spaulding D. Teenage mothers and breastfeeding: does paternal age make a difference? *J Hum Lact.* 2004;20(4):404-408.

Harrison Y. The relationship between daytime exposure to light and night-time sleep in 6-12-week-old infants. *J Sleep Res.* 2004;13(4):345-352.

Hartlaub PP, Wolkenstein AS, Laufenburg HF. Obtaining informed consent: it is not simply asking "do you understand?" *J Fam Pract.* 1993;36(4):383-384.

Hartmann K, Viswanathan M, Palmieri R, Gartlehner G, Thorp J Jr, Lohr KN. Outcomes of routine episiotomy: a systematic review. *JAMA.* 2005;293(17):2141-2148.

Hartmann P, Cregan M. Lactogenesis and the effects of insulin-dependent diabetes mellitus and prematurity. *J Nutr.* 2001;131(11):3016S-3020S.

Hartmann PE, Cregan MD, Ramsay DT, Simmer K, Kent JC. Physiology of lactation in preterm mothers: initiation and maintenance. *Pediatr Ann.* 2003;32(5):351-355.

Hartmann PE, Kulski JK. Changes in the composition of the mammary secretion of women after abrupt termination of breastfeeding. *J Physiol (Lond).* 1977;74:509-510.

Hartmann SU, Berlin CM, Howett MK. Alternative modified infant-feeding practices to prevent postnatal transmission of human immunodeficiency virus type 1 through breast milk: past, present, and future. *J Hum Lact.* 2006;22(1):75-88; quiz 89-93.

Hartmann SU, Berlin CM, Howett MK. Response to heat treating breast milk as an infant feeding option. *J Hum Lact.* 2006;22(3):268.

Hashira S, Okitsu-Negishi S, Yoshino K. Interleukin 8 in the human colostrum. *Biol Neonate.* 2002;82(1):34-38.

Hassett P. Taking on racial and ethnic disparities in health care: the experience at Aetna. *Health Aff (Millwood).* 2005;24(2):417-420.

Hattevig G, Kjellman B, Sigurs N, Bjorksten B, Kjellman NI. Effect of maternal avoidance of eggs, cow's milk and fish during lactation upon allergic manifestations in infants. *Clin Exp Allergy.* 1989;19(1):27-32.

Hauck FR, Moore CM, Herman SM, et al. The contribution of prone sleeping position to the racial disparity in sudden infant death syndrome: the Chicago Infant Mortality Study. *Pediatrics.* 2002;110(4):772-780.

Heck KE, Schoendorf KC, Chavez GF, Braveman P. Does postpartum length of stay affect breastfeeding duration? A population-based study. *Birth.* 2003;30(3):153-159.

Hediger ML, Overpeck MD, Kuczmarski RJ, Ruan WJ. Association between infant breastfeeding and overweight in young children. *JAMA.* 2001;285(19):2453-2460.

Heinig MJ, Francis J, Pappagianis D. Mammary candidosis in lactating women. *J Hum Lact.* 1999;15(4):281-288.

Heinig MJ. Closet consulting and other enabling behaviors [editor's note]. *J Hum Lact.* 1998;14(4):281-282.

Henderson JJ, Dickinson JE, Evans SF, McDonald SJ, Paech MJ. Impact of intrapartum epidural analgesia on breast-feeding duration. *Aust N Z J Obstet Gynaecol.* 2003;43(5):372-377.

Hill DJ, Roy N, Heine RG, et al. Effect of a low-allergen maternal diet on colic among breastfed infants: a randomized, controlled trial. *Pediatrics.* 2005;116(5):e709-e715.

Hill PD, Aldag JC, Chatterton RT, Zinaman M. Psychological distress and milk volume in lactating mothers. *West J Nurs Res.* 2005;27(6):676-693.

Hill PD, Aldag JC, Demirtas H, Zinaman M, Chatterton RT. Mood states and milk output in lactating mothers of preterm and term infants. *J Hum Lact.* 2006;22(3):305-314.

Hill PD, Aldag JC. Milk volume on day 4 and income predictive of lactation adequacy at 6 weeks of mothers of nonnursing preterm infants. *J Perinat Neonatal Nurs.* 2005;19(3):273-282.

Hill PD, Hanson KS, Mefford AL. Mothers of low birthweight infants: breastfeeding patterns and problems. *J Hum Lact.* 1994;10:169-176.

Hill PD, Humenick S. The occurrence of breast engorgement. *J Hum Lact.* 1994;10(2):79-86.

Hillis SD, Anda RF, Dube SR, Felitti VJ, Marchbanks PA, Marks JS. The association between adverse childhood experiences and adolescent pregnancy, long-term psychosocial consequences, and fetal death. *Pediatrics.* 2004;113(2):320-327.

Hogan M, Westcott C, Griffiths M. Randomized, controlled trial of division of tongue-tie in infants with feeding problems. *J Paediatr Child Health.* 2005;41(5-6):246-250.

Holiday KE, Allen JR, Waters DL, Gruca MA, Thompson SM, Gaskin KJ. Growth of human milk-fed and formula fed infants with cystic fibrosis. *J Pediatr Gastroenterol Nutr.* 1991;118:77-79.

Hollis BW, Wagner CL. Assessment of dietary vitamin D requirements during pregnancy and lactation. *Am J Clin Nutr.* 2004;79(5):717-726.

Hollis BW, Wagner CL. Vitamin D requirements during lactation: high-dose maternal supplementation as therapy to prevent hypovitaminosis D for both the mother and the nursing infant. *Am J Clin Nutr.* 2004;80(6):1752S-1758S.

Hollis BW. Circulating 25-hydroxyvitamin D levels indicative of vitamin D sufficiency: implications for establishing a new effective dietary intake recommendation for vitamin D. *J Nutr.* 2005;135(2):317-322.

Holmes W, Phillips J, Thorpe L. Initiation rate and duration of breast-feeding in the Melbourne aboriginal community. *Aust N Z J Public Health.* 1997;21(5):500-503.

Holmes W, Thorpe L, Phillips J. Influences on infant-feeding beliefs and practices in an urban aboriginal community. *Aust N Z J Public Health.* 1997;21(5):504-510.

Hooker E, Ball HL, Kelly PJ. Sleeping like a baby: attitudes and experiences of bedsharing in northeast England. *Med Anthropol.* 2001;19(3):203-222.

Hoppe C, Molgaard C, Vaag A, Barkholt V, Michaelsen KF. High intakes of milk, but not meat, increase s-insulin and insulin resistance in 8-year-old boys. *Eur J Clin Nutr.* 2005;59(3):393-398.

Howard C, Howard F, Lawrence R, Andresen E, DeBlieck E, Weitzman M. Office prenatal formula advertising and its effect on breast-feeding patterns. *Obstet Gynecol.* 2000;95(2):296-303.

Howard CR, Howard FM, Lanphear B, deBlieck EA, Eberly S, Lawrence RA. The effects of early pacifier use on breastfeeding duration. *Pediatrics.* 1999;103(3):E33.

Howard CR, Howard FM, Lanphear B, et al. Randomized clinical trial of pacifier use and bottle-feeding or cupfeeding and their effect on breastfeeding. *Pediatrics.* 2003;111(3):511-518.

Howard CR, Howard FM. Management of breastfeeding when the mother is ill. *Clin Obstet Gynecol.* 2004;47(3):683-695.

Howard L, Webb R, Abel K. Safety of antipsychotic drugs for pregnant and breastfeeding women with non-affective psychosis. *BMJ.* 2004;329(7472):933-934.

Howie PW, Forsyth JS, Ogston SA, Clark A, Florey CD. Protective effect of breast feeding against infection. *BMJ.* 1990;300(6716):11-16.

Hunziker UA, Barr RG. Increased carrying reduces infant crying: a randomized controlled trial. *Pediatrics.* 1986;77:641-648.

Hurst NM, Meier PP, Engstrom JL, Myatt A. Mothers performing in-home measurement of milk intake during breastfeeding of their preterm infants: maternal reactions and feeding outcomes. *J Hum Lact.* 2004;20(2):178-187.

Ibe OE, Austin T, Sullivan K, Fabanwo O, Disu E, Costello AM. A comparison of kangaroo mother care and conventional incubator care for thermal regulation of infants < 2000 g in Nigeria using continuous ambulatory temperature monitoring. *Ann Trop Paediatr.* 2004;24(3):245-251.

Ilett KF, Hale TW, Page-Sharp M, Kristensen JH, Kohan R, Hackett LP. Use of nicotine patches in breast-feeding mothers: transfer of nicotine and cotinine into human milk. *Clin Pharmacol Ther.* 2003;74(6):516-524.

Ingram J, Johnson D, Greenwood R. Breastfeeding in Bristol: teaching good positioning, and support from fathers and families. *Midwifery.* 2002;18(2):87-101.

Ingram J, Woolridge M, Greenwood R. Breastfeeding: it is worth trying with the second baby. *Lancet.* 2001;358(9286):986-987.

Innocenti Declaration on the Protection, Promotion, and Support of Breastfeeding. Florence, Italy: 1990; revised 2005.

Institute of Medicine (Subcommittee on Nutrition During Lactation, Food and Nutrition Board). *Nutrition During Lactation.* Washington, DC: National Academy of Sciences; 1991.

Institute of Medicine. *Nutrition During Pregnancy.* Washington, DC: National Academy of Sciences; 1991.

International Code of Marketing of Breast-Milk Substitutes. Geneva, Switzerland: World Health Organization; 1981.

Jarjou LM, Prentice A, Sawo Y, et al. Randomized, placebo-controlled, calcium supplementation study in pregnant Gambian women: effects on breast-milk calcium concentrations and infant birth weight, growth, and bone mineral accretion in the first year of life. *Am J Clin Nutr.* 2006;83(3):657-666.

Jarvinen KM, Laine ST, Jarvenpaa AL, Suomalainen HK. Does low IgA in human milk predispose the infant to development of cow's milk allergy? *Pediatr Res.* 2000;48(4):457-462.

Jensen RG. *Handbook of Milk Composition.* San Diego: Academic Press; 1995.

Johnson AN. Kangaroo holding beyond the NICU. *Pediatr Nurs.* 2005;31(1):53-56.

Jones E, Dimmock PW, Spencer SA. A randomised controlled trial to compare methods of milk expression after preterm delivery. *Arch Dis Child Fetal Neonatal Ed.* 2001;85(2):F91-F95.

Jones TF, Ingram LA, Fullerton KE, Marcus R, Anderson BJ, McCarthy PV, et al. A case-control study of the epidemiology of sporadic salmonella infection in infants, 2006:2380-2387.

Jordan S, Emery S, Bradshaw C, Watkins A, Friswell W. The impact of intrapartum analgesia on infant feeding. *BJOG.* 2005;112(7):927-934.

Kadam S, Binoy S, Kanbur W, Mondkar JA, Fernandez A. Feasibility of kangaroo mother care in Mumbai. *Indian J Pediatr.* 2005;72(1):35-38.

Kahn A, Mozin MJ, Rebuffat E, et al. Milk intolerance in children with persistent sleeplessness: a prospective double-blind crossover evaluation. *Pediatrics.* 1989;84(4):595-602.

Kahn B, Lumey LH, Zybert PA, et al. Prospective risk of fetal death in singleton, twin, and triplet gestations: implications for practice. *Obstet Gynecol.* 2003;102(4):685-692.

Kassing D. Bottle-feeding as a tool to reinforce breastfeeding. *J Hum Lact.* 2002;18(1):56-60.

Kawada M, Okuzumi K, Hitomi S, Sugishita C. Transmission of *Staphylococcus aureus* between healthy, lactating mothers and their infants by breastfeeding. *J Hum Lact.* 2003;19(4):411-417.

Kendall-Tackett KA, Sugarman M. The social consequences of long-term breastfeeding. *J Hum Lact.* 1995;11(3):179-183.

Kendall-Tackett KA. *Depression in New Mothers: Causes, Consequences and Treatment Alternatives.* Binghamton, NY: Haworth Press; 2005.

Kendall-Tackett KA. *Handbook of Women, Stress and Trauma.* New York: Brunner-Routledge/Taylor & Francis Group; 2005.

Kennell J, Klaus M, McGrath S, Robertson S, Hinkley C. Continuous emotional support during labor in a U.S. hospital: a randomized controlled trial. *JAMA.* 1991;265(17):2197-2201.

Kennell JH. Randomized controlled trial of skin-to-skin contact from birth versus conventional incubator for physiological stabilization in 1200 g to 2199 g newborns. *Acta Paediatr.* 2006;95(1):15-16.

Kent JC, Mitoulas LR, Cregan MD, Ramsay DT, Doherty DA, Hartmann PE. Volume and frequency of breastfeedings and fat content of breast milk throughout the day. *Pediatrics.* 2006;117(3):e387-e395.

Kent JC, Ramsay DT, Doherty D, Larsson M, Hartmann PE. Response of breasts to different stimulation patterns of an electric breast pump. *J Hum Lact.* 2003;19(2):179-186; quiz 87-88, 218.

Kirsten GF, Bergman NJ, Hann FM. Kangaroo mother care in the nursery. *Pediatr Clin North Am.* 2001;48(2):443-452.

Kitzinger S. *Women as Mothers: How They See Themselves in Different Cultures.* New York: Vintage Books; 1978.

Klaus MH, Kennell JH, Klaus PH. *Bonding: Building the Foundations of Secure Attachment and Independence.* St. Louis: Mosby; 1995.

Kleinman RE, ed. *Pediatric Nutrition Handbook.* 5th ed. Elk Grove Village, IL: American Academy of Pediatrics; 2003.

Koletzko B, Shamir R. Standards for infant formula milk. *BMJ.* 2006;332(7542):621-622.

Koletzko B. Long-term consequences of early feeding on later obesity risk. *Nestle Nutr Workshop Ser Pediatr Program.* 2006(58):1-18.

Kramer MS, Barr RG, Dagenais S, et al. Pacifier use, early weaning, and cry/fuss behavior: a randomized controlled trial. *JAMA.* 2001;286(3):322-326.

Kramer MS, Chalmers B, Hodnett ED, et al. Promotion of breastfeeding intervention trial (PROBIT): a randomized trial in the Republic of Belarus. *JAMA.* 2001;285(4):413-420.

Kramer MS, Chalmers B, Hodnett ED, et al. Promotion of breastfeeding intervention trial (PROBIT): a cluster-randomized trial in the Republic of Belarus: design, follow-up, and data validation. *Adv Exp Med Biol.* 2000;478:327-345.

Kramer MS, Guo T, Platt RW, et al. Breastfeeding and infant growth: biology or bias? *Pediatrics.* 2002;110(2 pt 1):343-347.

Kramer MS, Kakuma R. Optimal duration of exclusive breastfeeding. *Cochrane Database Syst Rev.* 2002(1):CD003517.

Kramer MS, Kakuma R. The optimal duration of exclusive breastfeeding: a systematic review. *Adv Exp Med Biol.* 2004;554:63-77.

Kroeger M, Smith LJ. *Impact of Birthing Practices on Breastfeeding: Protecting the Mother and Baby Continuum.* Sudbury, MA: Jones & Bartlett Publishers; 2004.

Kruse L, Denk CE, Feldman-Winter L, Mojta Rotondo F. Comparing sociodemographic and hospital influences on breastfeeding initiation. *Birth.* 2005;32(2):81-85.

Kumar SP, Mooney R, Wieser LJ, Havstad S. The LATCH scoring system and prediction of breastfeeding duration. *J Hum Lact.* 2006;22(4):391-397.

Kunz C, Lonnerdal B. Re-evaluation of the whey protein/casein ratio of human milk. *Acta Paediatr.* 1992;81(2):107-112.

Labarere J, Bellin V, Fourny M, Gagnaire JC, Francois P, Pons JC. Assessment of a structured in-hospital educational intervention addressing breastfeeding: a prospective randomised open trial. *BJOG.* 2003;110(9):847-852.

Labarere J, Gelbert-Baudino N, Ayral AS, et al. Efficacy of breastfeeding support provided by trained clinicians during an early, routine, preventive visit: a prospective, randomized, open trial of 226 mother–infant pairs. *Pediatrics.* 2005;115(2):e139-e146.

Labbok M, Krasovek K. Toward consistency in breastfeeding definitions. *Stud Fam Plann.* 1990;21:226-230.

Labbok MH, Clark D, Goldman AS. Breastfeeding: maintaining an irreplaceable immunological resource. *Nat Rev Immunol.* 2004;4(7):565-572.

Labbok MH, Hendershot GE. Does breastfeeding protect against malocclusion? An analysis of the 1981 child health supplement to the National Health Interview Survey. *Am J Prev Med.* 1987;3(4):227-232.

Labbok MH, Wardlaw T, Blanc A, Clark D, Terreri N. Trends in exclusive breastfeeding: findings from the 1990s. *J Hum Lact.* 2006;22(3):272-276.

LaGasse LL, Messinger D, Lester BM, et al. Prenatal drug exposure and maternal and infant feeding behaviour. *Arch Dis Child Fetal Neonatal Ed.* 2003;88(5):F391-F399.

Lahr MB, Rosenberg KD, Lapidus JA. Bedsharing and maternal smoking in a population-based survey of new mothers. *Pediatrics.* 2005;116(4):e530-e542.

Lalakea ML, Messner AH. Ankyloglossia: the adolescent and adult perspective. *Otolaryngol Head Neck Surg.* 2003;128(5):746-752.

LaMar K, Dowling DA. Incidence of infection for preterm twins cared for in cobedding in the neonatal intensive-care unit. *J Obstet Gynecol Neonatal Nurs.* 2006;35(2):193-198.

Lang S. *Breastfeeding Special Care Babies.* London: Balliere Tindall; 1997.

Larnkjaer A, Schack-Nielsen L, Michaelsen KF. Fat content in human milk according to duration of lactation. *Pediatrics.* 2006;117(3):988-989; author reply 989-990.

Laubereau B, Brockow I, Zirngibl A, et al. Effect of breast-feeding on the development of atopic dermatitis during the first 3 years of life—results from the GINI-birth cohort study. *J Pediatr.* 2004;144(5):602-607.

Lauer JA, Betran AP, Barros AJ, de Onis M. Deaths and years of life lost due to suboptimal breast-feeding among children in the developing world: a global ecological risk assessment. *Public Health Nutr.* 2006;9(6):673-685.

Lauritzen L, Hoppe C, Straarup EM, Michaelsen KF. Maternal fish oil supplementation in lactation and growth during the first 2.5 years of life. *Pediatr Res.* 2005;58(2):235-242.

Lawoyin TO, Atwood S, Olawuyi JF. A rapid assessment of breastfeeding status using current status data. *Afr J Med Med Sci.* 2001;30(1-2):23-25.

Lawrence R. *A Review of the Medical Benefits and Contraindications to Breastfeeding in the United States* (Maternal and Child Health Technical Information Bulletin). Arlington, VA: National Center for Education in Maternal and Child Health; October 1997.

Lawrence RA. Lactation support when the infant will require general anesthesia: assisting the breast-feeding dyad in remaining content through the preoperative fasting period. *J Hum Lact.* 2005;21(3):355-357.

Lawrence RA. Lower breastfeeding rates among supplemental nutrition program for women, infants, and children participants: a call for action. *Pediatrics.* 2006;117(4):1432-1433.

Lawrence RA. Mastitis while breastfeeding: old theories and new evidence. *Am J Epidemiol.* 2002;155(2):115-116.

Lawrence RA. Peer support: making a difference in breast-feeding duration. *CMJ.* 2002;166(1):42-43.

Leake RD, Weitzman RE, Fisher DA. Oxytocin concentrations during the neonatal period. *Biol Neonate.* 1981;39(3-4):127-131.

Leighton BL, Halpern SH. The effects of epidural analgesia on labor, maternal, and neonatal outcomes: a systematic review. *Am J Obstet Gynecol.* 2002;186(5 suppl nature):S69-S77.

Lewallen LP, Dick MJ, Flowers J, Powell W, Zickefoose KT, Wall YG, et al. Breastfeeding support and early cessation. *J Obstet Gynecol Neonatal Nurs.* 2006;35(2):166-172.

Li R, Darling N, Maurice E, Barker L, Grummer-Strawn LM. Breastfeeding rates in the United States by characteristics of the child, mother, or family: the 2002 National Immunization survey. *Pediatrics.* 2005;115(1):e31-e37.

Lieberman E, Davidson K, Lee-Parritz A, Shearer E. Changes in fetal position during labor and their association with epidural analgesia. *Obstet Gynecol.* 2005;105(5 pt 1):974-982.

Lieberman E, Lang J, Richardson DK, Frigoletto FD, Heffner LJ, Cohen A. Intrapartum maternal fever and neonatal outcome. *Pediatrics.* 2000;105(1 pt 1):8-13.

Lieberman E, O'Donoghue C. Unintended effects of epidural analgesia during labor: a systematic review. *Am J Obstet Gynecol.* 2002;186(5 suppl nature):S31-S68.

Lovelady CA, Hunter CP, Geigerman C. Effect of exercise on immunologic factors in breast milk. *Pediatrics.* 2003;111(2):E148-E152.

Lucas A, Morley R, Cole TJ, Gore SM, Davis JA, Bamford MF, et al. Early diet in preterm babies and developmental status in infancy. *Arch Dis Child.* 1989;64(11):1570-1578.

Lucas A, Morley R, Cole TJ, Gore SM, Lucas PJ, Crowle P, et al. Early diet in preterm babies and developmental status at 18 months. *Lancet.* 1990;335(8704):1477-1481.

Lucas A, Morley R, Cole TJ, Gore SM. A randomised multicentre study of human milk versus formula and later development in preterm infants. *Arch Dis Child Fetal Neonatal Ed.* 1994;70(2):F141-146.

Lucas A, Morley R, Cole TJ, Lister G, Leeson-Payne C. Breast milk and subsequent intelligence quotient in children born preterm. *Lancet.* 1992;339(8788):261-264.

Lucas A, Morley R, Cole TJ. Randomised trial of early diet in preterm babies and later intelligence quotient. *BMJ.* 1998;317(7171):1481-1487.

Luder E, Kattan M, Tanzer-Torres G, Bonforte RJ. Current recommendations for breastfeeding in cystic fibrosis centers. *Am J Public Health.* 1992;82:1380-1382.

Ludington-Hoe SM, Golant SK. *Kangaroo Care: The Best You Can Do to Help Your Preterm Infant.* New York: Bantam Books; 1993.

Ludington-Hoe SM, Lewis T, Morgan K, Cong X, Anderson L, Reese S. Breast and infant temperatures with twins during shared kangaroo care. *J Obstet Gynecol Neonatal Nurs.* 2006;35(2):223-231.

Ludington-Hoe SM, Nguyen N, Swinth JY, Satyshur RD. Kangaroo care compared to incubators in maintaining body warmth in preterm infants. *Biol Res Nurs.* 2000;2(1):60-73.

Lvoff NM, Klaus MH. Effect of the Baby-Friendly initiative on infant abandonment in a Russian hospital. *Arch Pediatr Adolesc Med.* 2000;154(5):474-477.

Maisels MJ. What's in a name? Physiologic and pathologic jaundice: the conundrum of defining normal bilirubin levels in the newborn. *Pediatrics.* 2006;118(2):805-807.

Malec MA. *Essential Statistics for Social Research.* Philadelphia: J.B. Lippincott; 1977.

Mandel D, Lubetzky R, Dollberg S, Barak S, Mimouni FB. Fat and energy contents of expressed human breast milk in prolonged lactation. *Pediatrics.* 2005;116(3):e432-e435.

Mannel R, Mannel RS. Staffing for Hospital Lactation Programs: Recommendations from a tertiary care teaching hospital. *J Hum Lact.* 2006;22(4):409-417.

Marinelli KA, Burke GS, Dodd VL. A comparison of the safety of cupfeedings and bottlefeedings in premature infants whose mothers intend to breastfeed. *J Perinatol.* 2001;21(6):350-355.

Marquis GS, Penny ME, Diaz JM, Marin RM. Postpartum consequences of an overlap of breastfeeding and pregnancy: reduced breast milk intake and growth during early infancy. *Pediatrics.* 2002;109(4):e56.

Martens PJ, Phillips SJ, Cheang MS, Rosolowich V. How Baby-Friendly are Manitoba hospitals? The Provincial Infant Feeding study. *Can J Public Health.* 2000;91(1):51-57.

Martens PJ. Does breastfeeding education affect nursing staff beliefs, exclusive breastfeeding rates, and Baby-Friendly Hospital Initiative compliance? The experience of a small, rural Canadian hospital. *J Hum Lact.* 2000;16(4):309-318.

Martin J. Is nipple piercing compatible with breastfeeding? *J Hum Lact.* 2004;20(3):319-321.

Martinez JC, Maisels MJ, Otheguy L, Garcia H, Savorani M, Mogni B, et al. Hyperbilirubinemia in the breastfed newborn: a controlled trial of four interventions. *Pediatrics.* 1993;91:470-473.

Mascarenhas ML, Albernaz EP, da Silva MB, da Silveira RB. Prevalence of exclusive breastfeeding and its determiners in the first 3 months of life in the south of Brazil. *J Pediatr (Rio J).* 2006;82(4):289-294.

Matthiesen AS, Ransjo-Arvidson AB, Nissen E, Uvnas-Moberg K. Postpartum maternal oxytocin release by newborns: effects of infant hand massage and sucking. *Birth.* 2001;28(1):13-19.

McCabe L, Ernest AE, Neifert MR, Yannicelli S, Nord AM, Garry PJ, et al. The management of breastfeeding among infants with phenylketonuria. *J Inherit Metal Dis.* 1989;12:467-474.

McClure VS. *Infant Massage: A Handbook for Loving Parents.* New York: Bantam Books; 1989.

McElwain NL, Booth-Laforce C. Maternal sensitivity to infant distress and nondistress as predictors of infant–mother attachment security. *J Fam Psychol.* 2006;20(2):247-255.

McFadden A, Toole G. Exploring women's views of breastfeeding: a focus group study within an area with high levels of socio-economic deprivation. *Matern Child Nutr.* 2006;2(3):156-168.

McGarvey C, McDonnell M, Chong A, O'Regan M, Matthews T. Factors relating to the infant's last sleep environment in sudden infant death syndrome in the Republic of Ireland. *Arch Dis Child.* 2003;88(12):1058-1064.

McGarvey C, McDonnell M, Hamilton K, O'Regan M, Matthews T. An 8-year study of risk factors for SIDS: bed-sharing versus non-bed-sharing. *Arch Dis Child.* 2006;91(4):318-323.

McKenna JJ, McDade T. Why babies should never sleep alone: a review of the co-sleeping controversy in relation to SIDS, bedsharing and breast feeding. *Paediatr Respir Rev.* 2005;6(2):134-152.

McNeill PM, Kerridge IH, Henry DA, Stokes B, Hill SR, Newby D, et al. Giving and receiving of gifts between pharmaceutical companies and medical specialists in Australia. *Intern Med J.* 2006;36(9):571-578.

McVeagh P. The World Health Organization Code of Marketing of Breast-Milk Substitutes and subsequent resolutions (the WHO code). *N S W Public Health Bull.* 2005;16(3-4):67-68.

Meier P, Hurst N, Rodriguez N, et al. Comfort and effectiveness of the Symphony breast pump for mothers of preterm infants: comparison of three suction patterns. *Adv Exp Med Biol.* 2004;554:321-323.

Meier P. Concerns regarding industry-funded trials. *J Hum Lact.* 2005;21(2):121-123.

Meier PP, Brown LP, Hurst NM, et al. Nipple shields for preterm infants: effect on milk transfer and duration of breastfeeding. *J Hum Lact.* 2000;16(2):106-114.

Merewood A MS, Chamberlain LB, Philipp BL, Bauchner H. Breastfeeding rates in US Baby-Friendly hospitals: results of a national survey. *Pediatrics.* 2005;116(3):628-634.

Merewood A, Heinig J. Efforts to promote breastfeeding in the United States: development of a national breastfeeding awareness campaign. *J Hum Lact.* 2004;20(2):140-145.

Merewood A, Philipp BL, Chawla N, Cimo S. The Baby-Friendly Hospital Initiative increases breastfeeding rates in a US neonatal intensive care unit. *J Hum Lact.* 2003;19(2):166-171.

Merewood A, Philipp BL. Becoming Baby-Friendly: Overcoming the issue of accepting free formula. *J Hum Lact.* 2000;16(4):279-282.

Merewood A, Philipp BL. Implementing change: becoming Baby-Friendly in an inner city hospital. *Birth.* 2001;28(1):36-40.

Merewood A, Philipp BL. Peer counselors for breastfeeding mothers in the hospital setting: trials, training, tributes, and tribulations. *J Hum Lact.* 2003;19(1):72-76.

Merten S, Ackermann-Liebrich U. Exclusive breastfeeding rates and associated factors in Swiss Baby-Friendly hospitals. *J Hum Lact.* 2004;20(1):9-17.

Merten S, Dratva J, Ackermann-Liebrich U. Do Baby-Friendly hospitals influence breastfeeding duration on a national level? *Pediatrics.* 2005;116(5):e702-e708.

Messner AH, Lalakea ML, Aby J, Macmahon J, Bair E. Ankyloglossia: incidence and associated feeding difficulties. *Arch Otolaryngol Head Neck Surg.* 2000;126(1):36-39.

Mestecky J, ed. *Immunology of Milk and the Neonate.* New York: Plenum Press; 1991.

Metaj M, Laroia N, Lawrence RA, Ryan RM. Comparison of breast- and formula-fed normal newborns in time to first stool and urine. *J Perinatol.* 2003;23(8):624-628.

Meyer DE, de Oliveira DL. Breastfeeding policies and the production of motherhood: a historical-cultural approach. *Nurs Inq.* 2003;10(1):11-18.

Mezzacappa ES, Katlin ES. Breast-feeding is associated with reduced perceived stress and negative mood in mothers. *Health Psychol.* 2002;21(2):187-193.

Michaelsen KF, Skafte L, Badsberg JH, Jorgensen M. Variation in macronutrients in human bank milk: influencing factors and implications for human milk banking. *J Pediatr Gastroenterol Nutr.* 1990;11(2):229-239.

Michie C, Lockie F, Lynn W. The challenge of mastitis. *Arch Dis Child.* 2003;88(9):818-821.

Miller V, Riordan J. Treating postpartum breast edema with areolar compression. *J Hum Lact.* 2004;20(2):223-226.

Miller, Alice. *For Your Own Good: Hidden Cruelty in Child-Rearing and the Roots of Violence.* New York: Farrar, Straus, Giroux; 1984.

Mitchell EA, Blair PS, L'Hoir MP. Should pacifiers be recommended to prevent sudden infant death syndrome? *Pediatrics.* 2006;117(5):1755-1758.

Mitchell EA, Williams SM. Does circadian variation in risk factors for sudden infant death syndrome (SIDS) suggest there are two (or more) SIDS subtypes? *Acta Paediatr.* 2003;92(9):991-993.

Mitoulas LR, Gurrin LC, Doherty DA, Sherriff JL, Hartmann PE. Infant intake of fatty acids from human milk over the first year of lactation. *Br J Nutr.* 2003;90(5):979-986.

Mitoulas LR, Kent JC, Cox DB, Owens RA, Sherriff JL, Hartmann PE. Variation in fat, lactose and protein in human milk over 24 h and throughout the first year of lactation. *Br J Nutr.* 2002;88(1):29-37.

Mitoulas LR, Lai CT, Gurrin LC, Larsson M, Hartmann PE. Effect of vacuum profile on breast milk expression using an electric breast pump. *J Hum Lact.* 2002;18(4):353-360.

Mitoulas LR, Lai CT, Gurrin LC, Larsson M, Hartmann PE. Efficacy of breast milk expression using an electric breast pump. *J Hum Lact.* 2002;18(4):344-352.

Mitoulas LR, Ramsay DT, Kent JC, Larsson M, Hartmann PE. Identification of factors affecting breast pump efficacy. *Adv Exp Med Biol.* 2004;554:325-327.

Mitra AK, Khoury AJ, Carothers C, Foretich C. Evaluation of a comprehensive loving support program among state Women, Infants, and Children (WIC) program breast-feeding coordinators. *South Med J.* 2003;96(2):168-171.

Mizuno K, Aizawa M, Saito S, Kani K, Tanaka S, Kawamura H, et al. Analysis of feeding behavior with direct linear transformation. *Early Hum Dev.* 2006;82(3):199-204.

Mizuno K, Kani K. Sipping/lapping is a safe alternative feeding method to suckling for preterm infants. *Acta Paediatr.* 2005;94(5):574-580.

Mizuno K, Mizuno N, Shinohara T, Noda M. Mother-infant skin-to-skin contact after delivery results in early recognition of own mother's milk odour. *Acta Paediatr.* 2004;93(12):1640-1645.

Mizuno K, Ueda A, Takeuchi T. Effects of different fluids on the relationship between swallowing and breathing during nutritive sucking in neonates. *Biol Neonate.* 2002;81(1):45-50.

Mizuno K, Ueda A. Changes in sucking performance from nonnutritive sucking to nutritive sucking during breast- and bottle-feeding. *Pediatr Res.* 2006;59(5):728-731.

Mizuno K, Ueda A. Neonatal feeding performance as a predictor of neurodevelopmental outcome at 18 months. *Dev Med Child Neurol.* 2005;47(5):299-304.

Mizuno K, Ueda A. The maturation and coordination of sucking, swallowing, and respiration in preterm infants. *J Pediatr.* 2003;142(1):36-40.

Mohammadzadeh A, Farhat A, Esmaeily H. The effect of breast milk and lanolin on sore nipples. *Saudi Med J.* 2005;26(8):1231-1234.

Montagne P, Cuilliere ML, Mole C, Bene MC, Faure G. Changes in lactoferrin and lysozyme levels in human milk during the first twelve weeks of lactation. *Adv Exp Med Biol.* 2001;501:241-247.

Montagu, Ashley. *Touching: The Human Significance of the Skin.* 3rd ed. New York: Harper & Row; 1986.

Montgomery SM, Ehlin A, Sacker A. Breast feeding and resilience against psychosocial stress. *Arch Dis Child.* 2006.

Moon RY, Oden RP, Grady KC. Back to sleep: an educational intervention with women, infants, and children program clients. *Pediatrics.* 2004;113(3 pt 1):542-547.

Moon RY, Sprague BM, Patel KM. Stable prevalence but changing risk factors for sudden infant death syndrome in child care settings in 2001. *Pediatrics.* 2005;116(4):972-977.

Morgan KH, Groer MW, Smith LJ. The controversy about what constitutes safe and nurturant infant sleep environments. *J Obstet Gynecol Neonatal Nurs.* 2006;35(6):684-691.

Moriceau S, Sullivan RM. Neurobiology of infant attachment. *Dev Psychobiol.* 2005;47(3):230-242.

Morrill JF, Heinig MJ, Pappagianis D, Dewey KG. Risk factors for mammary candidosis among lactating women. *J Obstet Gynecol Neonatal Nurs.* 2005;34(1):37-45.

Morris S, Meyer Palmer M. *The Normal Acquisition of Oral Feeding Skills: Implications for Assessment and Treatment.* New York: Therapeutic Media; 1982.

Morrison B, Ludington-Hoe S, Anderson GC. Interruptions to breastfeeding dyads on postpartum day 1 in a university hospital. *J Obstet Gynecol Neonatal Nurs.* 2006;35(6):709-716.

Morrow AL, Guerrero ML, Shults J, et al. Efficacy of home-based peer counselling to promote exclusive breastfeeding: a randomised controlled trial. *Lancet.* 1999;353(9160):1226-1231.

Moscone SR, Moore MJ. Breastfeeding during pregnancy. *J Hum Lact.* 1993;9(2):83-88.

Mosley C, Whittle C, Hicks C. A pilot study to assess the viability of a randomised controlled trial of methods of supplementary feeding of breast-fed pre-term babies. *Midwifery.* 2001;17(2):150-157.

Mukai S, Nitta M. Correction of the glosso-larynx and resultant positional changes of the hyoid bone and cranium. *Acta Otolaryngol.* 2002;122(6):644-650.

Muraro A, Dreborg S, Halken S, et al. Dietary prevention of allergic diseases in infants and small children. Part III: Critical review of published peer-reviewed observational and interventional studies and final recommendations. *Pediatr Allergy Immunol.* 2004;15(4):291-307.

Naarding MA, Ludwig IS, Groot F, et al. Lewis X component in human milk binds DC-SIGN and inhibits HIV-1 transfer to CD4 T lymphocytes. *J Clin Invest.* 2005;115(11):3256-3264.

Narayanan I, Mehta, Dhoudhury DK, Jain BK. Sucking on the emptied breast: non-nutritive sucking with a difference. *Arch Dis Child.* 1991;66(2):241-244.

Nassar E, Marques IL, Trindade Jr AS, Bettiol H. Feeding-facilitating techniques for the nursing infant with Robin Sequence. *Cleft Palate Craniofac J.* 2006;43(1):55-60.

Nelson EA, Taylor BJ, Jenik A, et al. International Child Care Practices study: infant sleeping environment. *Early Hum Dev.* 2001;62(1):43-55.

Nelson EA, Yu LM, Williams S. International Child Care Practices study: breastfeeding and pacifier use. *J Hum Lact.* 2005;21(3):289-295.

Nickell WB, Skelton J. Breast fat and fallacies: more than 100 years of anatomical fantasy. *J Hum Lact.* 2005;21(2):126-130.

Nikki L. Breastfeeding difficulty and pacifier use. *Breastfeed Rev.* 2002;10(1):11-13.

Nussenblatt V, Lema V, Kumwenda N, et al. Epidemiology and microbiology of subclinical mastitis among HIV-infected women in Malawi. *Int J STD AIDS.* 2005;16(3):227-232.

Nyqvist KH, Lutes LM. Co-bedding twins: a developmentally supportive care strategy. *J Obstet Gynecol Neonatal Nurs.* 1998;27(4):450-456.

Nyqvist KH. Breast-feeding in preterm twins: Development of feeding behavior and milk intake during hospital stay and related caregiving practices. *J Pediatr Nurs.* 2002;17(4):246-256.

Nystedt A, Edvardsson D, Willman A. Epidural analgesia for pain relief in labour and childbirth—a review with a systematic approach. *J Clin Nurs.* 2004;13(4):455-466.

Oddy WH, Li J, Landsborough L, Kendall GE, Henderson S, Downie J. The association of maternal overweight and obesity with breastfeeding duration. *J Pediatr.* 2006;149(2):185-191.

Oddy WH, Pal S, Kusel MM, Vine D, de Klerk NH, Hartmann P, et al. Atopy, eczema and breast milk fatty acids in a high-risk cohort of children followed from birth to 5 yr. *Pediatr Allergy Immunol.* 2006;17(1):4-10.

Oddy WH, Scott JA, Graham KI, Binns CW. Breastfeeding influences on growth and health at one year of age. *Breastfeed Rev.* 2006;14(1):15-23.

Onyango AW, Receveur O, Esrey SA. The contribution of breast milk to toddler diets in western Kenya. *Bull World Health Organ.* 2002;80(4):292-299.

Osterman KL, Rahm VA. Lactation mastitis: bacterial cultivation of breast milk, symptoms, treatment, and outcome. *J Hum Lact.* 2000;16(4):297-302.

Overpeck MD, Brenner RA, Cosgrove C, Trumble AC, Kochanek K, MacDorman M. National under-ascertainment of sudden unexpected infant deaths associated with deaths of unknown cause. *Pediatrics.* 2002;109(2):274-283.

Palmer G. *The Politics of Breastfeeding.* 2nd ed. London: Pandora Press; 1993.

Palmer MM. Recognizing and resolving infant suck difficulties. *J Hum Lact.* 2002;18(2):166-167.

Palmer MM. *The Normal Acquisition of Oral Feeding Skills; Implications for Assessment and Treatment.* New York: Theraputic Media; 1982.

Patel RR, Liebling RE, Murphy DJ. Effect of operative delivery in the second stage of labor on breast-feeding success. *Birth.* 2003;30(4):255-260.

Pattinson RC, Arsalo I, Bergh AM, Malan AF, Patrick M, Phillips N. Implementation of kangaroo mother care: a randomized trial of two outreach strategies. *Acta Paediatr.* 2005;94(7):924-927.

Pearce MS, Thomas JE, Campbell DI, Parker L. Does increased duration of exclusive breastfeeding protect against *Helicobacter pylori* infection? The Newcastle Thousand Families Cohort study at age 49-51 years. *J Pediatr Gastroenterol Nutr.* 2005;41(5):617-620.

Perez-Escamilla R, Guerrero ML. Epidemiology of breastfeeding: advances and multidisciplinary applications. *Adv Exp Med Biol.* 2004;554:45-59.

Philipp BL, Brown E, Merewood A. Pumps for peanuts: leveling the field in the neonatal intensive care unit. *J Perinatol.* 2000;20(4):249-250.

Philipp BL, Malone KL, Cimo S, Merewood A. Sustained breastfeeding rates at a US Baby-Friendly hospital. *Pediatrics.* 2003;112(3 pt 1):e234-e236.

Philipp BL, Merewood A, Gerendas EJ, Bauchner H. Breastfeeding information in pediatric textbooks needs improvement. *J Hum Lact.* 2004;20(2):206-210.

Philipp BL, Merewood A, Miller LW, et al. Baby-Friendly Hospital Initiative improves breastfeeding initiation rates in a US hospital setting. *Pediatrics.* 2001;108(3):677-681.

Philipp BL, Merewood A, O'Brien S. Methadone and breastfeeding: new horizons. *Pediatrics.* 2003;111(6 pt 1):1429-1430.

Philipp BL, Merewood A. The Baby-Friendly way: the best breastfeeding start. *Pediatr Clin North Am.* 2004;51(3):761-783, xi.

Phillips RM, Chantry CJ, Gallagher MP. Analgesic effects of breast-feeding or pacifier use with maternal holding in term infants. *Ambul Pediatr.* 2005;5(6):359-364.

Piper S, Parks PL. Use of an intensity ratio to describe breastfeeding exclusivity in a national sample. *J Hum Lact.* 2001;17(3):227-232.

Pisacane A, Continisio GI, Aldinucci M, D'Amora S, Continisio P. A controlled trial of the father's role in breastfeeding promotion. *Pediatrics.* 2005;116(4):e494-e498.

Polit DF, Hungler BP. *Nursing Research Principles and Methods.* 5th ed. Philadelphia: J.B. Lippincott; 1995.

Pollard K, Fleming P, Young J, Sawczenko A, Blair P. Night-time non-nutritive sucking in infants aged 1 to 5 months: relationship with infant state, breastfeeding, and bed-sharing versus room-sharing. *Early Hum Dev.* 1999;56(2-3):185-204.

Popper BK. *The Hospitalized Nursing Baby.* Schaumburg, IL: La Leche League International; 1998. Lactation Consultant Series II, Unit 1.

Porter J, Schach B. Treating sore, possibly infected nipples. *J Hum Lact.* 2004;20(2):221-222.

Porter RH. The biological significance of skin-to-skin contact and maternal odours. *Acta Paediatr.* 2004;93(12):1560-1562.

Prescott SL, Tang ML. The Australasian Society of Clinical Immunology and Allergy position statement: summary of allergy prevention in children. *Med J Aust.* 2005;182(9):464-467.

Pridham KF, Schroeder M, Brown R, Clark R. The relationship of a mother's working model of feeding to her feeding behaviour. *J Adv Nurs.* 2001;35(5):741-750.

Priya JJ. Kangaroo care for low birth weight babies. *Nurs J India.* 2004;95(9):209-212.

Pugh LC, Milligan RA, Frick KD, Spatz D, Bronner Y. Breastfeeding duration, costs, and benefits of a support program for low-income breastfeeding women. *Birth.* 2002;29(2):95-100.

Quillin SI, Glenn LL. Interaction between feeding method and co-sleeping on maternal-newborn sleep. *J Obstet Gynecol Neonatal Nurs.* 2004;33(5):580-588.

Radzyminski S. Neurobehavioral functioning and breastfeeding behavior in the newborn. *J Obstet Gynecol Neonatal Nurs.* 2005;34(3):335-341.

Radzyminski S. The effect of ultra low dose epidural analgesia on newborn breastfeeding behaviors. *J Obstet Gynecol Neonatal Nurs.* 2003;32(3):322-331.

Rajan L. The impact of obstetric procedures and analgesia/anaesthesia during labour and delivery on breast feeding. *Midwifery.* 1994;10(2):87-103.

Ramsay DT, Kent JC, Hartmann RA, Hartmann PE. Anatomy of the lactating human breast redefined with ultrasound imaging. *J Anat.* 2005;206(6):525-534.

Ramsay DT, Kent JC, Owens RA, Hartmann PE. Ultrasound imaging of milk ejection in the breast of lactating women. *Pediatrics.* 2004;113(2):361-367.

Ramsay DT, Mitoulas LR, Kent JC, et al. Milk flow rates can be used to identify and investigate milk ejection in women expressing breast milk using an electric breast pump. *Breastfeeding Med.* 2006;1(1):14-23.

Ramsay DT, Mitoulas LR, Kent JC, Larsson M, Hartmann PE. The use of ultrasound to characterize milk ejection in women using an electric breast pump. *J Hum Lact.* 2005;21(4):421-428.

Ramsay M, Gisel EG, McCusker J, Bellavance F, Platt R. Infant sucking ability, non-organic failure to thrive, maternal characteristics, and feeding practices: a prospective cohort study. *Dev Med Child Neurol.* 2002;44(6):405-414.

Ransjo-Arvidson AB, Matthiesen AS, Lilja G, Nissen E, Widstrom AM, Uvnas-Moberg K. Maternal analgesia during labor disturbs newborn behavior: effects on breastfeeding, temperature, and crying. *Birth.* 2001;28(1):5-12.

Rao H, May C, Hannam S, Rafferty GF, Greenough A. Survey of sleeping position recommendations for prematurely born infants on neonatal intensive care unit discharge. *Eur J Pediatr.* 2006.

Rapp D. *Is This Your Child? Discovering and Treating Unrecognized Allergies in Children and Adults.* New York: Quill William Morrow; 1991.

Rapp D. *Is This Your Child's World?* New York: Bantam Books; 1996.

Rasmussen KM, Kjolhede CL. Prepregnant overweight and obesity diminish the prolactin response to suckling in the first week postpartum. *Pediatrics.* 2004;113(5):e465-e471.

Rasmussen KM, Lee VE, Ledkovsky TB, Kjolhede CL. A description of lactation counseling practices that are used with obese mothers. *J Hum Lact.* 2006;22(3):322-327.

Rea MF, Marcolino FF, Colameo AJ, Trevellin LA. Protection of breastfeeding, marketing of human milk substitutes and ethics. *Adv Exp Med Biol.* 2004;554:329-332.

Rea MF. The Brazilian National Breastfeeding Program: a success story. *Int J Gynaecol Obstet.* 1990;31(suppl 1):79-82; discussion 83-84.

Rechtman DJ, Lee ML, Berg H. Effect of environmental conditions on unpasteurized donor human milk. *Breastfeeding Med.* 2006;1(1):24-26.

Rempel LA. Factors influencing the breastfeeding decisions of long-term breastfeeders. *J Hum Lact.* 2004;20(3):306-318.

Renfrew MJ, Dyson L, Wallace LM, D'Souza L, McCormick F, Spiby H. Breastfeeding for longer: what works? *J R Soc Health.* 2005;125(2):62-63.

Righard L. Making childbirth a normal process. *Birth.* 2001;28(1):1-4.

Riordan J, Bibb D, Miller M, Rawlins T. Predicting breastfeeding duration using the LATCH breast-feeding assessment tool. *J Hum Lact.* 2001;17(1):20-23.

Riordan J, Gill-Hopple K, Angeron J. Indicators of effective breastfeeding and estimates of breast milk intake. *J Hum Lact.* 2005;21(4):406-412.

Riordan J. *Breastfeeding and Human Lactation.* 3rd ed. Sudbury, MA: Jones & Bartlett Publishers; 2005.

Riva E. et al. Early breastfeeding is linked to higher intelligence quotient scores in dietary treated phenylketonuric children. *Acta Pediatr.* 1996;85:56-58.

Rocha NM, Martinez FE, Jorge SM. Cup or bottle for preterm infants: effects on oxygen saturation, weight gain, and breastfeeding. *J Hum Lact.* 2002;18(2):132-138.

Romond JL, Baker IT. Squatting in childbirth: a new look at an old tradition. *J Obstet Gynecol Neonatal Nurs.* 1985;14(5):406-411.

Ronayne de Ferrer PA, Baroni A, Sambucetti ME, Lopez NE, Ceriani Cernadas JM. Lactoferrin levels in term and preterm milk. *J Am Coll Nutr.* 2000;19(3):370-373.

Rowe-Murray HJ, Fisher JR. Baby-Friendly hospital practices: cesarean section is a persistent barrier to early initiation of breastfeeding. *Birth.* 2002;29(2):124-131.

Rowe-Murray HJ, Fisher JR. Operative intervention in delivery is associated with compromised early mother-infant interaction. *BJOG.* 2001;108(10):1068-1075.

Royal College of Midwives. *Successful Breastfeeding.* 3rd ed. London: Churchill Livingstone; 2002.

Rubin R. *Maternal Identity and the Maternal Experience.* New York: Spring Publishing; 1984.

Ryan AS, Zhou W. Lower breastfeeding rates persist among the special supplemental nutrition program for women, infants, and children participants, 1978-2003. *Pediatrics.* 2006;117(4):1136-1146.

Ryser FG. Breastfeeding attitudes, intention, and initiation in low-income women: the effect of the best start program. *J Hum Lact.* 2004;20(3):300-305.

Saarela T, Kokkonen J, Koivisto M. Macronutrient and energy contents of human milk fractions during the first six months of lactation. *Acta Paediatr.* 2005;94(9):1176-1181.

Saarinen KM, Juntunen-Backman K, Jarvenpaa AL, et al. Breast-feeding and the development of cows' milk protein allergy. *Adv Exp Med Biol.* 2000;478:121-130.

Saarinen KM, Juntunen-Backman K, Jarvenpaa AL, et al. Supplementary feeding in maternity hospitals and the risk of cow's milk allergy: a prospective study of 6209 infants. *J Allergy Clin Immunol.* 1999;104(2 pt 1):457-461.

Saarinen KM, Savilahti E. Infant feeding patterns affect the subsequent immunological features in cow's milk allergy. *Clin Exp Allergy.* 2000;30(3):400-406.

Sachs M, Dykes F, Carter B. Weight monitoring of breastfed babies in the United Kingdom—interpreting, explaining and intervening. *Matern Child Nutr.* 2006;2(1):3-18.

Sachs M, Dykes F, Carter B. Weight monitoring of breastfed babies in the UK—centile charts, scales and weighing frequency. *Matern Child Nutr.* 2005;1(2):63-76.

Salsberry PJ, Reagan PB. Dynamics of early childhood overweight. *Pediatrics.* 2005;116(6):1329-1338.

Sanches MT. Clinical management of oral disorders in breastfeeding. *J Pediatr (Rio J).* 2004;80(5 suppl):S155-S62. [Translated from Spanish]

Satter E. *Child of Mine: Feeding with Love and Good Sense.* Palo Alto, CA: Bull Publishing; 1983.

Satter E. *How to Get Your Kid to Eat … but Not Too Much.* Palo Alto, CA: Bull Publishing; 1987.

Scammon RE, Doyle LO. Observations on the capacity of the stomach in the first ten days of postnatal life. *Am J Dis Child.* 1920;20:516-538.

Scariati PD, Grummer-Strawn LM, Fein SB. A longitudinal analysis of infant morbidity and the extent of breastfeeding in the US. *Pediatrics.* 1997;99(6):e5.

Schaal B, Doucet S, Sagot P, Hertling E, Soussignan R. Human breast areolae as scent organs: morphological data and possible involvement in maternal-neonatal coadaptation. *Dev Psychobiol.* 2006;48(2):100-110.

Schack-Nielsen L, Larnkjaer A, Michaelsen KF. Long term effects of breastfeeding on the infant and mother. *Adv Exp Med Biol.* 2005;569:16-23.

Schafer E, Vogel MK, Viegas S, Hausafus C. Volunteer peer counselors increase breastfeeding duration among rural low-income women. *Birth.* 1998;25(2):101-106.

Schanler RJ, Lau C, Hurst NM, Smith EOB. Randomized trial of donor human milk versus preterm formula as substitutes for mothers' own milk in the feeding of extremely premature infants. *Pediatrics.* 2005;116(2):400-406.

Schulte-Hobein B, Schwartz-Bickenbach D, Abt S, Plum C, Nau H. Cigarette smoke exposure and development of infants throughout the first year of life: influence of passive smoking and nursing on cotinine levels in breast milk and infant's urine. *Acta Paediatr.* 1992;81(6-7):550-557.

Schwartz K, D'Arcy HJ, Gillespie B, Bobo J, Longeway M, Foxman B. Factors associated with weaning in the first 3 months postpartum. *J Fam Pract.* 2002;51(5):439-444.

Scott JA, Binns CW, Oddy WH, Graham KI. Predictors of breastfeeding duration: evidence from a cohort study. *Pediatrics.* 2006;117(4):e646-e655.

Sherman TI, Greenspan JS, St Clair N, Touch SM, Shaffer TH. Optimizing the neonatal thermal environment. *Neonatal Netw.* 2006;25(4):251-60.

Shields LBE, Hunsaker DM, Muldoon S, Corey TS, Spivack BS. Risk factors associated with sudden unexplained infant death: a prospective study of infant care practices in Kentucky. *Pediatrics.* 2005;116(1):e13-e20.

Sievers E, Haase S, Oldigs HD, Schaub J. The impact of peripartum factors on the onset and duration of lactation. *Biol Neonate.* 2003;83(4):246-252.

Sievers E, Oldigs HD, Schultz-Lell G, Schaub J. Faecal excretion in infants. *Eur J Pediatr.* 1993;152(5):542-454.

Sikorski J, Renfrew MJ, Pindoria S, Wade A. Support for breastfeeding mothers: a systematic review. *Paediatr Perinat Epidemiol.* 2003;17(4):407-417.

Siltanen M, Kajosaari M, Poussa T, Saarinen KM, Savilahti E. A dual long-term effect of breastfeeding on atopy in relation to heredity in children at 4 years of age. *Allergy.* 2003;58(6):524-530.

Sinha A, Madden J, Ross-Degnan D, Soumerai S, Platt R. Reduced risk of neonatal respiratory infections among breastfed girls but not boys. *Pediatrics.* 2003;112(4):e303.

Sisk PM, Lovelady CA, Dillard RG, Gruber KJ. Lactation counseling for mothers of very low birth weight infants: effect on maternal anxiety and infant intake of human milk. *Pediatrics.* 2006;117(1):e67-e75.

Slykerman RF, Thompson JM, Becroft DM, Robinson E, Pryor JE, Clark PM, et al. Breastfeeding and intelligence of preschool children. *Acta Paediatr.* 2005;94(7):832-837.

Smith JP, Thompson JF, Ellwood DA. Hospital system costs of artificial infant feeding: estimates for the Australian Capital Territory. *Aust N Z J Public Health.* 2002;26(6):543-551.

Smith LJ. A score sheet for evaluating breastfeeding educational materials. *J Hum Lact.* 1995;11:307-311.

Snowden HM, Renfrew MJ, Woolridge MW. Treatments for breast engorgement during lactation. *Cochrane Database Syst Rev.* 2001(2):CD000046.

Sorensen HJ, Mortensen EL, Reinisch JM, Mednick SA. Early weaning and hospitalization with alcohol-related diagnoses in adult life. *Am J Psychiatry.* 2006;163(4):704-709.

Spatz DL, Goldschmidt KA. Preserving breastfeeding for the rehospitalized infant: a clinical pathway. *MCN Am J Matern Child Nurs.* 2006;31(1):45-51; quiz 52-53.

Spitz AM, Lee NC, Peterson HB. Treatment for lactation suppression: little progress in one hundred years. *Am J Obstet Gynecol.* 1998;179(6):1485-1490.

St James-Roberts I, Alvarez M, Csipke E, Abramsky T, Goodwin J, Sorgenfrei E. Infant crying and sleeping in London, Copenhagen and when parents adopt a "proximal" form of care. *Pediatrics.* 2006;117(6):e1146-1155.

Stevens B, Yamada J, Ohlsson A. Sucrose for analgesia in newborn infants undergoing painful procedures. *Cochrane Database Syst Rev.* 2004(3):CD001069.

Stuart-Macadam P, Dettwyler KA. *Breastfeeding: Biocultural Perspectives.* New York: Aldine De Gruyter; 1995.

Stuebe AM, Rich-Edwards JW, Willett WC, Manson JE, Michels KB. Duration of lactation and incidence of type 2 diabetes. *JAMA.* 2005;294(20):2601-2610.

Sullivan ML, Leathers SJ, Kelley MA. Family characteristics associated with duration of breastfeeding during early infancy among primiparas. *J Hum Lact.* 2004;20(2):196-205.

Svensson K, Matthiesen AS, Widstrom AM. Night rooming-in: who decides? An example of staff influence on mother's attitude. *Birth.* 2005;32(2):99-106.

Swanson V, Power KG. Initiation and continuation of breastfeeding: theory of planned behaviour. *J Adv Nurs.* 2005;50(3):272-282.

Swift K, Janke J. Breast binding... is it all that it's wrapped up to be? *J Obstet Gynecol Neonatal Nurs.* 2003;32(3):332-339.

Tait P. Nipple pain in breastfeeding women: causes, treatment, and prevention strategies. *J Midwifery Women's Health.* 2000;45(3):212-215.

Tappero EP, Honeyfield ME. *Physical Assessment of the Newborn.* Petaluma, CA: NICU Ink; 1993.

Tappin D. Bedsharing, roomsharing, and sudden infant death syndrome in Scotland: a case-control study. *J Pediatrics.* 2005;147(1):32.

Taveras EM, Capra AM, Braveman PA, Jensvold NG, Escobar GJ, Lieu TA. Clinician support and psychosocial risk factors associated with breastfeeding discontinuation. *Pediatrics.* 2003;112(1 pt 1):108-115.

Taveras EM, Li R, Grummer-Strawn L, et al. Mothers' and clinicians' perspectives on breastfeeding counseling during routine preventive visits. *Pediatrics.* 2004;113(5):e405-e411.

Taveras EM, Li R, Grummer-Strawn L, et al. Opinions and practices of clinicians associated with continuation of exclusive breastfeeding. *Pediatrics.* 2004;113(4):e283-e290.

Taveras EM, Scanlon KS, Birch L, Rifas-Shiman SL, Rich-Edwards JW, Gillman MW. Association of breastfeeding with maternal control of infant feeding at age 1 year. *Pediatrics.* 2004;114(5):e577-e583.

Taylor JS, Kacmar JE, Nothnagle M, Lawrence RA. A systematic review of the literature associating breastfeeding with type 2 diabetes and gestational diabetes. *J Am Coll Nutr.* 2005;24(5):320-326.

Taylor MM. *Transcultural Aspects of Breastfeeding—USA.* Wayne, NJ: Avery Publishing Group; 1985. Lactation Consultant Series, Unit 2.

Thorley V. Latch and the fear response: overcoming an obstacle to successful breastfeeding. *Breastfeed Rev.* 2005;13(1):9-11.

Uvnas-Moberg K. *The Oxytocin Factor.* Cambridge, MA: Da Capo Press/Perseus Books Group; 2003.

Valiante AG, Barr RG, Zelazo PR, Papageorgiou AN, Young SN. A typical feeding enhances memory for spoken words in healthy 2- to 3-day-old newborns. *Pediatrics.* 2006;117(3):e476-e486.

Van der Wijden C, Kleijnen J, Van den Berk T. Lactational amenorrhea for family planning. *Cochrane Database Syst Rev.* 2003(4):CD001329.

Van Esterik P. *Risks, Rights and Regulations: Communicating about Risks and Infant Feeding.* Penang, Malaysia: World Alliance for Breastfeeding Action (WABA); 2002.

Van Esterik P. *Women, Work, and Breastfeeding.* North York, Ontario: York University Press; 1994.

Van Esterik, P. *Beyond the Breast-Bottle Controversy.* New Brunswick, NJ: Rutgers University Press; 1989.

van Odijk J, Kull I, Borres MP, et al. Breastfeeding and allergic disease: a multidisciplinary review of the literature (1966-2001) on the mode of early feeding in infancy and its impact on later atopic manifestations. *Allergy.* 2003;58(9):833-843.

Varendi H, Porter RH, Winberg J. The effect of labor on olfactory exposure learning within the first postnatal hour. *Behav Neurosci.* 2002;116(2):206-211.

Viggiano D, Fasano D, Monaco G, Strohmenger L. Breast feeding, bottle feeding, and non-nutritive sucking; effects on occlusion in deciduous dentition. *Arch Dis Child.* 2004;89(12):1121-1123.

Vogl SE, Worda C, Egarter C, Bieglmayer C, Szekeres T, Huber J, et al. Mode of delivery is associated with maternal and fetal endocrine stress response. *BJOG.* 2006;113(4):441-445.

Vohr BR, Poindexter BB, Dusick AM, McKinley LT, Wright LL, Langer JC, et al. Beneficial effects of breast milk in the neonatal intensive care unit on the developmental outcome of extremely low birth weight infants at 18 months of age. *Pediatrics.* 2006;118(1):e115-123.

Volmanen P, Valanne J, Alahuhta S. Breast-feeding problems after epidural analgesia for labour: a retrospective cohort study of pain, obstetrical procedures and breast-feeding practices. *Int J Obstet Anesth.* 2004;13(1):25-29.

Wailoo M, Ball H, Fleming P, Ward Platt MP. Infants bed-sharing with mothers. *Arch Dis Child.* 2004;89(12):1082-1083.

Walker M. *Breastfeeding Management for the Clinician: Using the Evidence.* Sudbury MA: Jones & Bartlett Publishers, 2006.

Walker M. *Mastitis in Lactating Women.* Schaumburg, IL: La Leche League International; 1999. Lactation Consultant Series II, Unit 2.

Wall V, Glass R. Mandibular asymmetry and breastfeeding problems: experience from 11 cases. *J Hum Lact.* 2006;22(3):328-334.

Wallace LM, Kosmala-Anderson J. A training needs survey of doctors' breastfeeding support skills in England. *Mat Child Nutr.* 2006;2(4):217-231.

Wang ML, Dorer DJ, Fleming MP, Catlin EA. Clinical outcomes of near-term infants. *Pediatrics.* 2004;114(2):372-376.

Wang RY, Bates MN, Goldstein DA, et al. Human milk research for answering questions about human health. *J Toxicol Environ Health A.* 2005;68(20):1771-1801.

Weatherly-White RC, Kuehn DP, Mirrett P, Gilman JI, Weatherley-White CC. Early repair and breast-feeding for infants with cleft lip. *Plast Reconstr Surg.* 1987;79:879-885.

Weaver LT, Ewing G, Taylor LC. The bowel habit of milk-fed infants. *J Pediatr Gastroenterol Nutr.* 1998;7(4):568-571.

Weed S. *Wise Woman Herbal: The Childbearing Year.* New York: Ash Tree Publishing; 1996.

Whaley LF, Wong DL. *Nursing Care of Infants and Children,* 4th ed. St. Louis: Mosby; 1991. Unit II.

Whitehead E, Dodds L, Joseph KS, et al. Relation of pregnancy and neonatal factors to subsequent development of childhood epilepsy: a population-based cohort study. *Pediatrics.* 2006;117(4):1298-1306.

WHO. *Global Strategy for Infant and Young Child Feeding.* Geneva, Switzerland: World Health Organization; 2003.

WHO/UNICEF. *Protecting, Promoting and Supporting Breastfeeding: The Special Role of Maternity Services* [a joint WHO/UNICEF statement]. Geneva, Switzerland: World Health Organization Nutrition Unit; 1989.

Wiberg B, Humble K, de Chateau P. Long-term effect on mother-infant behavior of extra contact during the first hour post partum V. Follow-up at three years. *Scand J Soc Med.* 1989;17:181-191.

Willumsen JF, Filteau SM, Coutsoudis A, et al. Breastmilk RNA viral load in HIV-infected South African women: effects of subclinical mastitis and infant feeding. *AIDS.* 2003;17(3):407-414.

Wilson-Clay B, Rourke JW, Bolduc MB, Stagg JD, Flatau G, Vaugh B. Learning to lobby for probreast-feeding legislation: the story of a Texas bill to create a breastfeeding-friendly physician designation. *J Hum Lact.* 2005;21(2):191-198.

Winberg J. Mother and newborn baby: mutual regulation of physiology and behavior—a selective review. *Dev Psychobiol.* 2005;47(3):217-229.

Winecker RE, Goldberger BA, Tebbett IR, et al. Detection of cocaine and its metabolites in breast milk. *J Forensic Sci.* 2001;46(5):1221-1223.

Winnicott DW. *Babies and Their Mothers.* Reading, MA: Addison-Wesley; 1987.

Wolf JH. Low breastfeeding rates and public health in the United States. *Am J Public Health.* 2003;93(12):2000-2010.

Worku B, Kassie A. Kangaroo mother care: a randomized controlled trial on effectiveness of early kangaroo mother care for the low birthweight infants in Addis Ababa, Ethiopia. *J Trop Pediatr.* 2005;51(2):93-97.

Wright CM, Parkinson K, Scott J. Breast-feeding in a UK urban context: who breast-feeds, for how long and does it matter? *Public Health Nutr.* 2006;9(6):686-691.

Wright CM, Parkinson KN, Drewett RF. How does maternal and child feeding behavior relate to weight gain and failure to thrive? Data from a prospective birth cohort. *Pediatrics.* 2006;117(4):1262-1269.

Yamauchi Y, Yamanouchi I. Breastfeeding frequency during the first 24 hours after birth in full-term neonates. *Pediatrics.* 1990;86(2):171-175.

Yamazaki A, Lee KA, Kennedy HP, Weiss SJ. Sleep-wake cycles, social rhythms, and sleeping arrangement during Japanese childbearing family transition. *J Obstet Gynecol Neonatal Nurs.* 2005;34(3):342-348.

Yap PL, McKiernan J, Mirtle CL, McClelland DB. The development of mammary secretory immunity in the human newborn. *Acta Paediatr Scand.* 1981;70(4):459-465.

Yeung CY, Lee HC, Lin SP, Yang YC, Huang FY, Chuang CK. Negative effect of heat sterilization on the free amino acid concentrations in infant formula. *Eur J Clin Nutr.* 2006;60(1):136-141.

Young EWD. *Alpha and Omega: Ethics at the Frontier of Life and Death.* Reading, MA: Addison-Wesley; 1989.

Zanardo V, Nicolussi S, Carlo G, et al. Beta endorphin concentrations in human milk. *J Pediatr Gastroenterol Nutr.* 2001;33(2):160-164.

Zanardo V, Nicolussi S, Cavallin S, et al. Effect of maternal smoking on breast milk interleukin-1alpha, beta-endorphin, and leptin concentrations and leptin concentrations. *Environ Health Perspect.* 2005;113(10):1410-1413.

Zanardo V, Nicolussi S, Favaro F, et al. Effect of postpartum anxiety on the colostral milk beta-endorphin concentrations of breastfeeding mothers. *J Obstet Gynaecol.* 2001;21(2):130-134.

Zanardo V, Nicolussi S, Giacomin C, Faggian D, Favaro F, Plebani M. Labor pain effects on colostral milk beta-endorphin concentrations of lactating mothers. *Biol Neonate.* 2001;79(2):87-90.

Zangen S, Di Lorenzo C, Zangen T, Mertz H, Schwankovsky L, Hyman PE. Rapid maturation of gastric relaxation in newborn infants. *Pediatr Res.* 2001;50(5):629-632.

Zeskind PS, Gingras JL. Maternal cigarette-smoking during pregnancy disrupts rhythms in fetal heart rate. *J Pediatr Psychol.* 2005:jsj031.

Zollner MS, Jorge AO. Candida spp. occurrence in oral cavities of breastfeeding infants and in their mothers' mouths and breasts. *Pesqui Odontol Bras.* 2003;17(2):151-155.

A. INTERNATIONAL BOARD OF LACTATION CONSULTANT EXAMINERS EXAM INFORMATION & PREPARATION[1]

The International Board of Lactation Consultant Examiners (IBLCE) provides the following for information only. No member of the IBLCE board of directors or staff has contributed or been consulted in the development of this text. The IBLCE does not endorse the content, accuracy, completeness, or usefulness of any information contained in this text, nor of any training course provided by the author.

For current and complete information regarding the IBLCE certification exam, please visit the IBLCE website at www.iblce.org or send e-mail to iblce@iblce.org.

WHAT IS THE IBLCE?

IBLCE stands for **I**nternational **B**oard of **L**actation **C**onsultant **E**xaminers, the organization that administers the world's first truly international certification program.

The annual exam to credential IBCLCs has been offered in 13 languages and at numerous sites all over the world, building bridges across language and geographical borders.

The IBLCE is a nonprofit organization with a policy-making board of directors with broad professional, organizational, and geographic representation. IBLCE has its international headquarters in the USA, regional offices in Australia and Austria, and honorary local coordinators in countries where there are groups of IBCLCs and regular exam sites.

IBLCE's primary purpose is to certify individuals who provide quality care to babies and mothers worldwide. There are over 15,000 currently certified IBCLCs worldwide, in 65 countries; their names are listed in on-line registries.

The IBLCE is very proud to be accredited by the U.S. National Commission for Certifying Agencies (NCCA), which sets stringent guidelines for health certifying organizations and accredits those who meet the criteria. The IBLCE has utilized these criteria since its inception and has maintained this important accreditation, reapplying every 5 years.

WHAT IS AN IBCLC, RLC?

International **B**oard **C**ertified **L**actation **C**onsultants (IBCLCs) are health care providers who, by meeting eligibility requirements and by passing an independent examination, are certified to possess the necessary skills, knowledge, and attitudes to provide quality breastfeeding assistance to babies and mothers.

In North America, IBCLCs may also use the designation **R**egistered **L**actation **C**onsultant, shown as (IBCLC, RLC).

IBCLC, RLCs are valuable members of the health care team who find recognition and career opportunities that may not be available to others who have studied lactation, but are not board certified. There are now

[1]© 2006 International Board of Lactation Consultant Examiners. Reproduced with permission of the IBLCE.

many designated positions for IBCLC, RLCs. They work in hospitals, maternal and child health, the community, and private practice.

As more health care facilities make a commitment to improving their breastfeeding practices and success rates, education of staff has been identified as a crucial step in this procedure. Health facilities that encourage and support their staff to become board certified find that the exam provides them with a strong incentive to extend their study and skills. Some hospitals now require all clinical staff who help mothers with breastfeeding to work toward IBCLC certification.

INTERNATIONAL BOARD OF LACTATION CONSULTANT EXAMINERS

The IBLCE mission is to develop the internationally recognized certification standard and award credentials to individuals who demonstrate competence in providing breastfeeding assistance to mothers and children worldwide.

IBLCE EXAM BLUEPRINT (2000)

All exam questions have both *discipline* and *chronological* parameters. The range for the possible number of questions that will be related to each *discipline* or *chronological period* appears in parentheses after each topic. For example, there will be 19–33 anatomy questions and 9–17 questions that refer to babies 4–6 months old. See the *Sample Exam Questions* in this appendix for examples of how the blueprint is applied.

Note: This blueprint gives you an indication of the breadth of information you need to know for the exam. The examples given are for guidance only; they are not inclusive of all aspects covered under each learning discipline. The disciplines are expanded into chapters in ILCA's *Core Curriculum for Lactation Consultant Practice* (Walker, ed., Sudbury, MA: Jones & Bartlett; 2002 and 2007).

Disciplines

A. Maternal and infant **ANATOMY** (19–33 questions); e.g., breast and nipple structure and development; blood, lymph, innervation, mammary tissue; infant oral anatomy and reflexes; assessment; anatomical variations

B. Maternal and infant normal **PHYSIOLOGY** and **ENDOCRINOLOGY** (19–33 questions); e.g., hormones; lactogenesis; endocrine/autocrine control of milk supply; induced lactation; fertility; infant hepatic, pancreatic, and renal function; metabolism; effect of complementary feeds; digestion and GI tract; voiding and stooling patterns

C. Maternal and infant normal **NUTRITION** and **BIOCHEMISTRY** (10–16 questions); e.g., breast milk synthesis and composition; milk components, function and effect on baby; comparison with other products/milks; feeding patterns and intake over time; variations of maternal diet; ritual and traditional foods; introduction of solids

D. Maternal and infant **IMMUNOLOGY** and **INFECTIOUS DISEASE** (10–16 questions); e.g., antibodies and other immune factors; cross infection; bacteria and viruses in milk; allergies and food sensitivity; long-term protective factors

E. Maternal and infant **PATHOLOGY** (19–33 questions); e.g., acute/chronic abnormalities and diseases, both local and systemic; breast and nipple problems and pathology; endocrine pathology; mother/child physical and neurological disabilities; congenital abnormalities; oral pathology; neurological immaturity; failure to thrive; hyperbilirubinemia and hypoglycemia; impact of pathology on breastfeeding

F. Maternal and infant **PHARMACOLOGY** and **TOXICOLOGY** (10–16 questions); e.g., environmental contaminants; maternal use of medication, OTC preparations, social or recreational drugs and their effect on the infant on milk composition and on lactation; galactagogues/suppressants; effects of medications used in labor; contraceptives; complementary therapies

G. **PSYCHOLOGY, SOCIOLOGY**, and **ANTHROPOLOGY** (10–16 questions); e.g., counseling and adult education skills; grief, postnatal depression and psychosis; effect of socio-economic, lifestyle, and employment issues on breastfeeding; maternal–infant relationship; maternal role adaptation; parenting skills; sleep patterns; cultural beliefs and practices; family; support systems; domestic violence; and mothers with special needs, e.g., adolescents, migrants

H. **GROWTH PARAMETERS** and **DEVELOPMENTAL MILESTONES** (10–16 questions); e.g., fetal and preterm growth; breastfed and artificially fed growth patterns; recognition of normal and delayed physical, psychological and cognitive developmental markers; breastfeeding behaviors to 12 months and beyond; weaning

I. **INTERPRETATION OF RESEARCH** (4–8 questions); skills required to critically appraise and interpret research literature, lactation consultant educational material, and consumer literature; understanding terminology used in research and basic statistics; reading tables and graphs; surveys and data collection

J. **ETHICAL and LEGAL ISSUES** (4–8 questions); e.g., IBLCE *Code of Ethics*; ILCA *Standards of Practice*; practicing within scope of practice; referrals and interdisciplinary relationships; confidentiality; medical-legal responsibilities; charting and report writing skills; record keeping; informed consent; battery; maternal/infant neglect and abuse; conflict of interest; ethics of equipment rental and sales

K. **BREASTFEEDING EQUIPMENT** and **TECHNOLOGY** (10–16 questions); e.g., identification of breastfeeding devices and equipment, their appropriate use, and technical expertise to use them properly; handling and storing human milk, including human milk banking protocols

L. **TECHNIQUES** (19–33 questions); e.g., breastfeeding techniques, including positioning and latch; assessing milk transfer; breastfeeding management; normal feeding patterns; milk expression

M. **PUBLIC HEALTH** (4–8 questions); e.g., breastfeeding promotion and community education; working with groups with low breastfeeding rates; creating and implementing clinical protocols; international tools and documents; WHO Code; BFHI implementation; prevalence, surveys, and data collection for research purposes

Chronological Periods

1. Preconception (2–7 questions)

2. Prenatal (9–17 questions)

3. Labor/birth (perinatal) (9–17 questions)

4. Prematurity (9–17 questions)

5. 0–2 days (19–31 questions)

6. 3–14 days (19–31 questions)

7. 15–28 days (19–31 questions)

8. 1–3 months (9–17 questions)

9. 4–6 months (9–17 questions)

10. 7–12 months (2–7 questions)

11. Beyond 12 months (2–7 questions)

12. General principles (40–53 questions)

EXAM INFORMATION

Exam Content

The exam is composed of 200 multiple choice questions. The degree of difficulty is set at postgraduate university level. Since effective lactation consultation requires assessment and decision-making skills, the questions are primarily designed to test the application of knowledge, rather than the pure recall of facts. Application questions are more realistic and enhance the validity of the exam.

The exam is administered in two sessions of 100 questions each. Of the 200 questions, 125 are *cognitive*, based on word scenarios, and 75 are based on photos. They are all combined for classification into *disciplines* and *chronological periods*.

The *IBLCE Exam Blueprint* in this appendix gives more information about the *disciplines* and *chronological periods*, with the number of anticipated exam questions for each shown in brackets. This outline helps you determine the relative emphasis of the exam and reflects average lactation consultant practice, based on an extensive role delineation survey. For example, *Pathology (19–33)* means that there will be a minimum of 19 questions and a maximum of 33 questions that address infant and maternal pathological conditions relevant to lactation consultant practice.

Checking your knowledge and skills off against the *IBLCE Exam Blueprint* will help you to identify areas you need to address and help you focus your study.

The sample test questions in this appendix were selected as examples of the type of multiple choice questions that may be expected on the *cognitive* portion of the exam. Since they are limited in scope, they should not be regarded as representative of the full range of material that will be tested or the degree of difficulty.

The *photo* section has 75 questions based on color photographs that illustrate various situations and clinical conditions relevant to lactation consultant practice. Typically, candidates are asked to evaluate whether or not a problem is present, the nature of the problem, or how it should be managed. Each candidate will be provided with a booklet of color pictures to use for this part of the exam.

Although the exam is administered in two sessions, the scores for the both sessions are added together to determine each candidate's overall score and pass/fail designation. Candidates pass or fail the examination as a whole. A higher score in one area can compensate for a lower score in another area, so the candidate passes the overall exam.

Exam Question Referencing

All examination questions are referenced to the technical/medical literature, usually to literature published within the last 5 years. Older scientific studies may be used if they are still quoted as reputable references in current texts. Each exam question is referenced to printed materials, not to statements made at conferences. Anecdotal material, controversial information, authors' opinions, and areas where the major texts give conflicting information are all avoided. References are current to the end of the calendar year prior to the exam.

IBLCE Exam Committee

The exam committee, chaired by a director of the IBLCE board, works under the direction of a PhD in psychometrics, who is a health professions certification examination consultant. The following groups will typically be represented on the exam committee to give a range of professional expertise: IBCLCs in hospital and in community practice, lactation educators, IBCLCs trained primarily through the mother support system, IBCLCs who trained through traditional health professions, medical practitioners experienced in supporting mothers and babies, a PhD-level researcher in lactation, and the highest scorer from the previous year's exam. As far as possible, the committee reflects the geographic distribution of IBCLCs, including Europe and the Asia/Pacific region.

The exam committee meets over several days to prepare, review, edit, and select test items, which are then compiled into a draft exam based on the blueprint. The committee draws from previously used questions and from new questions submitted by IBCLCs and other experts worldwide. All questions are written in a sophisticated multiple choice format. The final exam goes through several editing and approval stages before being translated into other languages, according to demand.

Exam Confidentiality

Each year, the IBLCE uses a percentage of previously used questions on the current exam, for validity testing. It is therefore considered unethical to divulge any questions on the IBLCE exam or to request information from previous candidates. If a candidate who had received inside information were to pass the exam unfairly, it would be to the detriment of breastfeeding babies and mothers and to the profession itself.

Exam Questions

Each question in the exam has an introductory sentence or paragraph (stem). All the information necessary to answer the question is given in the stem or the accompanying picture. Candidates can be assured there are no additional complicating circumstances if they are not mentioned.

Many items refer to a clinical situation involving the mother and/or baby and ask what "you" should do. In these items, "you" means you in your role as a lactation consultant. If you have another professional role that authorizes you to perform additional functions (such as a doctor with prescribing rights), do not include these functions in the role of the lactation consultant for the purposes of this exam. See ILCA's *Standards of Practice for Lactation Consultants* to better understand the LC role.

Each item contains a specific question that you should read carefully to know what is being asked. The key word is capitalized. Some questions may ask for "the MOST appropriate intervention" or "which of the following would NOT be appropriate to recommend." The purpose of these questions is not to mislead or trick you, but to represent the types of decisions that lactation consultants often face.

For example, a mother may benefit from any of several interventions, but the lactation consultant should know the intervention that is MOST likely to be effective in her situation and why other interventions might not be as effective. At other times, there are several interventions that may be effective, but there is one that should NOT be recommended.

There may also be questions which ask for "the MOST (or LEAST) likely cause or explanation." These questions test knowledge of the general principles that apply to clinical practice, which candidates acquire through their experience.

Each item has three to five responses, most commonly four. There is only one correct answer,

and knowledgeable candidates will be able to identify why this response is correct and why the other answers are not correct. IBLCE does not use true/false questions or such options as "all of the above," "none of the above," "a and c," etc. because these types of questions are not psychometrically valid.

The Critique Form

IBLCE is unusual in that we give you a critique form to use during the exam. Comments on individual questions should be restricted only to those which you have good reason to believe may be faulty and must include an explanation or they will not be collated and considered by the post-exam review committee. You should also state which answer you chose—many comments merely tell us why an incorrect answer is incorrect.

Your comments are entirely optional and will not affect your individual score in any way.

Common misconceptions and outdated ideas are often included among the incorrect responses. Candidates should not worry that these responses are intended to be correct. The exam has been checked by experts.

How the Exam Is Scored

The pass/fail cutoff score is determined according to the Nedelsky-Gross technique, which measures the degree of difficulty of each question, based on the number of sophisticated responses that might distract candidates from the correct response. The level of difficulty of the overall exam is, therefore, based on averaging a myriad of individual analyses of each question. The more difficult the exam, the lower the pass/fail cutoff score, and vice versa.

The Nedelsky-Gross technique ensures that there is no arbitrary number or percentage of candidates who pass the exam each year, and that candidates are not competing against each other. It also ensures that variations in the degree of difficulty of the exam from one year to another will not affect an individual candidate's likelihood of passing or failing the exam. Over the years, the pass/fail cutoff has ranged between 61% and 68%.

All answer sheets are computer-scanned and scored by a consultant psychometrician. Each sheet is checked for stray marks and possible double counting where a response has been erased and replaced. Every year, a number of answer sheets are hand scored to check accuracy.

There is only one correct answer to each question. Each item receives 1 point if correct, 0 if incorrect. Points are not deducted for incorrect answers, so candidates should attempt all questions.

After all answer sheets have been initially scored, each question is individually analyzed in the post-exam review process, using performance data from all (approximately 2500) candidates. This identifies any questions that did not perform as expected or were ambiguous. If there were to be a faulty question, this post-exam review is most likely to identify it. Questions are also reviewed on the basis of comments that candidates have made on their critique forms. Questions determined to have been flawed, e.g., any with 2 correct answers, are deleted from scoring for all candidates so no one is disadvantaged. All candidates' scores are then recomputed. This quality control procedure enhances reliability, validity, and fairness.

Each year, a number of previously used questions are included in the current exam, and the performance of the current candidates on those questions is compared with how the question performed when it was previously used. This procedure enhances validity by providing a check on whether the competence level of the candidate body has changed.

The IBLCE exam has a low failure rate, yet the highest scores are typically in the mid-80% range and the mean scores in the low- to mid-70% range. This result demonstrates a well-prepared, well-screened candidate body and a challenging exam.

SUMMARY OF IBLCE EXAM ADMINISTRATION PROCEDURES

1. **INQUIRY:** You download or are sent a copy of the *Candidate Information Guide* and the *Application Supplement* specific to the exam year and your country. If you decide to do the exam in another year, you will need to request the *Application Supplement* for that year.

2. **APPLICATION:** You complete *all* pages of the application form *and* enclose the necessary documentation. You send it to us with the appropriate exam fee, postmarked by the early, regular, or late deadlines. Closing dates are strictly adhered to. You keep a copy of all your application materials. We check that your application is complete, establish your file on the database, and determine your eligibility. We confirm information, as necessary. Incomplete applications are followed up and additional fees charged. Applications are processed in the order in which they are received. In busy periods, it may take 4 to 6 weeks before your application is processed. All applications except those requiring late fees should have been checked by the end of May. We send each candidate a receipt and a letter confirming acceptance as a candidate. We notify ineligible applicants.

3. **CHANGES/ERRORS:** Check the accuracy of your name and address on correspondence you receive from us. Be sure the spelling and presentation of your name are as you wish them to appear on your admission ticket and certificate, and that the address is correct for receiving your admission package and exam results. Please notify us in writing of any changes or corrections. We update your entry in the database if there are changes or corrections. Candidate details in the database are used to coordinate administration and organization of the exam. They are confidential to IBLCE and are never released to any third party.

4. **SITE ALLOCATION:** Your preliminary site allocation is noted in your confirmation letter. If you are later notified of a change of site, contact us *immediately* if the change creates a problem. If you want a site change, inform us *immediately*. Candidate numbers at each site determine the size of the exam room, the number of proctors contracted, and the number of exam materials dispatched. If you request a site change after mid June, we may not be able to accommodate you. Initially, we place each candidate at the exam site stated on her/his application form, but we note any preference for a more convenient site. Once candidate numbers are finalized, decisions are made about which sites, if any, must be cancelled or moved and whether we will offer additional sites.

5. **ADMISSION PACKET:** Early in July, we send your exam admission packet containing your admission ticket, information about the exam site and its location, plus exam rules and arrangements for the day.

6. **SEND OUTSTANDING DOCUMENTATION:** If you had incomplete BC or education hours at the time of your application, you must complete these hours *before* the exam. You send us the documentation of completion, preferably before the exam, but in any case no later than 2 weeks after the exam (or your results may be delayed).

7. **EXAM ADMINISTRATION AND SCORING:** You take the exam. We send your answer sheets to be computer scored by IBLCE's psychometrician. This process is time consuming, since the validity of each question is checked by a number of procedures. The exam review committee meets and some questions are deleted from scoring before all answer sheets are rescored. The exam as a whole is also validated.

8. **EXAM RESULTS:** We mail your exam results to you in mid-October. We mail all pass and fail letters on the same day, but experience has shown that some candidates receive their letters on a different day than other candidates, even in the same city. On the same day as the results are mailed, we also post them on the website, using a unique code number issued to each candidate. If you did not complete your BC or education hours before the exam, or if you did not send the documentation to us, your exam results will not be issued. If you have failed the exam, we send you your score report; your details remain confidential to IBLCE. If you have passed the exam, we send you your certificate, score report, your IBCLC ID card, and your copy of *The IBCLC Handbook.*

PREPARING FOR THE EXAM

Study Strategies

Because each candidate's background and experience are different, you are expected to determine your own strengths and weaknesses in the relevant *disciplines* and *chronological periods* and to organize your own program of study. The following information may help you organize your study, and it may be used in conjunction with other sections of this appendix: *IBLCE Exam Blueprint* and *Clinical Competencies Checklist*; the Suggested Reading List (http://www.iblce.org/reading%20list.htm) and also ILCA's *Standards of Practice.*

Plan your study program ahead and determine how you study best. Do you learn better on your own or when you can discuss material with colleagues? You may want to organize a study group or find a study partner, then take turns in preparing and presenting topics. Some people learn well from working through a textbook cover-to-cover; others prefer to choose a topic and study different sources of information.

Identify areas where your background has given you little experience and ensure you cover these areas in your preparation. For example, if you have worked only in a hospital postnatal area, you may have little experience with breastfeeding beyond the early period. Use the *Checklist of Suggested Activities* in this appendix as a checklist to see how well prepared you are.

We strongly suggest that you check off the *IBLCE Exam Blueprint* and the *Clinical Competencies Checklist* and be sure you have addressed all areas. Typically, candidates' exam scores are lower in the disciplines that are less clinical (G, H, I, J, and M), and yet practicing lactation consultants consider that these are important aspects of their work. To gain a better understanding of the roles and skills required, try to spend time with experienced IBCLCs working in various settings.

Allow time to integrate your new knowledge and skills into your practice. Two thirds of the exam questions will test your application of knowledge.

In determining how deeply to study a subject area, you need to ask yourself what a lactation consultant might need to know. As you study each topic, ask yourself how the information might fit into the broad scope of an IBCLC's practice. The practical application of your knowledge is the ultimate purpose of your study.

IBLCE Recognition Statement about Mother-to-Mother Support Organizations

The International Board of Lactation Consultant Examiners recognizes the critical role served by mother-to-mother support organizations such as La Leche League and the Australian Breastfeeding Association in support of mothers and babies in the initiation and duration of breastfeeding. These organizations also serve a vital role in providing the experiential base for developing the breastfeeding expertise of mother-to-mother support group leaders/counselors and lactation consultants. In addition, these organizations provide essential continuing education for leaders/ counselors/lactation consultants and others, disseminating knowledge and information based upon empirical research and clinical experience.

---

www.iblce.org

This is the address for the IBLCE website. This is where you can find further information about the IBLCE, the exam, recertification and CERPs, and where you can download the *Guide* and the *Application Form*. This is where you can find out more about the IBLCE board and the administrative team. This is where you can find the registry of names of currently certified IBCLCs. This is where you can find the latest information in the news section. This is where you can read the most recently published statistical report on the IBLCE exam. This is where you will find links to the lactation consultant professional associations. This is where you can find information about professional standards, including the *Code of Ethics for IBCLCs* and the *Clinical Competencies Checklist.*

CHECKLIST OF SUGGESTED ACTIVITIES

The *IBLCE Exam Blueprint* covers many *disciplines* and *chronological periods.* The experiences in each candidate's background may not address all areas listed. For example, someone who works on a postpartum ward may have little experience with older breastfeeding babies. An accredited mother support counselor may have little experience with premature or special care babies. A candidate with children of her or his own may have a better knowledge of child development.

It is vital that lactation consultants are thoroughly familiar with normal breastfeeding. This puts abnormal situations and experiences into perspective.

The following suggested activities may help broaden the scope of your professional development. You should seek to observe areas that are not part of your everyday work experience. Although most of these activities will not be applicable toward your clinical practice hours, they will help to make you aware of deficiencies in your background and increase the efficiency of your preparation. This list is in no particular order and is a starting point only; you may think of other activities that will augment your general breastfeeding consultant experience.

As you prepare for the exam, tick the boxes on this checklist to measure the breadth of your experiences.

☐ Work with or observe a lactation consultant to study her or his experiences and client interactions.

☐ Expand your professional education to a broad spectrum of programs. Consider attending a childbirth conference, a seminar conducted by a professional association, or sessions presented by a lawyer, a dietician, or a human relations counselor. Although only lactation topics meet the exam eligibility requirement, other professional education opportunities are also valuable.

☐ Study the anatomy and physiology of the breast in detail, including how milk is synthesized. A course may help. A thorough knowledge of the underlying structures and functions of the breast is essential, as it will enable you to assess each mother and her problems on an individual basis and will help you develop a management plan specific to the mother and her baby.

☐ Learn about infant oral anatomy and development.

☐ Offer to present a session to your colleagues on the biochemistry of human milk, or a similar challenging topic. Presenting a topic usually requires you to develop a real understanding of the subject matter you are talking about.

☐ Observe the interaction of a mother and baby continuously for the first 2 hours after birth. Compare the baby of a mother who used no medication during labor with the baby of a mother who used pain-relief medication.

☐ Study the interactions of newborns with their mothers.

☐ Attend a variety of mother-to-mother support meetings to observe mothers and babies and to learn breastfeeding techniques. Note how counselors listen, ask questions, practice ethics, etc.

☐ Observe the developmental milestones of babies and young children in a casual setting. You might spend time at a playground, a play group, or a mother support gathering watching the interactions of mothers and babies/toddlers. Try to guess the ages of babies/toddlers by observing their developmental activity level. Ask the mother her child's age to see if you have determined correctly.

☐ Do a study of the normal growth, development, and breastfeeding behavior of a single baby over a 6-month period. Describe the first few days and weeks. How do these differ from breastfeeding at 6 months?

☐ Have an IBCLC observe your consultations or interactions with mothers. Ask her or him to critique different things at different times—your counseling skills, your problem-solving skills, your practical skills, or your breastfeeding knowledge in the clinical situation.

☐ Become a mother support group newsletter subscriber. These publications are generally full of mothers' personal experiences.

☐ Sit with an IBCLC who is staffing a breastfeeding phone counseling line. Listen to her/his counseling techniques.

☐ Attend a Baby-Friendly Hospital Initiative course. Review hospital practices to see how breastfeeding friendly they are. What types of breastfeeding problems might poor hospital practices generate? How might these be prevented?

☐ Seek out a professional lactation consultant organization for support, information, and educational opportunities.

While these suggestions are not mandatory, they will help you to broaden your perspective, enhance your skills, and focus your studies in this multidisciplinary field. You may think you are going to use the credential only in your current practice setting, but IBCLCs are qualified and accountable for competence in all practice settings.

We are continually trying to improve the materials we publish. So, if you have any suggestions to help us when next we revise the *Candidate Information Guide,* the *Application Form,* or the *Application Supplement,* please let us know. The easiest way is to send us a message by email, at: exam@iblce.org.

SAMPLE EXAM QUESTIONS FROM IBLCE *CANDIDATE'S GUIDE* 2006

These sample questions are indicative of the *types* of questions you can expect in the exam. They are not representative of the overall degree of difficulty, so "passing" this exam is not an indication that you are ready to pass the IBLCE exam. These questions are from old exams and more likely to be easier because they are testing more basic knowledge. The number and letter in parentheses after each question indicates the *chronological period* and the *discipline* on the *IBLCE Exam Blueprint*. The answers are shown in a box at the end.

1. A woman interrupts your breastfeeding class to ask you about breastfeeding an anticipated adopted baby. She has been using an electric pump and has generated a 1 oz (30 ml) per day supply. What should you do FIRST?

   A. Praise her for her interest and offer to meet with her later to discuss it further.

   B. Ask how she plans to provide nutrition for the baby beyond her own 1 oz (30 ml) per day production.

   C. Thank her for attending and ease her out the door as quickly as possible.

   D. Inform her that it is unlikely she will bring in more milk. **[1-G]**

2. A pregnant woman contacts you after attending a prenatal class on infant feeding. The instructor has been very positive about breastfeeding, but emphasized that lactation hormones may affect sexual functioning. You should tell her that lactation hormones usually:

   A. reduce libido.

   B. increase libido.

   C. reduce vaginal lubrication.

   D. increase vaginal lubrication.

   E. do not affect libido or vaginal lubrication.

   [2-B]

3. Which of the following techniques minimizes the risk of causing nipple trauma?

   A. Position the infant on his back in his mother's arms and elicit the rooting reflex; when the infant turns his head, place the nipple in his mouth.

   B. Support the breast using the first and second fingers on either side of the areola.

   C. Prevent the nipple from coming in contact with the infant's soft palate to decrease the incidence of tongue thrusting.

   D. Position the infant so that his entire body faces the mother, and much of the areolar tissue is in the infant's mouth. **[5-L]**

4. The MOST advantageous moment for the first breastfeed of a premature infant is when the baby is:

   A. awake and in an alert state.

   B. crying from a recently performed procedure and needing comfort.

   C. relaxed, peaceful, and drowsy.

   D. in a deep sleep and unable to resist an attempt to put the breast into his mouth.

   [4-L]

5. The definitive symptom of incorrect positioning of a baby at the breast is:

   A. nipple pain.

   B. irritated, inflamed nipple epithelium.

   C. stabbing pain when the baby latches on.

   D. a compression stripe across the nipple.

   E. blanching of the whole nipple after feeding.

   [6-L]

6. You are a lactation consultant in private practice. A mother reports that she feels rejected by her 2-week-old infant's refusal to breastfeed, and she wants to hit him. How should this conversation be handled for documentation purposes?

   A. Do not write any notes, since they can be subpoenaed.

   B. Write her statement as a quote and urgently phone the physician or an appropriate social service agency.

   C. Contact a lawyer.

   D. Take written notes and require that the mother initial them.

   [12-J]

7. A mother had been expressing to maintain her milk supply for her very sick baby. You have been seeing her weekly and her son is now 4 months old and has been hospitalized since birth. When told 3 days ago that her son would be in the hospital for a year, she stopped expressing. You should:

   A. begin intensive counseling to convince her to relactate.

   B. discontinue meeting with her.

   C. meet with her a final time to explain how to dry up her milk.

   D. send her a leaflet on breastfeeding, bringing her attention to drying up one's milk.

   E. continue to meet with her until both of you feel comfortable with ending the appointments.

   [9-G]

8. A mother contacts you complaining of overall aching and fatigue and has a fever of 103°F (39.4°C). Her breast is sore and has red streaks. Her baby refuses to breastfeed. The MOST important thing you should advise her to do is:

   A. go to bed and get plenty of rest, arranging for the father to give the baby a bottle of formula at night.

   B. breastfeed frequently, offering the affected side first.

   C. see her doctor to discuss antibiotic treatment.

   D. offer the unaffected breast only.   [12-E]

9. For babies, objects and people do not exist when out of sight. In which of the following age ranges is this perception most likely to change?

   A. 3–5 months

   B. 6–9 months

   C. 10–13 months

   D. 14–17 months   [10-H]

10. A mother is found to be HIV positive as a result of artificial insemination. She breastfed her baby, who is now 6 months old, for the first 6 weeks. The child will MOST likely have:

    A. no symptoms of AIDS and no HIV antibodies.

    B. no symptoms of AIDS, but he may have HIV antibodies.

    C. symptoms of AIDS and no HIV antibodies.

    D. symptoms of AIDS and HIV antibodies.

    [9-D]

A statistical report on the most recent exam is published each year by IBLCE's psychometrician, Dr. Leon Gross. The report can be read on the IBLCE website and is updated each year, usually in early December. Please visit **www.iblce.org**

11. The mother of a 19-month-old baby is concerned because he wants to breastfeed at naptime and bedtime, and he appears to have little appetite for other foods. The doctor considered him to be very healthy at his 18-month checkup, but the mother still worries that his continued breastfeedings are preventing him from eating enough solid foods. Your BEST response is:

    A. Toddlers who drink too much milk and do not eat enough solid foods can develop "milk anemia."

    B. Many toddlers have small appetites, whether they are weaned or not.

    C. Human milk is all he needs.

    D. Human milk has very little nutritional value for a 19-month-old child. [11-H]

12. You are working with an obstetrician in conducting a study of pregnant women who have inverted nipples. The study requires photo documentation of the women's breasts. What is the MOST appropriate legal and ethical procedure in taking these photographs?

    A. Obtain written release from the women before photographing them.

    B. Obtain written release from the women after photographing them.

    C. Obtain written release from the women only if the photographs are to be submitted for publication.

    D. Offer written assurance to share any royalties from the use of the photographs. [2-J]

Negative Stem Question Construction

The following questions are samples of certain kinds of construction forms with which some candidates may be unfamiliar. Because this type of question requires a "mental shift" to think in negative terms after answering a series of positive questions, candidates sometimes interpret them as ambiguous or tricky. However, in spite of these concerns, the construction forms below are psychometrically valid and they represent skills that lactation consultants use. As familiarity and practice may help allay candidate concerns, these questions are grouped according to three common construction types. Work through them carefully and the interpretation shift will become evident. You will be alerted to the groups of negative stem questions on the exam and you should take special care to make the mental shift.

The "NOT" Construction

13. A 9-day-old infant with cleft palate defects should NOT be positioned for feedings with its body:

    A. in the cradle or across-the-front position.

    B. semi-upright or upright.

    C. in the clutch/underarm position.

    D. prone. [6-E]

14. Which of the following is NOT a developmental indicator for introducing solid foods?

    A. baby shows interest in table foods.

    B. baby has the fine motor skills to grasp food with the thumb and fingers.

    C. baby swallows without tongue protrusion.

    D. baby can hold and drink from a cup with few spills. [9-H]

15. Which of the following is NOT a part of normal sucking technique?

    A. tongue darting in and out

    B. tongue covering the gum line

    C. tongue curved around the breast

    D. jaws rhythmically compressing the areola

    E. lips flanged [5-L]

16. Which of the following foods is NOT a good source of calcium?

    A. natural cheese

    B. red meat

    C. almonds

    D. dark green, leafy vegetables [12-C]

The "LEAST Likely" Construction

17. A mother contacts you because she is concerned that her 3-month-old baby is suddenly waking up more frequently at night, in spite of being breastfed at least every 3 hours during the day. Which of the following would be the LEAST appropriate response?

    A. The baby may be experiencing a growth spurt.

    B. The baby may be experiencing the discomforts of early teething.

    C. The baby may have a chronic or low-grade infection and should be examined by the doctor.

    D. The baby does not need feedings at night at this age and is using you as a pacifier. [8-G]

18. After several years of planning, a hospital will be implementing a new breastfeeding protocol. Which of the following components of the protocol is LEAST LIKELY to promote breastfeeding success?

    A. early initiation of breastfeeding

    B. progressive lengthening of time at the breast

    C. nighttime breastfeeding

    D. supplements only when medically indicated [5-M]

19. A mother, 4 months postpartum, has a large lump at the 12:00 position on the areola. She can express a yellowish, thick fluid from the corresponding nipple pore. The LEAST LIKELY cause of this lump is:

    A. a plugged milk duct.

    B. a galactocele.

    C. a neoplasm.

    D. an abscess. [9-E]

20. A woman is ready to be discharged from the hospital. She will be returning to work when her baby is 8 weeks old. She wants to express milk at work and have her milk fed to her baby by her child care provider. She asks you what she can do during those first few weeks to promote a smooth transition back to work. Which of the following suggestions is LEAST LIKELY to help her?

    A. Try to arrange a longer maternity leave.

    B. Be sure that she has a child care provider who is supportive of breastfeeding, and that she freezes some extra breast milk for the first few days when her return to work will likely cause her milk supply to diminish.

    C. Breastfeed the baby exclusively for 4–6 weeks and then start bottle feeding expressed breast-milk several times per week, so that the baby will take a bottle when she leave.

    D. Introduce the bottle during the first week in order to accustom the baby to it. [5-H]

The "EXCEPT" Construction

21. Actual drug passage to breast milk is dependent upon all of the following EXCEPT:

    A. milk pH.

    B. drug teratogenicity.

    C. drug solubility.

    D. drug ionization.

    E. lipid solubility. [12-F]

22. You should expect breastfeeding problems with a baby who has a cleft defect to include all of the following EXCEPT:

    A. forming a seal.

    B. maintaining a vacuum.

    C. positioning his tongue over his gum line.

    D. preventing aspiration. **[6-E]**

23. All of the following can be responsible for sub-optimal milk production EXCEPT:

    A. short frequent feedings.

    B. insufficient mammary glandular tissue.

    C. lower than normal prolactin level.

    D. retained placental fragment. **[12-B]**

Exam Strategies

Both the morning and afternoon sections are 3 hours each. This is sufficient for even slow test takers and candidates doing the exam in a second language to finish. During the afternoon session there will be 75 questions that correspond to clinical photographs in the exam booklet.

There are no penalties for incorrect answers, so attempt every question, even those of which you are not sure. This strategy will increase your

---

Exam Strategies (continued)

chance of passing and prevent mismatching subsequent questions with the wrong numbers on your answer sheet. You may mark in your test booklet the questions you wish to reconsider and return to them later. If you change an answer, be sure to erase your original answer completely.

Questions with a negative stem construction (see samples shown previously) are grouped together on the exam with a note advising you when they start. These are not trick questions, but they need careful attention.

Questions are not arranged in order of difficulty or subject matter. Therefore, you can work out how many questions you should complete within a chosen time interval and pace yourself accordingly.

Answers to Sample Questions

1. A	2. C	3. D	4. A	5. A	6. B
7. E	8. C	9. B	10. B	11. B	12. A
13. D	14. D	15. A	16. B	17. D	18. B
19. C	20. D	21. B	22. C	23. A	

CODE OF ETHICS FOR IBCLCs 2004

PREAMBLE

It is in the best interests of the profession of lactation consultants and the public it serves that there be a Code of Ethics to provide guidance to lactation consultants in their professional practice and conduct. These ethical principles guide the profession and outline commitments and obligations of the lactation consultant to self, client, colleagues, society, and the profession.

The purpose of the International Board of Lactation Consultant Examiners (IBLCE) is to assist in the protection of the health, safety, and welfare of the public by establishing and enforcing qualifications of certification and for issuing voluntary credentials to individuals who have attained those qualifications. The IBLCE has adopted this Code to apply to all individuals who hold the credential of International Board Certified Lactation Consultant.

Principles of Ethical Practice

The International Board Certified Lactation Consultant shall act in a manner that safeguards the interests of individual clients, justifies public trust in her/his competence, and enhances the reputation of the profession.

The International Board Certified Lactation Consultant is personally accountable for her/his practice and, in the exercise of professional accountability, must:

1. Provide professional services with objectivity and with respect for the unique needs and values of individuals.

2. Avoid discrimination against other individuals on the basis of race, creed, religion, gender, sexual orientation, age, and national origin.

3. Fulfill professional commitments in good faith.

4. Conduct herself/himself with honesty, integrity, and fairness.

5. Remain free of conflict of interest while fulfilling the objectives and maintaining the integrity of the lactation consultant profession.

6. Maintain confidentiality.

7. Base her/his practice on scientific principles, and on current research and information.

8. Take responsibility and accept accountability for personal competence in practice.

9. Recognize and exercise professional judgment within the limits of her/his qualifications. This principle includes seeking counsel and making referrals to appropriate providers.

10. Inform the public and colleagues of his/her services by using factual information. An International Board Certified Lactation Consultant shall not advertise in a false or misleading manner.

11. Provide sufficient information to enable clients to make informed decisions.

12. Provide information about appropriate products in a manner that is neither false nor misleading.

13. Permit use of her/his name for the purpose of certifying that lactation consultant services have been rendered only if she/he provided those services.

14. Present professional qualifications and credentials accurately, using "IBCLC" only when certification is current and authorized by the IBLCE, and complying with all requirements when seeking initial or continued certification from the IBLCE. The lactation consultant is also subject to disciplinary action for aiding another person in violating any IBLCE requirements or aiding another person in representing herself/himself as an IBCLC when she/he is not.

15. Report to an appropriate person or authority when it appears that the health or safety of colleagues is at risk, as such circumstances may compromise standards of practice and care.

16. Refuse any gift, favor, or hospitality from patients or clients currently in her/his care that might be interpreted as seeking to exert influence to obtain preferential consideration.

17. Disclose any financial or other conflicts of interest in relevant organizations providing goods or services. Ensure that professional judgment is not influenced by any commercial considerations.

18. Present substantiated information and interpret controversial information without personal bias, recognizing that legitimate differences of opinion exist.

19. Withdraw voluntarily from professional practice if she/he has engaged in any substance abuse that could affect her/his practice; has been adjudged by a court to be mentally incompetent; or has an emotional or mental disability that affects her/his practice in a manner that could harm the client.

20. Obtain maternal consent to photograph, audiotape, or videotape a mother and/or her infant(s) for educational or professional purposes.

21. Submit to disciplinary action under the following circumstances: if convicted of a crime under the laws of the practitioner's country that is a felony or a misdemeanor, an essential element of which is dishonesty, and that is related to the practice of lactation consulting; if disciplined by a national, state, province, or local government or authority, and at least one of the grounds for the discipline is the same or substantially equivalent to these principles; if committed an act of misfeasance or malfeasance which is directly related to the practice of the profession as determined by a court of competent jurisdiction, a licensing board, or an agency of a governmental body; or if violated a Principle set forth in the *Code of Ethics for International Board Certified Lactation Consultants* that was in force at the time of the violation.

22. Accept the obligation to protect society and the profession by upholding the *Code of Ethics for International Board Certified Lactation Consultants* and by reporting alleged violations of the Code through the defined review process of the IBLCE.

23. Require and obtain consent to share clinical concerns and information with the medical practitioner or other primary health care provider before initiating a consultation.

24. Adhere to those provisions of the *International Code of Marketing of Breast-Milk Substitutes* and subsequent WHA resolutions that pertain to health workers.

25. Understand, recognize, respect, and acknowledge intellectual property rights, including but not limited to copyrights (which apply to written material, photographs, slides, illustrations, etc.), trademarks, service marks, and patents.

Effective December 1, 2004

TO LODGE A COMPLAINT

IBCLCs shall act in a manner that justifies public trust in their competence, enhances the reputation of the profession, and safeguards the interests of individual clients.

To protect the credential and to assure responsible practice by its certificants, the IBLCE depends on IBCLCs, members of the coordinating and supervising health professions, employers, and the public to report incidents that may require action by the IBLCE Discipline Committee.

Only signed, written complaints will be considered. Anonymous correspondence will be discarded. The IBLCE will become involved only in matters that can be factually determined, and will provide the accused party with every opportunity to respond in a professional and legally defensible manner.

Complaints that appear to fit the scope of the Discipline Committee's responsibilities should be sent to:

> **IBLCE, Chair of the Discipline Committee**
> **7245 Arlington Boulevard, Suite 200**
> **Falls Church VA 22042-3217 USA**

Inquiries may be directed to ethics@iblce.org.

COMPETENCY STATEMENTS

The following competency statements identify and summarize the special knowledge and skills included in the role of an International Board Certified Lactation Consultant (IBCLC), Registered Lactation Consultant (RLC).

The International Board Certified Lactation Consultant, Registered Lactation Consultant will:

1. Possess the skills, knowledge, and attitudes to provide competent comprehensive consultation and education in routine and special circumstance lactation, from pre-conception to beyond 12 months.

2. Integrate additional knowledge from the following disciplines in providing care for breastfeeding families: maternal and infant anatomy; physiology and endocrinology; nutrition and biochemistry; immunology and infectious disease; pathology; pharmacology and toxicology; psychology, sociology, and anthropology; growth parameters and developmental milestones; interpretation of research; ethical and legal issues; breastfeeding equipment and technology; techniques; and public health.

3. Utilize knowledge of personality, counseling skills, and family and group theory when providing breastfeeding support.

4. Integrate cultural, psychosocial, nutritional, and pharmacological aspects of breastfeeding into lactation consultant practice.

5. Utilize appropriate communication skills in interactions with clients and health care providers.

6. Maintain a collaborative, supportive relationship with clients, emphasizing individualized family care, client autonomy, informed decision making, and optimal health care.

7. Act as an advocate for breastfeeding in the community, in the workplace, and within the health care professions.

8. Utilize adult learning principles when providing educational experiences for clients, health care providers, and the community.

9. Interpret current research findings to determine appropriateness for application to practice.

10. Function and contribute as a member of the healthcare team, provide follow-up plans, and make appropriate referrals to other health care providers and community support resources.

11. Maintain comprehensive client records.

12. Follow a professional code of ethics, local laws and codes, and maintain appropriate standards of hygiene.

13. Observe the guidelines for health workers outlined in the WHO International Code of Marketing of Breast-Milk Substitutes.

14. Maintain and enhance knowledge and skills with appropriate and regular continuing education.

A more detailed description of the role and skills of a lactation consultant is provided in *Standards of Practice for Lactation Consultants,* published by the International Lactation Consultant Association (ILCA).

> website: www.ilca.org
> email: info@ilca.org

CLINICAL COMPETENCIES CHECKLIST[2]

Much of the clinical practice of the International Board Certified Lactation Consultant (IBCLC) consists of systematic problem solving in collaboration with breastfeeding mothers and other members of the health care team. This checklist includes most of the clinical/practical skills that an entry-level IBCLC needs in order to be satisfactorily proficient to provide safe and effective care for breastfeeding mothers and babies. The list is designed to encompass common breastfeeding situations and the challenges that are encountered most frequently by lactation consultants. This checklist can help you identify areas where you have less experience or knowledge, and you are encouraged to try to focus your professional education on these aspects. Clinical instructors can use this checklist as an appropriate guide in providing individualized education.

Communication and Counseling Skills

In all interactions with mothers, families, health care professionals, and peers, the student will demonstrate effective communication skills to maintain collaborative and supportive relationships. *The student will:*

- ☐ Identify factors that might affect communication (i.e., age, cultural/language differences, hearing or visual impairment, mental ability, etc.)
- ☐ Demonstrate appropriate body language (i.e., position in relation to the other person, comfortable eye contact, appropriate tone of voice for the setting, etc.)
- ☐ Demonstrate knowledge of and sensitivity to cultural differences
- ☐ Elicit information using effective counseling techniques (i.e., asking open-ended questions, summarizing the discussion, and providing emotional support)

---

[2] IBLCE thanks ILCA and the IBCLCs from all over the world who worked on developing these clinical competencies.

☐ Make appropriate referrals to other health care professionals and community resources

The student will provide individualized breastfeeding care with an emphasis on the mother's ability to make informed decisions. *The student will:*

☐ Assess mother's psychological state and provide information appropriate to her situation

☐ Include those family members or friends the mother identifies as significant to her

☐ Obtain the mother's permission for providing care to her or her baby

☐ Ascertain the mother's knowledge about and goals for breastfeeding

☐ Use adult education principles to provide instruction to the mother that will meet her needs

☐ Select appropriate written information and other teaching aids

History Taking and Assessment Skills

The student will be able to:

☐ Obtain a pertinent history
☐ Perform a breast evaluation related to lactation
☐ Develop a breastfeeding risk assessment
☐ Assess and evaluate the infant's ability to breastfeed
☐ Assess effective milk transfer

Documentation and Communication Skills with Health Professionals

The student will:

☐ Communicate effectively with other members of the health care team, using written documents appropriate to the location, facility, and culture in which the student is being trained, such as consent forms, care plans, charting forms/clinical notes, pathways/care maps, and feeding assessment forms

☐ Use appropriate resources for research to provide information to the health care team on conditions and medications that affect breastfeeding and lactation

☐ Write referrals and follow-up documentation/letters to referring and/or primary health care providers that illustrate the student's ability to identify:

☐ The mother's concerns or problems, planned interventions, evaluation of outcomes, and follow-up

☐ Situations in which immediate verbal communication with the health care provider is necessary, such as serious illness in the infant, child, or mother

☐ Report instances of child abuse or neglect to specific agencies as appropriate or legally required

Skills for the First Two Hours after Birth

The student will:

☐ Identify events that occurred during the labor and birth process that may adversely affect breastfeeding

☐ Identify and discourage practices that may interfere with breastfeeding

☐ Promote continuous skin-to-skin contact of the term newborn and mother until the first breastfeed

☐ Assist the mother and family to identify newborn feeding cues

☐ Help the mother and infant to find a comfortable position for latch-on/attachment during the first breastfeed after birth

☐ Identify correct latch-on/attachment

☐ Reinforce to mother and family the importance of:

☐ Keeping the mother and baby together
☐ Feeding the baby on cue—but at least 8 times in each 24-hour period

Postpartum Skills

Prior to a mother–baby dyad's discharge from care, the student will observe a breastfeed and effectively instruct the mother about:

☐ Assessment of adequate milk intake by the baby

☐ Normal infant sucking patterns

☐ How milk is produced and supply maintained, including discussion of growth/appetite spurts

☐ Normal newborn behavior, including why, when, and how to wake a sleepy newborn

☐ Avoidance of early use of a dummy/pacifier and bottle teat

☐ Importance of exclusive breast milk feeds and possible consequences of mixed feedings with cow's milk or soy

☐ Prevention and treatment of sore nipples

☐ Prevention and treatment of engorgement

☐ SIDS prevention behaviors

☐ Family planning methods and their relationship to breastfeeding

☐ Education regarding drugs (such as nicotine, alcohol, caffeine, and illicit drugs) and complementary remedies (such as herbal teas)

☐ Plans for follow-up care for breastfeeding questions, infant's medical, and mother's postpartum examinations

☐ Community resources for breastfeeding assistance

Problem-Solving Skills

The student will be able to:

☐ Identify problems

☐ Assess contributing factors and cause

☐ Develop an appropriate breastfeeding plan in consultation with the mother

☐ Assist the mother to implement the plan

☐ Evaluate effectiveness of the plan

Skills for Maternal Breastfeeding Challenges

The student will be able to assist mothers with the following challenges:

☐ Cesarean birth

☐ Flat/inverted nipples

☐ Thrush infections of breast, nipple, areola, and milk ducts

☐ Continuation of breastfeeding when mother is separated from her baby

    ☐ Milk expression techniques

    ☐ Maintaining milk production

    ☐ Collection, storage, and transportation of milk

☐ Cultural beliefs that are not evidence based and may interfere with breastfeeding (i.e., discarding colostrum, rigidly scheduled feedings, necessity of formula after every breastfeeding, etc.)

☐ Medical conditions that may impact on breastfeeding

☐ Adolescent mother

    ☐ Strategies for returning to school

    ☐ Maintaining milk production

☐ Nipple pain and damage

☐ Engorgement

☐ Blocked duct and/or nipple pore

☐ Mastitis

☐ Breast surgery/trauma

☐ Overproduction of milk

☐ Postpartum psychological issues including transient sadness ("baby blues") and postpartum depression

☐ Appropriate referrals

☐ Medications compatible with breastfeeding

☐ Insufficient milk supply, differentiating between perceived and real

☐ Weaning issues

☐ Safe formula preparation and feeding techniques

☐ Care of breasts

Skills for Infant Breastfeeding Challenges

The student will be able to assist mothers who have infants with the following challenges:
- ☐ Traumatic birth
- ☐ 35–38 weeks' gestation
- ☐ Small for gestational age (SGA) or large for gestational age (LGA)
- ☐ Multiple births
- ☐ Preterm birth, including the benefits of kangaroo care
- ☐ High risk for hypoglycemia
- ☐ Sleepy infant
- ☐ Excessive weight loss, slow/poor weight gain
- ☐ Hyperbilirubinemia (jaundice)
- ☐ Ankyloglossia (short frenulum)
- ☐ Thrush infection
- ☐ Colic/fussiness
- ☐ Gastric reflux
- ☐ Lactose overload
- ☐ Food intolerances
- ☐ Neurodevelopmental problems
- ☐ Teething and biting
- ☐ Breast refusal/early baby-led weaning
- ☐ Breastfeeding a toddler
- ☐ Breastfeeding through pregnancy
- ☐ Tandem feeding

Management Skills

The student will demonstrate the ability to:
- ☐ Perform a comprehensive breastfeeding assessment
- ☐ Assess milk transfer
- ☐ Calculate an infant's caloric/kilojoule and volume requirements
- ☐ Increase milk production

Skills for Use of Technology and Devices

The student will have up-to-date knowledge about breastfeeding-related equipment and demonstrate appropriate use and understanding of potential disadvantages or risks of the following:
- ☐ A device to evert nipples
- ☐ Nipple creams/ointments
- ☐ Breast shells
- ☐ Breast pumps
- ☐ Alternative feeding techniques
  - ☐ Tube feeding at the breast
  - ☐ Cup feeding
  - ☐ Spoon feeding
  - ☐ Eyedropper feeding
  - ☐ Finger feeding
  - ☐ Bottles and artificial nipples/teats
- ☐ Nipple shields
- ☐ Pacifiers/soothers
- ☐ Infant scales
- ☐ Use of herbal supplements for mother and/or infant

Skills for Breastfeeding Challenges That Are Encountered Infrequently

The following issues are encountered relatively infrequently and might not be seen during the student's training. The entry-level lactation consultant would not be expected to be proficient in these situations, but should have the basic skills to assist the mother and infant while seeking guidance from a more experienced IBCLC.

Infant:
- ☐ Infant with tonic bite/ineffective/dysfunctional suck

☐ Cranial-facial abnormalities, such as micronathia (receding lower jaw) and cleft lip and/or palate

☐ Down syndrome

☐ Cardiac problems

☐ Chronic medical conditions, such as cystic fibrosis, PKU, etc.

Mother:

☐ Induced lactation and relactation

☐ Coping with the death of an infant

☐ Chronic medical conditions, such as multiple sclerosis, lupus, seizures, etc.

☐ Disabilities that may limit mother's ability to handle the baby easily, such as rheumatoid arthritis, carpal tunnel syndrome, cerebral palsy, etc.

☐ HIV/AIDS: understanding of current recommendations

Skills for Meeting Professional Responsibilities

The student will demonstrate the following professional responsibilities:

☐ Conduct herself or himself in a professional manner, by complying with the IBLCE *Code of Ethics for International Board Certified Lactation Consultants* and the ILCA *Standards of Practice*; and by adhering to the *International Code of Marketing of Breast-Milk Substitutes* and its subsequent World Health Assembly resolutions.

☐ Practice within the laws of the setting in which s/he works, showing respect for confidentiality and privacy.

☐ Use current research findings to provide a strong evidence base for clinical practice, and obtain continuing education to enhance skills and obtain/maintain IBCLC certification.

☐ Advocate for breastfeeding families, mothers, infants and children in the workplace, community, and within the health care system.

☐ Use breastfeeding equipment appropriately and provide information about risks as well as benefits of products, maintaining an awareness of conflict of interest if profiting from the rental or sale of breastfeeding equipment.

Sites for Acquisition of Skills

The student may acquire clinical/practical skills in the following settings:

☐ Private practice IBCLC office

☐ Private obstetric, pediatric, family, or independent midwifery practice

☐ Public health department; Women, Infants and Children (WIC) Program (in the U.S.); maternal and child health services

☐ Hospital

  ☐ Lactation services

  ☐ Birthing center

  ☐ Postpartum unit

  ☐ Mother–baby unit

  ☐ Level II and level III nurseries: special care nursery, neonatal intensive care nursery

  ☐ Pediatric unit

☐ Home health (community nursing) services

☐ Outpatient follow-up breastfeeding clinics

☐ Breastfeeding telephone counseling services

☐ Prenatal and postpartum breastfeeding classes

☐ Home births (if legally permitted)

☐ Volunteer community support group meetings

B. STANDARDS OF PRACTICE FOR INTERNATIONAL BOARD CERTIFIED LACTATION CONSULTANTS[1]

PREFACE

This is the third edition of *Standards of Practice for International Board Certified Lactation Consultants* (IBCLCs) published by the International Lactation Consultant Association (ILCA). All individuals practicing as a currently certified IBCLC should adhere to ILCA's *Standards of Practice* and the International Board of Lactation Consultant Examiners' (IBLCE) *Code of Ethics for International Board Certified Lactation Consultants* in all interactions with clients, families, and other health care professionals. ILCA recognizes the certification conferred by the IBLCE as the worldwide professional credential for lactation consultants.

Quality practice and service are the core responsibilities of a profession to the public. Standards of practice are stated measures or levels of quality that are models for the conduct and evaluation of practice. Standards of practice:
- promote consistency by encouraging a common systematic approach
- are sufficiently specific in content to guide daily practice
- provide a recommended framework for the development of policies and protocols, educational programs, and quality improvement efforts
- are intended for use in diverse practice settings and cultural contexts

STANDARD 1. PROFESSIONAL RESPONSIBILITIES

The IBCLC has a responsibility to maintain professional conduct and to practice in an ethical manner, accountable for professional actions and legal responsibilities.
1.1 Adhere to these ILCA *Standards of Practice* and the IBLCE *Code of Ethics*
1.2 Practice within the scope of the *International Code of Marketing of Breast-Milk Substitutes* and all subsequent World Health Assembly resolutions
1.3 Maintain an awareness of conflict of interest in all aspects of work, especially when profiting from the rental or sale of breastfeeding equipment and services
1.4 Act as an advocate for breastfeeding women, infants, and children
1.5 Assist the mother in maintaining a breastfeeding relationship with her child
1.6 Maintain and expand knowledge and skills for lactation consultant practice by participating in continuing education
1.7 Undertake periodic and systematic evaluation of one's clinical practice
1.8 Support and promote well-designed research in human lactation and breastfeeding, and base clinical practice, whenever possible, on such research

---

1. Approved by the Board of Directors, October 2005. Copyright © 2005 International Lactation Consultant Association. Copies of the Standards of Practice document may be freely made, so long as the content remains unchanged, and they are distributed free-of-charge.

STANDARD 2. LEGAL CONSIDERATIONS

The IBCLC is obligated to practice within the laws of the geopolitical region and setting in which she/he works. The IBCLC must practice with consideration for rights of privacy and with respect for matters of a confidential nature.

2.1 Work within the policies and procedures of the institution where employed, or if self-employed, have identifiable policies and procedures to follow

2.2 Clearly state applicable fees prior to providing care

2.3 Obtain informed consent from all clients prior to:
  - assessing or intervening
  - reporting relevant information to other health care professional(s)
  - taking photographs for any purpose
  - seeking publication of information associated with the consultation

2.4 Protect client confidentiality at all times

2.5 Maintain records according to legal and ethical practices within the work setting

STANDARD 3. CLINICAL PRACTICE

The clinical practice of the IBCLC focuses on providing clinical lactation care and management. This is best accomplished by promoting optimal health, through collaboration and problem solving with the client and other members of the health care team. The role of the IBCLC includes:
- assessment, planning, intervention, and evaluation of care in a variety of situations
- anticipatory guidance and prevention of problems
- complete, accurate, and timely documentation of care
- communication and collaboration with other health care professionals

3.1 Assessment

3.1.1 Obtain and document an appropriate history of the breastfeeding mother and child

3.1.2 Systematically collect objective and subjective information

3.1.3 Discuss with the mother and document as appropriate all assessment information

3.2 Plan

3.2.1 Analyze assessment information to identify issues and/or problems

3.2.2 Develop a plan of care based on identified issues

3.2.3 Arrange for follow-up evaluation where indicated

3.3 Implementation

3.3.1 Implement the plan of care in a manner appropriate to the situation and acceptable to the mother

3.3.2 Utilize translators as needed

3.3.3 Exercise principles of optimal health, safety, and universal precautions

3.3.4 Provide appropriate oral and written instructions and/or demonstration of interventions, procedures, and techniques

3.3.5 Facilitate referral to other health care professionals, community services, and support groups as needed

3.3.6 Use equipment appropriately:
- refrain from unnecessary or excessive use
- assure cleanliness and good operating condition
- discuss the risks and benefits of recommended equipment, including financial considerations
- demonstrate the correct use and care of equipment
- evaluate safety and effectiveness of use

3.3.7 Document and communicate to health care providers as appropriate:
- assessment information
- suggested interventions
- instructions provided
- evaluations of outcomes
- modifications of the plan of care
- follow-up strategies

3.4 Evaluation

3.4.1 Evaluate outcomes of planned interventions

3.4.2 Modify the care plan based on the evaluation of outcomes

STANDARD 4. BREASTFEEDING EDUCATION AND COUNSELING

Breastfeeding education and counseling are integral parts of the care provided by the IBCLC.

4.1 Educate parents and families to encourage informed decision making about infant and child feeding

4.2 Utilize a pragmatic problem-solving approach, sensitive to the learner's culture, questions, and concerns

4.3 Provide anticipatory guidance (teaching) to:
- promote optimal breastfeeding practices
- minimize the potential for breastfeeding problems or complications

4.4 Provide positive feedback and emotional support for continued breastfeeding, especially in difficult or complicated circumstances

4.5 Share current evidence-based information and clinical skills in collaboration with other health care providers

C. THE INTERNATIONAL BOARD CERTIFIED LACTATION CONSULTANT: SCOPE OF PRACTICE AND EDUCATION GUIDELINES[1]

THE INTERNATIONAL BOARD CERTIFIED LACTATION CONSULTANT: SCOPE OF PRACTICE AND EDUCATION GUIDELINES

Introduction

The purpose of this document is to inform consumers, health care professionals, employers, health care policy makers, third-party payors, educators and students regarding the basic knowledge, skills, and competencies of an International Board Certified Lactation Consultant.* It also serves as the framework for evaluation and accreditation of International Board Certified Lactation Consultant education programs.

Role Definition

The International Board Certified Lactation Consultant is a health care professional whose scope of practice encompasses working collaboratively with primary care providers to assure appropriate clinical/practical management of breastfeeding and lactation in order to protect, promote and support breastfeeding. Such

---

1. Approved by the ILCA Board of Directors, 2001. Copyright © 2001 International Lactation Consultant Association.

practice includes providing education, counseling and clinical/practical management to allow breastfeeding to be seen as the expected way in which healthy newborns are to be fed as well as to prevent and solve breastfeeding problems. Education efforts extend to the community as well as to breastfeeding families and health care colleagues.

> *Note: The International Lactation Consultant Association (JLCA) recognizes the International Board Certified Lactation Consultant (IBCLC) credential as the appropriate certification for lactation consultants.

The role of the International Board Certified Lactation Consultant is dynamic and changes as the theory and practice of breastfeeding support and lactation management evolve to incorporate research findings and to adapt to societal needs. Practice is based on the principles outlined in this document, on the *Standards of Practice for IBCLC Lactation Consultants* and on the *International Board Certified Lactation Consultant Examiners (IBLCE) Code of Ethics.*

Certification

Lactation consultants who are certified by the IBLCE have the professional responsibility to maintain the IBLCE credential. Certification is evidence that the individual has achieved and maintains the knowledge, skills and wisdom required for the provision of competent breastfeeding care and services. International Board Certified Lactation Consultants are accountable for the outcomes of their practice and are responsible for complying with the laws within their practice jurisdictions.

Framework for Education and Practice

The theoretical framework for International Board Certified Lactation Consultant education derives from the health, biological and social sciences. Clinical/practical preparation involves acquiring the knowledge, judgment, and skills necessary to provide optimal, safe care for the breastfeeding mother and child. Acceptable clinical/practical practice and educational curricula are based on a foundation of fundamental principles, professional responsibilities, core knowledge, and competencies

Fundamental Principles

- Breastfeeding is a normal physiologic and developmental process for the majority of mothers and infants.
- Breastfeeding promotes optimal child health as well as optimal maternal health and is a vital component of public health policy.
- Every child has the right to receive human milk, and every woman has the right to breastfeed her child unless there is a medical contraindication.
- Every woman has the right to receive accurate, evidence-based information, support, and clinical/practical management for herself and her child.
- Mothers and infants have the right to receive, when needed, skilled assistance and clinical/practical management to breastfeed effectively.

Professional Responsibilities

International Board Certified Lactation Consultants have a professional responsibility to:

- Recognize that breastfeeding provides a foundation for optimal health outcomes and nurturing behaviors.
- Strive to support women to make informed decisions and take responsibility for their own well-being and that of their children.
- Work in respectful partnership with women and their chosen support systems.
- Advocate for the health and well-being of children by providing information about infant needs to guide mothers in informed decision making about infant and child feeding.
- Integrate observation, knowledge, and intuition in assessing mothers and children and in developing breastfeeding management strategies.
- Demonstrate clinical/practical competency, professional accountability, and legal responsibility.
- Facilitate the collaborative care of the mother and infant.
- Critically evaluate and incorporate research findings to provide and maintain evidenced-based practice.
- Participate in self-evaluation, peer review, continuing education, and other activities to ensure quality practice.
- Engage in professional conduct and practice in an ethical manner.
- Promote and protect breastfeeding through community outreach.
- Stay informed about the national and international issues and trends in maternal/newborn care and women's health.

Core Knowledge Outline (Subject areas from the IBLCE Examination Blueprint)

A. Anatomy

Mother
    General
    Breast and nipple (specific to lactation)
Infant
    General
    Head
      Oral
    Neck and shoulders
    Gastrointestinal

B. Physiology and Endocrinology

Mother
    General maternal hormones
    Milk synthesis and production
    Fertility/family planning
    Induced lactation and re-lactation
Infant
    General infant hormones
    Neuro-endocrine-gut reactions

Sucking, swallowing and breathing

Digestion

Elimination

C. Nutrition and Biochemistry

Mother

Principles of nutrition for women of childbearing age

Weight loss and gain

Cultural diet issues/ritual foods during post-partum period

Milk composition

Effect of maternal diet on milk composition

Infant

Guidelines for infant feeding

Comparison between human milk and artificial feeding products

Complementary and supplementary foods

Food sensitivities

Weaning/introduction of solids

D. Immunology and Infectious Disease

Protective properties of human milk

Immune system factors

Cells, antibodies and other immunoglobulins in human milk

Non-antibody factors — lactoferrin, bifidus factor, enzymes, hormones, growth factors, oligosaccharides, etc.

Decreased risk of infections and some chronic illnesses

Etiology

Manifestations

Prevention

Management

Decreased risk of allergies

Etiology

Manifestations

Prevention

Management

E. Pathology

Maternal

Labor and birth complications

Breast problems

Engorgement

Sore nipples

Yeast infections

Mastitis/abscesses

Plugged ducts

Insufficient glandular development

Breast surgery

Breast implants

Breast cancer

Acute illnesses

Chronic illnesses

Physical disabilities

Infant

Birth trauma

Inability to coordinate breathing/sucking/swallowing

Respiratory distress

Sucking problems

Swallowing difficulty

Preterm birth

Hyperbilirubinemia

Slow weight gain

Failure to thrive

Congenital anomalies/birth defects

Acute illnesses

Chronic illnesses

Oral pathology

Neurological impairment

F. Pharmacology and Toxicology

Pharmacology

Role of lactation consultant

Resources

Pharmacokinetics

Effects of drugs and substances commonly used during lactation

Over-the-counter medications

Alcohol

Tobacco

Management of lactation during drug therapy

Contraindications for breastfeeding

Pharmacologic family planning

Galactogogues/milk suppressants

Recreational/street drugs

Complementary therapies

Herbs

Homeopathic remedies

Acupuncture

Other toxicology

Environmental pollutants

G. Psychology, Sociology, and Anthropology

Adult learning
Counseling skills
Mother issues
  Incorporating breastfeeding into one's lifestyle
  Breastfeeding outside the home
  Maternal empowerment
  Employment
  Post-partum depression/psychosis
  Domestic violence/sexual abuse
Parenting role
  Mother–infant relationship
  Father–infant relationship
  Sibling–infant relationships
  Other family roles
  Single parenting
  Adolescent parenting
Alternative family styles
Cultural beliefs and practices
Support systems

H. Growth Parameters and Developmental Milestones

Social, adaptive, psychosocial and physical assessment of the child
  Prenatal growth
  Feeding cues
  Infant needs and temperament
  Feeding patterns and normal growth curves throughout breastfeeding
Developmental milestones of the early years
  Small and large motor development
  Cognitive development
  Markers of developmental delays
Developmental issues throughout breastfeeding
  Feeding and sleeping patterns
  Breastfeeding toddler
  Tandem breastfeeding
Weaning

I. Interpretation of Research

Critical reading and interpretation
  Study design
  Human rights issues
  Results

Application to lactation consultant practice

Lactation measurement tools

Research terminology

Basic statistics

Data collection for research purposes

J. Ethical and Legal Issues

Medical-legal responsibilities

Standards of Practice for IBCLC Lactation Consultants and other pertinent documents

IBLCE Code of Ethics and other pertinent documents

Evidence-based Guidelines for Breastfeeding Management During the First Fourteen Days

Confidentiality

Informed consent

Referrals

Charting and report writing

Ethical practice

Remaining current

Interdisciplinary relationships

Neglect, maternal/infant abuse cases

Expert witness role

Rental and sale of equipment

Evaluating practice

K. Breastfeeding Equipment and Technology

Identification of breastfeeding devices and equipment

Appropriate use of breastfeeding equipment

Alternatives to high-technology solutions

Milk collection, storage and use

Donor milk banking

L. Techniques

Breastfeeding techniques

Positioning

Latching on

Feeding management skills

Evaluating effectiveness of milk transfer

Typical feeding patterns

Multiple birth infants

Manual expression

M. Public Health

Community education

Health promotion activities

Work place issues

JBCLC lactation consultant as change agent

Creating and implementing protocols

International Code of Marketing of Breast-Milk Substitutes and other resolutions

The Innocenti Declaration

The Baby-Friendly Hospital Initiative

Affecting public policy

Nutrition programs providing for vulnerable populations

International Labor Organization (ILO) recommendations

International Board Certified Lactation Consultant Competencies

The International Board Certified Lactation Consultant demonstrates multiple competencies. It is essential that the International Board Certified Lactation Consultant:

· think critically and reflectively in order to affect the clinical/practical management of the mother–baby dyad.

· sustain an evidence-based practice.

· collaborate effectively with the client and in multidisciplinary health care teams.

· continually update knowledge and skills.

· maintain awareness of the need to promote breastfeeding.

PRACTICE GUIDELINES

I. Client Care Competencies

In order to provide appropriate care, a systematic process of assessment, management, and evaluation is used by the lactation consultant to:

1. Obtain an appropriate breastfeeding history for the mother and child.
2. Perform a comprehensive breastfeeding assessment of mother–infant dyad.
3. Evaluate all assessment data to develop a plan of care that is both appropriate for specific problems and acceptable to the client.
4. Function as a member of the interdisciplinary health care team by collaborative systematic problem solving. Effectively coordinate breastfeeding care by providing written reports of consultations and making appropriate referrals to other health care providers and community service/support resources.
5. Identify the need for and provide client teaching and anticipatory guidance appropriate to the client's age, developmental status, (dis)ability, culture, religion, ethnicity and support system.
6. Evaluate results of management using accepted outcome criteria, revise the plan accordingly, and consult and/or refer when needed.
7. Maintain comprehensive client records.
8. Provide safe care and understand the principles of universal precautions.

II. Lactation Consultant-Client Relationship Competencies

In order to establish a collaborative and supportive relationship with the client, the International Board Certified Lactation Consultant:

1. Promotes client autonomy, dignity, and self-determination by providing care that is non-judgmental and sensitive to client needs.
2. Establishes a partnership with the client to provide individualized optimal care consistent with the client's health belief system, and facilitates informed decision making and self-care.
3. Acknowledges personal values and cultural differences and recognizes their impact on the provider/client relationship.
4. Uses effective communication and counseling skills.
5. Provides a physically safe and confidential environment for care.
6. Offers comfort and emotional support to clients and their families.
7. Functions as an advocate for the mother and child within the family.
8. Advocates for the mother and child within the health care system.

III. Health Education and Counseling Competencies

In order to plan, develop, coordinate, and provide appropriate breastfeeding education and counseling in response to the needs of clients, including breastfeeding families, health care professionals, and the community, the International Board Certified Lactation Consultant:

1. Provides information that meets client needs, promotes informed choice, and is appropriate to culture, language, and literacy.
2. Uses adult learning principles when providing educational experiences for clients.
3. Shares current evidence-based information.
4. Evaluates teaching strategies and effectiveness.
5. Demonstrates techniques and appropriate use of equipment according to the needs of the client.
6. Works collaboratively with others providing support and assistance. i.e., paraprofessionals, volunteers with community breastfeeding support groups, peer counselors, etc.

IV. Professional Role Competencies

In order to contribute to the practice of lactation consulting and the advancement of the profession, the International Board Certified Lactation Consultant:

1. Maintains IBLCE certification.
2. Adheres to these Guidelines, the *ILCA Standards of Practice for IBCLC Lactation Consultants, and the IBLCE Code of Ethics.*
3. Practices within the scope of the *International Code of Marketing of Breast-Milk Substitutes* and subsequent relevant resolutions.
4. Works within the policies and procedures of the institution where employed, or if self-employed, has identifiable policies and procedures, including informing clients about fees, obtaining informed consent, protecting confidentiality, and maintaining appropriate client records.

5. Uses breastfeeding equipment in an appropriate manner, including discussing benefits and risks, assuring cleanliness and maintaining an awareness of conflict of interest when/if profiting from the rental or sale of breastfeeding equipment.

6. Maintains and expands knowledge and skills for lactation consultant practice by participating in continuing education programs and professional development activities in addition to reading current literature.

7. Evaluates own practice periodically and systematically in order to strive for improvement of care.

8. Supports and promotes well-designed research in human lactation and breastfeeding and bases clinical/practical practice on such research whenever possible.

9. Serves as a role model, preceptor, and mentor to other lactation consultants and students.

10. Seeks information about ethical, legal, and political issues regarding client advocacy and health care.

11. Participates in legislative and institutional policy-making activities related to breastfeeding.

12. Acts as an advocate for breastfeeding women, infants, and children in the community (including the media), the workplace, and within the health care system.

13. Interprets and promotes the role of the International Board Certified Lactation Consultant to consumers, other health care professionals, and the community.

14. Develops, uses, and maintains collaborative relationships with health care professionals to strengthen the role of the International Board Certified Lactation Consultant.

15. Maintains membership and participates in JLCA and local affiliate, if available.

EDUCATION GUIDELINES

I. Philosophy and Objectives

An International Board Certified Lactation Consultant education program is based upon a clearly articulated philosophy of what constitutes quality care for the breastfeeding mother–child dyad and the role of the lactation consultant in the provision of that care. An International Board Certified Lactation Consultant education program emphasizes individualized family care, client autonomy with informed decision making, and optimal health care through a collaborative, supportive relationship with clients and primary care providers. In order to provide care, support and services for breastfeeding families, practitioners must be able to clearly define both the necessary services and the role of the International Board Certified Lactation Consultant as the service provider.

The first objective of an International Board Certified Lactation Consultant education program is to prepare an individual for entry-level practice with emphasis on clinical/practical support and the management of normal breastfeeding and lactation. A secondary objective may be to provide continuing education opportunities for practicing International Board Certified Lactation Consultants. Such education is based upon understanding the interrelationship of many academic subject areas including: maternal and infant anatomy; physiology and endocrinology; nutrition and biochemistry; pathology; psychology, sociology, and anthropology; public health; normal growth and development; ethics and law; and evidence-based management principles. The body of scientific knowledge that forms the basis for the field of breastfeeding and human lactation results from a comprehension of the interrelationships between these subject areas and their impact on the care of a mother–infant dyad.

ILCA believes that the profession of lactation consulting is responsible for setting and maintaining the standards for the educational preparation of International Board Certified Lactation Consultants. ILCA further believes that professional education is a lifelong endeavor. The expanding body of knowledge of human lactation and breastfeeding coupled with corresponding changes in health care and society present a continuing challenge to International Board Certified Lactation Consultant educators and create a mandate for ongoing review of educational processes and outcomes.

II. Program Organization

Evaluation of any International Board Certified Lactation Consultant education programs is based on the following criteria:

1. The program has defined goals, measurable objectives, and adequate resources, in addition to appropriate curriculum, program design and faculty.

2. A complete International Board Certified Lactation Consultant education program includes at least 190 didactic hours of lactation/breastfeeding content and at least 250 hours of supervised clinical/practical practice for the student who has extensive experience and 500 hours for those with less experience, as required by the International Board of Lactation Consultant Examiners. Those students who are health care professionals must complete at least 45 hours of didactic lactation education and at least 250 hours of supervised clinical/practical practice. Students may attend a course offering a complete program or compile the same hours by attending several courses or partial programs.

3. The faculty of an International Board Certified Lactation Consultant program will offer expertise in breastfeeding and human lactation. It is also desirable that they be multidisciplinary and, where appropriate, culturally diverse. To serve as both mentors and role models, the majority of the faculty will possess current IBLCE credentials and maintain their competence through regular clinical/practical practice. The director of the program will be an International Board Certified Lactation Consultant prepared at the master level of formal education or higher in the USA or the equivalent in other countries.

4. Clinical/practical preceptors are qualified by education and experience in the management of the breastfeeding mother and child. They are also competent in clinical/practical instruction. The use of IBCLC practitioners as preceptors is preferred, whenever possible. A faculty/student ratio of no greater than 1:10 for supervised clinical/practical practice or a preceptor/student ratio of no greater than 1:2 is recommended.

5. The International Board Certified Lactation Consultant education program has clear admission criteria that may include specific content courses recommended by IBLCE for eligibility for certification. Qualified applicants are admitted without regard to gender, race, disability, marital status, ethnic origin, creed, age, or sexual orientation. Selection and admission criteria are established by the sponsoring institution and its lactation consultant education faculty. Programs encourage enrollment and retention of students from culturally diverse populations.

6. Adequate classroom and clinical/practical teaching facilities, administrative support, and teaching aids are designated for the program. Students have access to adequate library resources. Technology support is sufficient to maintain distance learning programs, where offered.

7. Student records and program data are maintained in a manner that ensures confidentiality, retrievability and permanence. Transcripts are available upon student request.

III. Program Curriculum

Evaluation of an International Board Certified Lactation Consultant education program curriculum is based on the following criteria:

1. Curriculum content prepares students to meet standards of practice and prepares students in total or in part to be eligible for international certification.

2. Teaching strategies are based on currently accepted theories and principles of adult education.

3. The curriculum content includes the fundamental principles, professional responsibilities, core knowledge, and competencies, as outlined in this document under *Framework for Education and Practice,* pages 2–10.

IV. Program Evaluation

Assessment of International Board Certified Lactation Consultant education programs is based on the following criteria:

1. The program employs a variety of evaluation strategies to measure student achievement of IBCLC lactation consultant competencies. These strategies may include written tests and reports; observation of the student in the classroom, laboratory, and clinical/practical settings; conferences with the faculty and/or clinical/practical mentors; peer review and self-assessments.

2. Evaluation is ongoing, and students review their progress regularly with a faculty mentor.

3. There are written policies regarding expected levels of achievement, probation, dismissal, and withdrawal. These policies include expectations for mentor/preceptorship and any time limits for completion of the program.

4. A formal student grievance procedure exists.

5. There is a regular, formal evaluation of the total educational program. Evaluation is an integral part of the planning process and allows for timely revisions. Formative and summative evaluations are suggested and could include the following: program philosophy and goals, curriculum objectives and content, clinical/practical settings and experience, student-to-faculty ratios, faculty and clinical/practical mentor/ preceptor performance, and student outcomes.

6. Surveys are conducted on both a short- and long-term basis to assess the impact of the program on career development and role satisfaction, as well as the impact of the graduates on the provision of breastfeeding/human lactation support and services. Sources of data and feedback to the program may include the following: students, preceptors, faculty, graduates, employers, funding sources, clients, and records of certification examination performance.

Accreditation is a voluntary external review process. It recognizes lactation consultant education programs that have achieved a level of quality that deserves the confidence of the student consumer and the public. Accreditation often is used as a criterion in decision making by funding organizations, state regulatory bodies, employers, third party payors, student loan/scholarship granting agencies and potential students. Because accreditation status is reviewed periodically, it encourages continuous self- study and improvement. This document outlines the basic knowledge, skills, and competencies of a practitioner and provides the basis for evaluation and approval of International Board Certified Lactation Consultant education programs by an official accreditation body.

Acknowledgements

The Professional Education Council of the International Lactation Consultant Association acknowledges the assistance of the Association of Women's Health, Obstetric and Neonatal Nurses (AWHONN) and the National Association of Nurse Practitioners in Reproductive Health (NANPRH). Their jointly prepared document, *The Women 's Health Nurse Practitioner: Guidelines for Practice and Education* served as a general model of clear, unified guidelines for practice and education. The Professional Education Council also thanks the North Carolina Nurses Association for their helpful discussion of multiple competencies in their North Carolina Nurses Association Position Paper, *Registered Nurse Education in the 21st Century.*

GENERAL PURPOSE - NCS® - ANSWER SHEET
SEE IMPORTANT MARKING INSTRUCTIONS ON SIDE 2

SIDE 2

GENERAL PURPOSE

NCS®

ANSWER SHEET

form no. 4521

Each answer row prints the choices A B C D E over the circles ① ② ③ ④ ⑤.

101 ①②③④⑤	111 ①②③④⑤	121 ①②③④⑤	131 ①②③④⑤	141 ①②③④⑤
102 ①②③④⑤	112 ①②③④⑤	122 ①②③④⑤	132 ①②③④⑤	142 ①②③④⑤
103 ①②③④⑤	113 ①②③④⑤	123 ①②③④⑤	133 ①②③④⑤	143 ①②③④⑤
104 ①②③④⑤	114 ①②③④⑤	124 ①②③④⑤	134 ①②③④⑤	144 ①②③④⑤
105 ①②③④⑤	115 ①②③④⑤	125 ①②③④⑤	135 ①②③④⑤	145 ①②③④⑤
106 ①②③④⑤	116 ①②③④⑤	126 ①②③④⑤	136 ①②③④⑤	146 ①②③④⑤
107 ①②③④⑤	117 ①②③④⑤	127 ①②③④⑤	137 ①②③④⑤	147 ①②③④⑤
108 ①②③④⑤	118 ①②③④⑤	128 ①②③④⑤	138 ①②③④⑤	148 ①②③④⑤
109 ①②③④⑤	119 ①②③④⑤	129 ①②③④⑤	139 ①②③④⑤	149 ①②③④⑤
110 ①②③④⑤	120 ①②③④⑤	130 ①②③④⑤	140 ①②③④⑤	150 ①②③④⑤

151 ①②③④⑤	161 ①②③④⑤	171 ①②③④⑤	181 ①②③④⑤	191 ①②③④⑤
152 ①②③④⑤	162 ①②③④⑤	172 ①②③④⑤	182 ①②③④⑤	192 ①②③④⑤
153 ①②③④⑤	163 ①②③④⑤	173 ①②③④⑤	183 ①②③④⑤	193 ①②③④⑤
154 ①②③④⑤	164 ①②③④⑤	174 ①②③④⑤	184 ①②③④⑤	194 ①②③④⑤
155 ①②③④⑤	165 ①②③④⑤	175 ①②③④⑤	185 ①②③④⑤	195 ①②③④⑤
156 ①②③④⑤	166 ①②③④⑤	176 ①②③④⑤	186 ①②③④⑤	196 ①②③④⑤
157 ①②③④⑤	167 ①②③④⑤	177 ①②③④⑤	187 ①②③④⑤	197 ①②③④⑤
158 ①②③④⑤	168 ①②③④⑤	178 ①②③④⑤	188 ①②③④⑤	198 ①②③④⑤
159 ①②③④⑤	169 ①②③④⑤	179 ①②③④⑤	189 ①②③④⑤	199 ①②③④⑤
160 ①②③④⑤	170 ①②③④⑤	180 ①②③④⑤	190 ①②③④⑤	200 ①②③④⑤

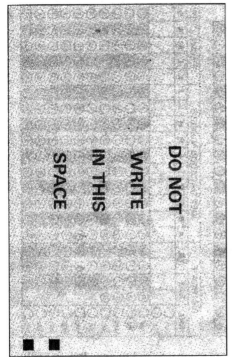

Trans-Optic® by NCS MPF-4521: 3231302928

Printed in U.S.A.

© 1977 by National Computer Systems, Inc.

EXAMPLES

WRONG
1 ① ⊗ ③ ④ ⑤

WRONG
2 ① ② ③ ④ ⑤ (③ marked with a check)

WRONG
3 ① ② ③ ④ ⑤ (④ partly filled)

RIGHT
4 ① ② ③ ● ⑤

IMPORTANT DIRECTIONS FOR MARKING ANSWERS

- Use #2 pencil only.
- Do NOT use ink or ballpoint pens.
- Make heavy black marks that fill the circle completely.
- Erase cleanly any answer you wish to change.
- Make no stray marks on the answer sheet.

DO NOT

WRITE

IN THIS

SPACE